Gerontological Concerns and Responses in India

Mala Kapur Shankardass
Editor

Gerontological Concerns and Responses in India

Springer

Editor
Mala Kapur Shankardass
Gurugram, Haryana, India

ISBN 978-981-16-4763-5 ISBN 978-981-16-4764-2 (eBook)
https://doi.org/10.1007/978-981-16-4764-2

This Springer imprint is published by the registered company Springer Nature Singapore Pte Ltd.
The registered company address is: 152 Beach Road, #21-01/04 Gateway East, Singapore 189721, Singapore

Acknowledgements

The idea of bringing out a book on Gerontological Concerns and Responses in India arose after I was approached a couple of years back by few publishing houses to edit a book on this important topic based on my specialization in this field. I discussed the idea with few colleagues across the country, and on their encouragement, I decided to compile this volume. I am grateful to them for their confidence in me to take this project forward.

India is moving forward with addressing various ageing issues, and it was an idea to collate these developments in a book which excited me. Fortunately, many of my reputed academic friends and colleagues working in the field of gerontology enthusiastically supported this project and agreed to contribute chapters for this publication. I thank them profusely for writing articles on topics given by me and thus making this special volume relevant for readers across the globe. Each of the contributions which focus on different developments and interests in gerontological studies is extremely valuable. I am grateful to each one of the contributors for their in-depth knowledge and sharing of their views in a comprehensive manner covering in very meaningful ways the context of the field of gerontology. They have eloquently touched on developments in the country related to their topic. Each one of the experts has discussed various important aspects related to interests of older people and highlighted the academic and research relevance to society. The various chapters have holistically dealt to engage the reader with gerontological discourses as they are increasing in ageing India and also in the world. I am restraining myself from individually identifying names of chapter contributors here as these appear in the table of contents. Each one of them unhesitatingly patiently supported this publication right from its inception to its outcome which due to unavoidable reasons got delayed in coming out in the market. As reputed experts, each one of them has a very busy schedule, but they took time out to make a success of this project. I do not have appropriate words to express my gratitude to each of them.

I am thankful to the publishing team of Springer Nature and especially to Mrs. Satvinder Kaur, Editor—Humanities and Social Sciences—for her interest in this project and coordinating with her team of Ramesh Kumaran and N. S. Pandian.

I would also like to take this opportunity of appreciating the support extended by my family in always being by my side in completion of this work. My husband, my son, daughter-in-law accommodated my commitments and stood by me. My three-year-old grandson provided the much-needed relaxation whenever I needed it. I am looking forward to the interactions with the readers and will be appreciative for their support and readership.

Gurugram, Haryana, India Mala Kapur Shankardass

Contents

Editor and Contributors

About the Editor

Mala Kapur Shankardass is a sociologist, gerontologist, and health and development social scientist. She recently retired as Associate Professor from University of Delhi, India. She is a writer, researcher, consultant, and an activist. She has been involved with ageing studies since 1992 when she started postdoctoral work on ageing issues. She has done prestigious assignments with United Nations agencies and international as well as national institutions covering gender issues, policy matters, health and well-being-related concerns, quality of life matters, enabling environments, societal responses, etc. She has participated in panel discussions, delivered key note addresses, and chaired sessions on ageing concerns with reputed organizations in both India and abroad. She has been recognized for her work and contributions in gerontology across the world. She is also associated with NGOs working on ageing issues and for the welfare of older people.

Contributors

Prof. Ashish Goel University College of Medical Sciences and Guru Teg Bahadur Hospital, Delhi, India

Kavim Bhatnagar World Food Programme, Dhaka, Bangladesh

Anupama Datta Head, Policy Research and Advocacy, HelpAge India, New Delhi, India

Avinash De Sousa Department of Psychiatry, Lokmanya Tilak Municipal Medical College, Mumbai, India;
Desousa Foundation, Mumbai, India

Retd Professor A. B. Dey Department of Geriatric Medicine, All India Institute of Medical Sciences, New Delhi, India

Reetika Dikshit Department of Psychiatry, Lokmanya Tilak Municipal Medical College, Mumbai, India

Saima Farhad Department of Social Work, University of Kashmir, Srinagar, Jammu and Kashmir, India

Prabhat Gautam Roy University College of Medical Sciences and Guru Teg Bahadur Hospital, Delhi, India

Sandhya Gupta Department of Mental Health Nursing, College of Nursing AIIMS, New Delhi, India

Jasbir Kaur MM College of Nursing, Solan, Himachal Pradesh, India

Vinod Kumar Emeritus President, Alzheimer's & Related Disorders Society of India, Delhi, India

Ankita Kumari International Institute for Population Sciences (IIPS), Mumbai, India

Pragya Lodha Clinical Psychologist, Private Practice, Mumbai, India

Shazia Manzoor Department of Social Work, University of Kashmir, Srinagar, Jammu and Kashmir, India

Anindya J. Mishra Indian Institute of Technology, Roorkee, India

R. Narendhar Alzheimer's and Related Disorders Society of India (ARDSI), New Delhi, India

Avanish Bhai Patel Alliance School of Law, Alliance University, Bengaluru, India

Meera Pattabiraman Alzheimer's and Related Disorders Society of India (ARDSI), New Delhi, India

Retd Professor Indira Jai Prakash Department of Psychology, Bangalore University, Bangalore, India

Anurag Priyadarshee Foundation for Holistic Vision, New Delhi, India

Kiran Puri Director, Development Welfare and Research Foundation (DWRF), New Delhi, India

S. Irudaya Rajan The International Institute of Migration and Development, Kerala, Thiruvananthapuram, India

Rakshit Bhardwaj University College of Medical Sciences and Guru Teg Bahadur Hospital, Delhi, India

Chandana Sarmah Department of Anthropolgy, Gauhati University, Guwahati, Assam, India

T. V. Sekher International Institute for Population Sciences (IIPS), Mumbai, India

Mala Kapur Shankardass Asia Representative, International Network for Prevention of Elder Abuse (INPEA); Managing Trustee, Development, Welfare and Research Foundation (DWRF), New Delhi, India

Vibha Singh Tata Institute of Social Science, Mumbai, India

S. Siva Raju Tata Institute of Social Science, Mumbai, India

S. Sunitha The International Institute of Migration and Development, Kerala, Thiruvananthapuram, India

Chapter 1
Understanding the Field of Gerontology in India

Mala Kapur Shankardass

Abstract Gerontology as a field has since last couple of decades of the twentieth century made a mark in India. Now it is a vast field, contributing theoretically and empirically as the study of ageing with experts from many fields involved with this specialization. Today gerontologists are contributing in many different ways to various interests of older people from a number of perspectives gearing towards their wellbeing. With the demographic and epidemiological transition taking place in the country, the resultant population ageing concerns require a scientific approach and a robust methodology to study responses emerging to understand the diverse dimensions affecting older people. Increasingly research on ageing issues is taking into account micro and macro studies as well as conducting longitudinal surveys to assess the impacts on older people of the changes happening in the society. Greater focus is being given to understanding the social, cultural, emotional, psychological and financial as well as health conditions of older people. Such findings are the ways and means to improve the situation and quality of life of older people, which is an important goal of gerontology. It is also emerging as a field linking policy and practice which can have a positive impact on the wellbeing of older people. As discipline gerontology provides solutions to ageing problems in different settings, cultural contexts and social environments and it is also the reason for its growing popularity in this century.

Keywords Gerontology · Wellbeing of older people · Theoretical and empirical underpinnings

Gerontology is a vast field that has come of age and recognized as a specialization in many countries. In India, it started making a mark around the last two decades of the twentieth century. As a subject, it has progressed steadily over the years and in this century has made inroads as a theoretical as well as an empirical study of ageing processes and age related diseases. Today gerontologists include researchers and practitioners from the fields of biology, nursing, medicine, criminology, dentistry,

M. K. Shankardass (✉)
Asia Representative, International Network for Prevention of Elder Abuse (INPEA); Managing Trustee, Development, Welfare and Research Foundation (DWRF), New Delhi, India

M. K. Shankardass (ed.), *Gerontological Concerns and Responses in India*,
https://doi.org/10.1007/978-981-16-4764-2_1

social work, physical and occupational therapy, psychology, psychiatry, sociology, economics, political science, architecture, geography, pharmacy, public health, housing and anthropology.

While it is true that the basic principle behind studying gerontology is to understand the ageing process and help those through it, its scope and opportunities are not limited to that only. As a field of study, it is broad including the anthropological, economic, health, historical, philosophical, political, psychological, religious and sociological as well as the gender issues of the older population. Over the years it is seen that the knowledge, understanding and expertise of a gerontologist make him/her a very valuable resource for any industry or field that's trying to create services and products for the elderly, contributing towards their wellbeing. The applications of gerontology overlap with many fields. Studies go beyond disciplinary boundaries, from social science perspectives to health and medicine. It has emerged as an integrative discipline, providing a deep understanding of processes of ageing and its inter-disciplinary linkages.

The contributions which gerontologists make to theory and research in the field of ageing is growing over the years (Samanta, 2017) and especially with growing numbers of older people, the demand for their work is rapidly increasing. Ageing research, theory, practice and policy are getting linked in many exciting, innovative ways as the demographic transition resulting in ageing of the populations is affecting many countries across the globe, including India. The body of theory and research is drawing from different disciplines, orientations and conceptual models which provide clarity and understanding to ageing processes. The research focus in the last twenty years or so has considerably expanded and different theoretical and methodological developments have taken place drawing from work being done in aged societies of Europe, America and some parts of Asia Pacific region (Alkema & Alley, 2006; Medeiros, 2014). At present, as part of growth of the discipline of gerontology, there are many empirical studies both small and large scale, generally through different kinds of surveys and based on demographic, epidemiological and population data at national and regional levels. The increasing emphasis on theory building in the study of ageing has come of age universally. It is now recognized that experience of ageing needs to be identified as social and cultural reality touching on various parameters transgressing through macro and micro level phenomena by establishing gerontology as a scientific discipline.

In this century in India gerontological imagination has been related to the effort to emphasize the importance of cultural, economic, epidemiological diversity in understanding the social process of age and ageing. Important contributions have been made to insights on health aspects, psychological concerns, family structures, intergenerational relationships, social cultural dimensions, income aspects, retirement, migration impacts, rural urban differences, abuse and neglect issues and in general with experiences of older adults (Geography and You, 2019; Giridhar, et al., 2014; Lamb, 2009; Samanta et al., 2015; Shankardass, 2020; Shankardass & Rajan, 2018). There is a growing emphasis on bringing focus on longitudinal studies within the country though not yet across countries. A significant study in the forthcoming full national scale longitudinal ageing study in India (LASI) being coordinated by the International Institute for Population Sciences in collaboration with Harvard School of Public Health and University of Southern California, USA. This project hopes to scientifically highlight with sound methodological rigour the health, economic, social dimensions and determinants and consequences of population ageing in the country. However, greater emphasis is being placed on the internationally harmonized instruments for studying demographic and epidemiological shifts taking place and in understanding their impacts. This is clearly leading to amassing empirical data as part of research projects of universities and institutions with limited attention to theory driven research, which no doubt requires adequate focus for the field of gerontology finding its due place as an academic subject.

Present data on gerontology in India reveals growing research emphasis on questions related to disease burdens, health care and disability, geriatric and nursing care practice, care giving aspects, emotional and economic security, work related and retirement options, living arrangements, housing requirements, gender differences, crime against the elderly, empowerment strategies, policy and programmatic responses and provision of enabling environments, to name some of the aspects. Researchers believe that these questions are important for understanding the social, cultural, emotional, psychological and financial as well as health conditions of older people. Such findings are the ways and means to improve the situation and quality of life of older people, which is an important goal of gerontology. The significance of empirical research studies is that they provide a pragmatic link to policy and practice. In the last decade, UNFPA as part of its programmatic exercise took up an important project on 'Building knowledge base on population ageing in India (BKPAI). In collaboration with Institute of Social and Economic Change (ISEC), Bangalore, Institute of Economic Growth, Delhi and Tata Institute of Social Sciences (TISS), Mumbai, the project focused on seven states to document different aspects of ageing. This is one of the first population based data from rural and urban areas to throw light on the various dimensions of the ageing scenario with state wise comparisons between Himachal Pradesh, Kerala, Maharashtra, Odisha, Punjab, Tamil Nadu and West Bengal.

Many social scientists in the country, like in other parts of the world too, involved with the discipline of gerontology are voicing need for developing sound theoretical orientation in the field of sociology, psychology, social work, economics, demography, criminology, family studies, community medicine, nursing and health sciences. There is a strong belief that theory driven research would lead to sound empirical generalizations with satisfactory explanations in understanding the ageing process. This would significantly contribute to building the knowledge base of the gerontology discipline and lead to its maturity and further development in the country. An appropriately and carefully designed theoretical framework is necessary for sound empirical research which provides deep insights into our understanding of ageing processes and its links with society. An orientation for explaining the reasons behind research questions such as why certain situations and circumstances arise, what is the outcome of emerging scenarios, where lie the solutions and how do we assess them and will they transform reality, are essential.

The popularity of the field and its expansion in the last few years is based on its ability to transform lives of older people to better conditions and experiences. The field of gerontology, as it has developed in the country and elsewhere since last few decades is becoming popular because it links policy and practice in all its sub fields and contributes towards the wellbeing of older people throughout the world. Across ageing countries, it provides solutions to ageing problems in different settings, cultural contexts and social environments. It leads to intellectual debates and discourses about how to age and retain aspects to celebrate age, remove ageism, minimize age related disabilities and problems and enhance quality of life.

The marriage between theory and research is essential for the growth of the discipline. Maximizing such links is significant for its scientific contributions in societies where the reality of ageing of populations can no longer be ignored. Both theoretical frameworks and empirical understanding of ageing experience can no doubt go along independently but harnessing the two is essential for enhancing the scope of gerontology in each country and universally. It would be safe to state that the rich field of gerontology will only survive when micro data is pitched in with macro analysis by bringing together theory and research and not limiting it to any sub field. However, the debates about gerontology being a distinct academic discipline or applied social science or even a hybrid of several disciplines has been continuing and will still do so as clearly it is a field concerned primarily with the changes that occur between the attainment of maturity and the death of the individual and with factors that influence these changes which cut across different disciplinary understandings (Shankardass, 2004).

Moving from late twentieth century to twenty-first century, the field of gerontology has gained momentum in India. It has gained importance along with the field of geriatrics which has gradually established in few medical institutions. Both the Indian Council of Social Science Research and the Indian Council of Medical Research have over the years contributed to the growth of gerontology and geriatrics, which is largely seen as being part of the broader field of gerontology. With support from these national institutions today there is right mix of research methodology that ensures breadth and rigour in understanding ageing issues scientifically. Experiences from Europe and America, where gerontology has longer history than in India, suggest that to unify research on ageing within cross-disciplinary, inter-disciplinary and multi-disciplinary perspectives entails enhancing both the capacity and reliability of scientific observation. As it had been pointed out by Achenbaum (1995) there has been a consequent emergence of an inter-disciplinary amalgam, resulting in the evolution of applied gerontology, critical gerontology, dialectical gerontology, educational gerontology, experimental gerontology, hermeneutic gerontology, qualitative gerontology, social gerontology, anthropological gerontology, financial gerontology—each imposing narrow boundaries on their subject. As it happened in the USA, in India too there has been a conceptual division in the field of ageing which has led to development of the biology of the senescence, geriatric medicine and the sociology of ageing population (Shankardass, 2004).

This book brings many experts from different fields together keeping the spirit of gerontological discourses being multi-disciplinary and inter-disciplinary intact.

It discusses various dimensions of older people's experience of ageing along with programs and initiatives in place to address issues and concerns related to population ageing. It is first of its kind volume putting various perspectives together in depth and with an understanding that promotes growth of Gerontology in India. It will enhance the reader's knowledge of the field and provide an integrative approach to study ageing processes, concepts, practices and ideas that influence development of Gerontology in India. I hope the pragmatic link it provides to policy and practice will be appreciated.

References

Achenbaum, A. W. (1995). *Crossing frontiers: Gerontology emerges as a science*. Cambridge University Press.

Alkema, G. E., Alley, D.E. (2006). Gerontology's future: an integrative model for disciplinary for disciplinary advancement. *The Gerontologist*, *46*(5), 574–582.

Ageing in India. (2019). *Geography and You.*

Giridhar, G., Sathyanarayana, K. M., Kumar, S., James, K. S., & Alam, M. (2014). *Population ageing in India*. Cambridge University Press.

Lamb, S. (2009). *Aging and the Indian diaspora: Cosmopolitan families in India and abroad*. Indiana University Press.

Medeiros, K. (2014). Who "owns" gerontology? The importance of thinking beyond the sciences. *The Gerontologist*, *54*(4).

Samanta, T., Chen, F., Vanneman, R. (2015). Living arrangements, and health of older adults in India. *Journals of Gerontology Series: Psychological and Social Sciences*, *706*, 937–947.

Samanta, T. (2017). Bridging the gap: Theory and research in social gerontology. In Samanta T (Ed.), *Cross-cultural and cross-disciplinary perspectives in social gerontology*. Springer.

Shankardass, M. K. (2004). The study of ageing. In A. Bose & M. K. Shankardass (Eds.), *Growing old in India: Voices reveal, statistics speak*. B R Publishing Corporation.

Shankardass, M. K., & Rajan, S.I. (Eds). (2018). *Abuse and neglect of the elderly in India*. Springer.

Shankardass, M. K. (2020). Reflections on elder abuse and mistreatment in India. In M. K. Shankardass (Ed.), *International handbook of elder abuse and mistreatment* (pp. 371–384). Springer.

Chapter 2
Growth of Geriatrics and Old Age Care in India

A. B. Dey

Abstract Old age care, as a speciality of medicine, existed before the recent development of "Geriatrics" in modern medicine. Demographic transition in an ageing society accompanied by epidemiological transition to a stage with high prevalence of chronic non-communicable diseases have necessitated a new speciality in the practice of medicine. As societies will move towards large ageing population in coming centuries, Geriatric Medicine is expected to emerge as a predominant discipline. The speciality has traversed a long way from "Workhouse Medicine" to a modern discipline in the last century. Health services for older people have changed substantially since middle of the twentieth century with the unravelling of many unknown diseases till date with a concomitant growth of ways and means of addressing them. Geriatric medicine has undergone significant changes from what it was a few decades back both in developed and developing countries, though a lot more needs to be done. Training and education are still evolving in the field. The strengths of this speciality include a multidisciplinary working team, comprehensive assessment, improved hospital environments, need for early intervention, rehabilitation, etc. Geriatric Medicine in countries with resource constraints is different from that practiced in the developed societies though the focus on retaining health and vitality till late life would be an important consideration globally.

Keywords Geriatrics · Old age care · Training · Education · Comprehensive assessment · Interventions

Introduction

Substantial rise in human longevity has been witnessed in the second half of the last century in India. However, enhanced longevity has not been accompanied by equally enhanced quality in the last phase of life. Complex health issues, pain, disability, failing mind, frailty are common terms used to describe the state of health in old age. As we live longer, many more health issues unravel which are otherwise not

---

A. B. Dey (✉)
Department of Geriatric Medicine, All India Institute of Medical Sciences, New Delhi, India

M. K. Shankardass (ed.), *Gerontological Concerns and Responses in India*,
https://doi.org/10.1007/978-981-16-4764-2_2

commonly encountered. The inadequacy of social support mechanisms coupled with poorly functioning health system renders older persons helpless. Old age for many in this country is a trying time to endure suffering. There is an urgent need for putting in place a care system that addresses health and welfare issues in old age.

Care of older members is a function of the family and society. For centuries old age care had existed and is not a novel concept. It has become a new challenge for society because of exponential growth in the number and proportion of the old and the very old population in successive censuses in the country since 1950. Along with the tremendous rise in numbers, it has become clear that the need for security pertaining to the socio-economic, health and emotional state of the older population have also grown substantially. Thus, there is a need for strengthening various institutions of civil society to make old age more secure.

Health system in India is limited by its capacity to face the challenges of the growing old population. Old age care must overcome the competing need for safe motherhood, healthy childhood, protection from potentially preventable, curable and communicable diseases; and profitable organ care through rapidly changing technology. Additionally, limited infrastructures, physically and economically inaccessible health care systems are managed by professionals with no training or exposure to complex health needs of the elderly and the situation becomes more critical because of the inadequate social support system.

Old age care is complex and needs involvement of multiple disciplines of medicine. This has not been an easy achievement and has taken more than half a century to put in place a discipline which addresses the health needs of older people. Under such circumstances, there is an urgent need for training health professionals to take care of older people at different levels of health system. This will help to alleviate the health and well-being concerns in later years of life. Development of academic discipline of geriatric medicine is an important intervention in old age care and this will help in producing trained health professionals.

Geriatrics or geriatric medicine is the branch of medicine concerned with diagnosis, treatment and prevention of diseases in older people and the problems specific to ageing population. This discipline of medicine exists as a standalone speciality in many countries and as a sub-speciality of internal medicine or family medicine in some countries. The discipline aims to promote good health in old age. However, it is important to note that geriatrics differs from gerontology. Geriatrics is derived from the Greek word *geron* meaning "old man" and *iatros* meaning "healing", gerontology refers to the study of ageing and covers a broader perspective than geriatrics. Geriatrics is also often referred to as medical gerontology.

Geriatric Medicine differs from standard adult medicine because it focuses on the unique needs of the older person. The older person is biologically different in structure and function from a young adult as most organ systems invariably decline in functionality with age. Health in old age is reflection of the events of life process and as a result, older people are heterogeneous. Principles of clinical and diagnostic reasoning used for young ailing adults do not apply to older patients. Geriatricians distinguish between diseases and the effects of normal ageing, take a holistic view of the diseases, aim at functionality and treat the whole person rather than organs or organ systems.

History of Old Age Care

The history of old age care is as ancient as human ageing. First descriptions of Geriatrics come from ancient Indian system of medicine—*Ayurveda* (>1500 BC). It is one of the most ancient medical sciences in the world and is a part of *(upveda)* of *Atharva Veda.* Based on the fundamental laws of nature, Ayurveda propagates the concept of rejuvenation as a solution to the challenges of ageing. After birth and growth; senility leading to death is an inevitable process. Ayurveda considers that ageing begins before birth and continues throughout life at different rates in different races and therefore, varies for different individuals and for different tissues of the body. It involves two opposite processes that simultaneously come into operation, namely, "evolution" and "involution", i.e. growth and atrophy. Ageing, thus, represents structural and functional changes of an organism over its entire life span.

Ayurveda has two main objectives namely, (1) to maintain the health of healthy individuals; and (2) to cure the diseases of the diseased persons. Accordingly, Ayurveda puts considerable emphasis on the science of gerontology and *rasayanacikitsa* (therapy). A prolonged life is closely linked with profound physical changes as well as the changes in the socio-economic conditions in which an individual is living. Each of these changes is studied under the sub disciplines of geriatrics and gerontology. Ayurveda considers the phenomenon of ageing from an entirely different angle. It elaborates a comprehensive clinical discipline called *rasayanatantra* exclusively devoted to the study of ageing and its prevention and care with the help of *rasayanacikitsa.* The *rasayanatantra* is one of the eight major clinical disciplines of *astangaayurveda.* The term does not only refer to a drug or a therapy but to a comprehensive discipline which may also include therapy. It is a multidimensional approach taking care of the body, mind and spirit, thus embracing the total well-being of an individual. Though mainly used for maintaining the health of healthy persons, *rasayanacikitsa* can be utilized for the care of the diseased also. *Rasayanacikitsa,* i.e. the rejuvenation therapy, provides comprehensive physiological and metabolic restoration.

In the western world, old age care developed slowly but definitively in medieval and pre-modern era. Arabic physician, Algizar (circa 898–980), wrote several books on health and health care of the elderly, sleep disorders, forgetfulness and improvement of memory and causes of mortality. Another Arabic physician Ishaqibn Hunayn of ninth and tenth century AD wrote Treaties on Drugs for Forgetfulness. An ancient treaties on medicine—"Medicine "of 1025 AD, was the first documentation of functional and structural changes in old age and strategies for good health through oil massage, exercises such as walking or horse-riding.

The term geriatrics was proposed by Nascher of Mount Sinai Hospital, New York. Modern geriatrics owes its origin to Dr. Marjorie Warren of the United Kingdom and is regarded as the "Mother" of Geriatrics. She emphasized the role of rehabilitation in the care of older people and aggressive strategy of diagnosis, treatment, care and support for older people living in care institutions for a long term. The practice of geriatrics evolved in the United Kingdom with application of the principles of "multi-disciplinary" team approach where all health professionals have equal stake and their contributions in optimizing the well-being and independence of older people are equally shared. Another British Geriatrician, Bernard Isaacs, described some of the crucial concepts of geriatrics.

Old age health care is very well developed in the United Kingdom with major state support through the National Health Services and the efficient general practice which came into existence after the Second World War. Geriatric Medicine is also developed in North America and Europe. Like most of the other services like education and research initiatives, geriatric medicine also got a boost in these nations in the post—Second World War era.

History of Professional Associations

The American Geriatrics Society (AGS) was founded in 1942 by a group of physicians "to encourage and promote the study of geriatrics". Initially, the AGS focused on improving clinical care for older adults. In 1953, the Society began publishing the Journal of the American Geriatrics Society—one of the top medical journals of the last century. Soon it started influencing biomedical research on ageing and health. The Society also published important books such as the Geriatrics Review Syllabus and Geriatrics at Your Fingertips and actively promotes medical education to meet the unique health care needs of older people. During the same time a group of American scientists, established the inter-disciplinary professional association, the Gerontological Society of America in 1945 devoted to research, education and practice in the field of ageing. On the other side of the Atlantic, the British Geriatrics Society (BGS) was established in 1947 to address the suffering and distress of the aged and infirm by the improvement of standards of medical care and publishing and distributing the results of research on old age and old age health care. Establishment of professional associations of health professionals engaged in care of older patients was not limited to the United States and the United Kingdom. Keeping pace with population ageing, countries in North America, Europe and Asia Pacific region, initiated services for older people and training of human resources; and formed societies and associations. In 1950, an international association of professional associations was formed as International Association of Gerontology (IAG) which in 2004, was converted to the International Association of Geriatrics and Gerontology (IAGG). Currently, IAGG has 73 member organizations from 65 countries worldwide with a combined membership of over 45,100 professionals.

Geriatric Medicine in Middle East, South East Asia and Pacific Countries

Geriatric Medicine is in poor shape in most of the countries in Middle East, South East Asia and Pacific Countries. Some of these countries have a low proportion of older people in the population. However, it has emerged as an important discipline in health care systems in Australia, Hong Kong, Japan, New Zealand, Republic of Korea and Singapore, reflecting the state of socio-economic development and efficiency in the functioning of the health system. There is special focus on developing human resources and long-term care in these countries. However, the health care expenditure related to old age care varies from state spending to insurance-based systems in the different countries across the globe. Old age care is evolving in countries like China, Indonesia, Malaysia, Oman, Sri Lanka and Thailand in response to the prevalent socio-economic and cultural conditions.

Geriatric Medicine in India

India like many other developing countries did not realize the impact of population ageing till 1970s. The need for Geriatric Medicine as a separate speciality was not appreciated and it had a late beginning. In the year 1978, the out-patient service in Geriatric Medicine was started at the Madras Medical College & Hospital in Chennai. The inpatient service was established after a decade in 1988 and the post-graduate programme in Geriatric Medicine started in 1996 under the aegis of Dr MGR Medical University of Tamil Nadu.

The National Policy on Older Persons (NPOP), adopted 1999, mandated establishment of Geriatric Medicine departments in all medical colleges in the country. Responding to the NPOP, the Medical Council of India developed the curriculum for post-graduate training in Geriatric Medicine in 1999 and the Madras Medical College was the first medical college to establish Postgraduate training in India. In 2004, a Post Graduate Diploma in Geriatric Medicine was launched by Indira Gandhi National Open University, Delhi to equip doctors with knowledge and skill in the field of Geriatrics and to enable them to deal with special problems faced by older patients. After initial enthusiasm, the programme lost its importance due to lack of hands on training facilities and non-recognition by the licensing authorities. Subsequently, Amrita Institute of Medical Science in Kochi, Kerala and Christian Medical College, Vellore, Tamil Nadu started a post-graduate training programme in Geriatric Medicine.

There is very limited exposure to old age care in undergraduate medical curriculum and nearly non-existent in nursing and para-professional training. To address these issues of poor skilling in old age care, Government of India launched an intensive training programme with financial assistance from the World Health Organization (WHO). The programme was managed by the All India Institute of Medical

Sciences (AIIMS), New Delhi and reached 100 medical colleges between 1998 and 2001. In addition, more than 2000 primary care physicians were trained in workshops conducted in medical colleges across the country. This initiative along with focused operational and epidemiological training in collaboration with the WHO led to the creation of the critical mass of teachers and specialists trained in old age care. However, evidence-base created through research hinted the requirement of a bigger initiative.

National Programme for Health Care of the Elderly (NPHCE) was launched in 2010 by the Ministry of Health and Family Welfare, the Government of India. The programme has two-pronged strategy namely, capacity building through postgraduate training in medical colleges and expansion of services from district hospitals to the dispensaries located in the farthest periphery. AIIMS, New Delhi has initiated fourth postgraduate training programme in 2012. Since then, two more departments with postgraduate training programmes have been established in Maharashtra; one each in the public and private sector. The pledge of establishing more departments and postgraduate training programmes in twenty Regional Geriatric Centres by 2017 is yet to be converted to reality.

Lack of interest bordering on hostile attitude on the part of internists, limited resources for medical education on the part of state governments and most importantly antagonistic attitude of the regulatory body, i.e. the Medical Council of India have contributed to failure of the NPHCE in expanding postgraduate training in Geriatric Medicine. The matter has been further complicated by present state focus on organ centric tertiary care than universal health coverage through strengthening of primary health care.

Training and Education in Geriatric Medicine

There is a substantial variation in the training and education in geriatric medicine across the globe. There is a global debate regarding position of Geriatric Medicine in undergraduate and postgraduate curriculum as to whether it should be a part of family medicine or internal medicine or it should be a standalone discipline. In the United States, geriatricians are primary-care physicians who are board-certified in either family medicine or internal medicine and also have additional training in geriatric medicine. In the United Kingdom, Geriatric Medicine is one of the largest specialties. The discipline provides an opportunity to maintain a generalist approach while also developing a sub-speciality interest and the chance to work both in community and hospital settings. Geriatricians have developed expanded expertize in the ageing process, the impact of ageing on illness patterns, drug therapy for seniors, health maintenance and rehabilitation. They serve in a variety of roles including hospital care, long-term care, home care and terminal care. They are frequently involved in ethics consultations to represent the unique health and diseases patterns seen in older population. The model of care practiced by geriatricians is heavily focused on working closely with other practitioners such as nurses, pharmacists, therapists and social workers. Indian system of Geriatric Medicine is still evolving and is likely to be British type of care system.

Minimum Geriatric Competencies

A need has been felt to create uniform training programs in geriatric medicine so that the standard of care remains the same for all older persons at all levels of health care system. This can be ensured by putting in place minimum competencies in geriatric education. The guiding principles for minimum geriatric competencies are as follows:

1. Focus on issues that are pertinent to the health outcomes for older patients;
2. Focus on taking care of the older masses;
3. Limited number of content domains and competencies with no more than 5 to 8 domains 3 to 5 competencies in each; and
4. A common system of teaching and evaluation at any medical school.

The domains of core competency are cognitive and behavioural disorders, medication management, self-care capacity, falls, balance, gait disorders, atypical presentation of disease, palliative care, hospital care for elders and health care planning and promotion.

Problems in Establishment of Academic Geriatric Medicine

The establishment of Academic Geriatric Medicine in medical curricula across the developing world is a difficult exercise because of the prevalent considerations. Many doctors do not believe that Geriatric Medicine needs special attention and insist that it is a part of internal medicine with little difference if any. Societies with low life expectancy believe that it is not relevant to teach students about care of older people because most of the population would not reach that age anyway. Geriatric medicine is perceived to be a low paying, non-glamorous branch of medicine associated with senile and old patients with poor prognosis and low returns.

It is important to clarify these concerns and make Geriatric Medicine relevant to the demographic requirement of developing countries. Some of the immediate actions in this direction would include the following:

1. Awareness programmes should be undertaken on active ageing to provide a positive image of ageing to medical graduates.
2. Primary health care needs to be strengthened in providing services to ensure active ageing for the population.

3. Substantial investment needs to be made in developing human resources and infrastructure for quality health care for older people.
4. Various paradigms of old age care need to be recognized and included in curriculum.
5. Education in geriatric medicine needs to be enhanced with definition of minimum competencies in doctors.

Conclusion

Geriatric Medicine is a futuristic discipline as the demographic trend across the globe points towards large ageing population in the coming centuries. It has come a long way since the days of early "Workhouse Medicine". Services for older people have improved to a great extent over the decades both in developed and developing countries. There is still much to be done. The strengths of this speciality include collaboration of a multidisciplinary team, comprehensive assessment, improved hospital environments, need for early intervention, rehabilitation and discharge them to their own homes thereby giving them good quality of life till death. The future of medicine certainly belongs to care of older people and it is important to identify areas of research in Geriatric Medicine. The multidisciplinary team approach adopted by Geriatric Medicine towards the comprehensive assessment and management of an older patient will become increasingly important and relevant in the twenty-first century practice of medicine.

Key Messages

- Old age care as a speciality of medicine existed in ancient times.
- Geriatric Medicine has emerged as a modern discipline in the last century. The training and education are still evolving.
- Geriatric Medicine in developing countries is different from that practiced in developed countries due to economic, social and cultural differences. In coming decades, the discipline will have a distinct existence in developing countries.

Chapter 3
Gerontological Nursing in India: Inception and Trends

Sandhya Gupta

Abstract Gerontological nursing is a new field which is a sub-speciality of nursing that focuses on health care of elderly by preventing and treating diseases and disabilities in older adults. Gerontological nursing is defined as the specialized nursing care of the older adults that occur in any setting in which the nurses use knowledge, expertise and caring abilities to promote optimal functioning, which means not only understanding their diseases and knowing who the support people are in their lives, but also creating a plan of care that includes their social, financial and personal goals. Effort to introduce geriatric competencies in the curriculum of nursing courses is done to formalize and sustain the presence of gerontological nursing. Gerontological nursing may be practiced in any setting, for example, the nursing home, the hospital, in community and the homes.

Keywords Nursing · Gerontological nursing · Older persons · Speciality nursing

Introduction

Gerontological nursing is one of the very sub-speciality in infancy still in India that focuses on health care of older persons by preventing and treating diseases and disabilities. Caring for elderly patients means understanding their diseases and also knowing who the support people are in their lives, in addition, create plan of care that includes their personal, social and financial goals.

Gerontological Nursing

Geriatric nursing is defined as the specialized care of the elderly that occur in any setting in which the nurses use knowledge, expertise and caring abilities to promote optimal functioning. Geriatric nursing will be well positioned to play a central role

S. Gupta (✉)
Department of Mental Health Nursing, College of Nursing AIIMS, New Delhi, India

M. K. Shankardass (ed.), *Gerontological Concerns and Responses in India*,
https://doi.org/10.1007/978-981-16-4764-2_3

in improving the health of elderly if established with infrastructure and professional academic background. Currently, nurses whether working independently, in collaborative practice with physicians, or as members of geriatric teams, nurses have shown to give ordinary care to elderly with basic input in their training.

History of Geriatric Nursing

The origins of gerontological nursing have begun when nursing council added the courses in geriatric in basic curriculum in the year 2007. Awareness of the need for education in gerontological nursing, as well as the need for improvement in care for institutionalized elderly is of greater value in nursing profession in India today.

Inception and Trends of Gerontological Nursing

The assessment of health and functional status of elderly, planning and providing appropriate nursing and other health care services, evaluating the effectiveness of such care is the scope of gerontological nursing practice. The emphasis is placed on optimizing the functional ability in the activities of daily living; promoting, maintaining and restoring health, including mental health; preventing and minimizing the disabilities of acute and chronic illness; and maintaining life in dignity and comfort until death. There could be multiple settings where gerontological nursing may be practiced, for example, the homes, community, the oldage homes. nursing home and hospital,

In addition to traditional nursing care responsibilities, the new roles of gerontological nurses include multidisciplinary team members and leaders. Due to the recent changes in health systems, new roles are evolving for nurses. For example, to develop innovative ways of resolving problems and resolving issues health promotion, quality assurance, education of staff as well as the older persons and prevention of hospitalization, in addition to early detection of acute illnesses and arranging consultation.

There are many gray areas of geriatric nursing, the first relates to the role of geriatric teams generally. Whereas care geriatric care team has consistently shown to substantially improve the outcome for elderly, geriatric health care professionals will flourish only in an environment that provides empirical evidence as well as clinical support. The second area relates to participation in making health policy, while the nurses have made inroads in influencing health care policy, the need for gerentologic nurses at the policy table is underrepresented and not valued. The effectiveness of gerentologic nurses to shape and direct policy on behalf of elderly will take much more time. Geriatric nursing aims to promote health by preventing and treating diseases and disabilities in elderly. Caring for older patients means not only understanding their diseases and knowing who the support people are in their lives, but also creating a plan of care that includes their financial, personal and social goals.

Currently, in collaborative practice alongside physicians, or as members of geriatric teams, generalist nurse practitioners along with one year specialized training have shown to improve care to elderly in the community, in hospitals and in specialized care facilities.

There is good evidence that, in the future, geriatric nursing will be a force for improvements in care to elderly during the next decade as the number of elderly will increase in number. The need for improving geriatric competencies for all practising nurses should accelerate as well as the curriculum revisions ensure geriatric competency in the future nursing workforce. Expanded efforts are needed in increasing the number of nurses armed with geriatric specialization above the current level and ensuring that all specialist nurses will complete their academic programs with adequate preparation in geriatric nursing. These efforts should also serve to ensure capacity in nurses who work with older patients who have comorbidities such as heart disease, cancer and neurological disorders.

Gerontology Nurse

A gerontology nurse is a nursing specialist who works directly with elderly to provide them with specialized care and high quality of life. In gerontological nursing, much of the tasks is done by nurse similar to that of a generalist nurse and additional care of age related problems and specialized treatments.

Health Issues of the Elderly—Needs to Be Addressed

Health problems in the elderly cannot be seen in isolation. Bigger and wider range of social, psycho-emotional and financial correlates determine the medical problems—and accordingly, needs have to be addressed.

Social Issues

- As industrialization resulting in children moving out to take up jobs in other places, which cause problems like isolation and lack of support for old parents and breaking of joint family support systems.
- Modernization of society causes increase in abuse of elderly leading to several psychological illnesses.
- Lack of pension and inadequate facilities for health care, rehabilitation and recreation.

Psycho-Emotional Aspects

- One of the Spouses may pass away
- Friend circle becomes restricted
- Retirement increases the isolation process
- Neglected by youth
- Not able to keep themselves occupied.

This complex interplay increases the risk of mental stress and also aggravates the impact of stress related diseases as ischemic heart disease and hypertension among elderly.

Issues Related to Health Care System

- The health care system lacks adequate number of trained medical, paramedical personnel in geriatric medicine which adversely affects the health care of the elderly.
- Mobile health services for the elderly and ambulance services are limited in the rural and peripheral areas making the health care facilities difficult to reach.
- Lack of health insurance system in our proactive measures to maintain health of geriatric population by adopting preventive strategies such as yoga and other day to day activity to prevent diseases related to inactivity can be stressed.
- At present, most of the geriatric OPD services are available at tertiary care hospitals and are urban based. At the primary care level, the overall infrastructure is grossly deficient.
- Low awareness among people regarding the services available.

Major Constraints for Geriatric Health Care

- Lack of specialized and trained manpower
- No dedicated health care infrastructure
- Gerontologic nursing not yet a popular speciality.

Role of the Gerontologic Nurse

A gerontologic nurse is a specialist that helps elderly patients recover from illness or injury by providing practical care based on care plans, also plan rehabilitation, conduct check-ups in specialized care facilities or long-term care facilities. While some specialists administer medication and do pain management and are also trained for preventative care so to avoid injuries and common medical conditions which usually develop most commonly in oldage.

A nurse will be required to perform a number of duties for aged population. For example, they are often responsible for

- measuring and recording vital signs;
- administering medications;
- exercising and massaging patients;
- watching for signs of elder abuse;
- transporting patients to clinics/hospital visits
- helping patients with their daily needs, such as bathing, dressing and using the bathroom.

Throughout all of this, the gerontologic nurses are also be required to keep accurate patient records and coordinate care with the physicians. The gerontologic nurses are responsible for the physical well-being, mental and emotional well-being. Mostly, elderly patients will seem morose or angry, due to various reasons such as their failing health, lack of independence and isolation from their loved ones. A gerontologic nurse is required to keep a close observation of these patients and to remain cheerful and compassionate, even during the most difficult times. When working as a gerontologic nurses, they have to also encourage to communicate with patients' family members. And need to explain a patient's care regimen or medications, or act as a liaison between the family members, the patient and the physician. A gerontologic nurses are also in an excellent position to give both patients and their loved ones advice on certain health and self-care ability related issues.

Additional Duties of Gerontologic Nurse Includes

- Conduct routine check-ups and screenings
- and to seek medical help immediately when sick.
- Develop patient care plans
- Administer medication
- Assist with pain management
- Teach not to take many medicines at one time
- Bathing and bedsore prevention
- Grooming
- Regularity in meals—To teach
  - to take small frequent meals and more of green leafy vegetables and fruits
  - to drink water in small quantities frequently even if not thirsty.
- Helping Patients keep their independence
  - Helping to become socially active
  - To remain busy by doing simple light work which is of interest.

- Exercises
  - Move all body joints and do whatever exercises possible.
  - To maintain body weight slightly below the desired weight.
- To avoid smoking and drinking alcohol
- Help rehabilitate patients after injuries.

Become a Nurse Manager

Advanced practice nurses who specialize in gerontology work in many different settings. Some of these settings include private practices, personal homes and old age homes (*yet to evolve this role in India*). Those nurses who have a passion for helping patients who need nursing care the most, this could be the most fulfilling path in future. With an optimistic attitude, we can say geriatric nursing is a multi-faceted field and nurse can grow as a specialist. This is to be foreseen in future in India, as there is some sporadic birth of long stay homes where nurses are employed. But most of the other facilities for elder's care are still managed with untrained staff as of now in India.

Advanced practice Gerontologic Nurses

The advanced practice gerontologic nurses work in collaboration with gerontologic physicians and social workers to render care to elderly and serve as faculty to prepare increasingly large numbers of gerontologic nurses. The majority of these elderly have a disproportionate number of untoward acute health events and chronic illnesses that require primary, acute and long-term care.

Evidence is strong that advanced practice gerontologic nurses, often as part of gerontologic teams, ensure quality care to elderly people and significantly improve health outcomes in ambulatory, acute and institutional long-term care.

Yet, despite a 30-year effort on the part of academic and professional nursing organizations, advanced practice gerentologic nurses do not exist in India still. As all elder facilities for elder's care are still managing with staff having basic training not yet trained the specialized gerentologic care as of now in India.

Adult and Family Advanced practice Nurses

Even though in India we are yet to start advance gerontologic nursing, there is growing interest within nursing fraternity for learning care for elderly. Thus, there are several new initiatives taken with the specific goal to teach best practice in gerentologic care basic nursing curriculum.

These initiatives include the development of curriculum competencies in gerentologic for all programs for post graduates. They also include the development of training materials, ongoing professional education and encourage the creation of specialist programs to acquire extra training in geriatric nursing.

Training for Gerontological Nursing

- **Gerontologicalizing the Generalist Nurse**

In addition to focusing on nurses for working with elderly during the past 10 years, the profession has slowly embraced a strategy to prepare all nurses with basic geriatric competencies as a way to ensure that elderly get appropriate nursing care. Virtually all nurses in the course of their careers care for elderly; providing preventive programs; manage multiple chronic conditions and deal with mental and physical frailty and facilitate a peaceful death. It is, therefore, imperative that these nurses have basic competence to care for elderly.

To date, there have been two initiatives to ensure geriatric competency in generalist nurses. The first is to ensure geriatric competency in all students who graduate from a nursing programme.

Basic Training in Nursing

Though all nursing schools have begun to include gerontologic nursing in their curricula and have gerontologic nursing as a significant and integral part. The second initiative, which is only now developing, involves preparing practising nurses and the pre-service fresh nurses each year with competency in gerontologic nursing.

From being a generalist to a specialist in the field of nursing still takes time hence therefore in the mean time the basic curriculum was revised for incorporating geriatric care in all the courses. Few short term training programs are planned frequently by ministry, in colleges of nursing in the country.

Specialized Training

- Specialized training can be done by taking up post basic one year speciality diploma of geriatric nursing in which the nurse will get the hands-on experience and get certified as post basic gerentologic nurse. The entry qualification is that

the nurse requires at least one year experience after the basic General Nursing Diploma or BSc Nursing degree.
- Also, MSc in gerontological nursing going to be initiated soon by few geriatric care centres in the country which are in making at present.
- Initial efforts to ensure geriatric competency in the practising nurse have focused on the organizations representing the elite group of professional nurses who have an interest and expertise in a specific area of nursing, such as geriatric competency in speciality nurses offers an opportunity to make substantial inroads into "gerontologizing" practising nurses.
- Effort to introduce geriatric competencies has involved presentations for geriatric presence at national level meetings, providing ready-made materials for use in organizations, journals and web sites and creating and/or supporting geriatric special interest group that allows for formalizing a sustained interest in gerentologic nursing.

National Programme for the Health Care of Elderly (NPCHE) (Directorate General of Health Services)

This programme was launched with the vision of: (1) to provide accessible, affordable and high-quality long-term, comprehensive and dedicated care services to an ageing population; (2) creating a new "architecture" for Ageing; (3) to build a framework to create an enabling environment for "a Society for all Ages;" (4) To promote the concept of Active and Healthy Ageing. Government has initiated the development of Modules for all nursing professionals working in Primary health care and in secondary and tertiary care settings.

Future of Gerontology Nursing

There will always be a demand for nurses in future, but it is especially high in gerentologic nursing. As Baby Boomers age and the number of people living well past 80 grows, the need for those with ageing expertise grows. This is a growing speciality that will have a very high demand now and in the future, this could be one of the most sought after choices in nursing specializations in future.

Conclusion

Gerontological nursing is going to be one of the most sought specialization keeping in view that most baby boomers of today will be in geriatric category after 50 years.

Bibliography

Alam, M., Karan, A. (2011). Elderly health in india: dimension, determinants and differentials. In *Working Paper No. 3, Building Knowledge Base on Ageing in India.* Bangalore: Institute for Social and Economic Change, New Delhi: United Nations Population Fund, Delhi: Institute of Economic Growth.

Balamurugan, J., Dr. Ramathirtham, G. (2012). Health problems of aged people. *International Journal of Research in Social Sciences*, *2*(3).

https://www.indiannursingcouncil.org/

Ford, P. (2004). *Nursing assessment and elderly people.* A Royal College of Nursing Tool Kit.

Government of India. (2011). *Ministry of health and family welfare.* Director General of Health Services, MOHFW. National Program for Health Care of the Elderly (NPHCE): Operational Guidelines 2011.

Royal College of Nursing. (2004). *What difference a nurse makes: A report on the benefits of expert nursing to the clinical outcomes for elderly people on continuing care* (2nd ed.).

Royal College of Nursing Caring in partnership: older people and nursing staff working towards the future. (2004).

WHO. (2015). *World report on ageing and health.*

World Health Organization Active and Healthy Ageing. Report of a Regional Consultation, Thiruvananthapuram, Kerala, India, December 6–8, 2007

Chapter 4
Ageing India: Psychological Concerns and Responses

Indira Jai Prakash

Abstract The proportion of older people in the population is growing rapidly in India. Absence of comprehensive health care delivery system along with socio-cultural and familial changes will compromise the quality of life of older Indians. Considerable physical morbidity, psychological distress and mental health problems are reported in the Indian elderly. Longevity brings with it increased chances of disability, dementia and long-term care crisis. Geriatrics and Gero-psychology research and practice are emerging slowly but steadily. Government of India has come up with several schemes and programmes for the wellbeing of senior citizens. Implementation and monitoring of such schemes and coverage have not been satisfactory. This paper examines health, morbidity, mental health issues in elderly, available resources and recommended measures to deal with the situation.

Keywords Physical morbidity · Psychological issues · Available resources and measures

Introduction

Ageing is a multilayered concept with biological, social, psychological, demographic and many other implications. While individuals age as they transit through their life cycle from birth onwards, populations age due to structural changes. Demographic ageing is a dynamic phenomenon where a proportion of older people in the population increases more rapidly than younger age groups. Usually, this is due to decline in both birth and death rates. While it is difficult to mark the exact threshold of old age, for most practical concerns, 60 years is taken as the cutoff point separating adults from the elderly. Since the beginning of recorded history, there used to be more young children than older people. But, driven by falling fertility rates and remarkable increases in life expectancy, population ageing will accelerate. Hence, in the last few decades, the number of older persons is increasing the world over. A World Health Organization report (2011) states that the number of people aged 65

I. J. Prakash (✉)
Department of Psychology, Bangalore University, Bangalore, India

M. K. Shankardass (ed.), *Gerontological Concerns and Responses in India*,
https://doi.org/10.1007/978-981-16-4764-2_4

will outnumber children under age 5. The older segment of 65+ is projected to grow from an estimated 524 million in 2010 to nearly 1.5 billion in 2050, with most of the increase in developing countries. If cutoff age is lowered to 60 instead of 65, then, the number will be higher than the projected figures in the WHO report.

Indian population is demographically still young as the proportion of its old has not yet reached the levels that are seen in European countries. But being a highly populous country, next only to China, even a small proportion translates to large absolute number. Any country that has more than 7% of elderly in its population is considered 'Greying' or 'Old'. India thus qualifies as a greying nation as it has already 8.6% of elderly in its population and the number is still growing. Demographers opine that the ageing process in India has been initiated from 'apex' rather than from 'base'. That is the increase in elderly population was more due to improvement of survival of those in old age range rather than any significant decline in fertility. India had been subjected to one-sided 'demographic modernization' which was confined to mortality decline. The effect of controlling fertility was felt only in the late eighties. Till recently the increase in the proportion of aged in the population was more due to an impressive decline in mortality (Roy, 2004).

In the future, a further decline in fertility rate and improvement in survival rates will push India closer to other developed countries in terms of demographic profile. Summary of the Government of India report on Indian Elderly (2016) provides the following information about profile of elderly.

- According to Population Census 2011, there are nearly 104 million elderly persons (aged 60 years or above) in India; 53 million females and 51 million males.
- Both the share and size of elderly population is increasing over time. From 5.6% in 1961 the proportion has increased to 8.6% in 2011. For males, it was marginally lower at 8.2%, while for females it was 9.0%.
- As regards rural and urban areas, 71% of elderly population resides in rural areas while 29% live in urban areas.
- The sex ratio among elderly people was as high as 1028 in 1951, subsequently, it dropped and again reached up to 1033 in 2011.
- The life expectancy at birth during 2009–13 was 69.3 for females as against 65.8 years for males. At the age of 60 years, average remaining length of life was found to be about 18 years (16.9 for males and 19.0 for females) and that at age 70, it was less than 12 years (10.9 for males and 12.3 for females).
- The old age dependency ratio climbed from 10.9% in 1961 to 14.2% in 2011 for India as a whole. For females and males, the value of the ratio was 14.9% and 13.6% in 2011. In rural areas, 66% of elderly men and 28% of elderly women were working, while in urban areas only 46% of elderly men and about 11% of elderly women were working.
- The percent of literates among elderly persons increased from 27% in 1991 to 44% in 2011. The literacy rate among elderly females (28%) is less than half of the literacy rate among elderly males (59%).
- Prevalence of heart diseases among elderly population was much higher in urban areas than in rural parts.

- Most common disability among the aged persons was locomotor disability and visual disability as per Census 2011.
- In the age group of 60–64 years, 76% of persons were married while 22% were widowed. Remaining 2% were either never married or divorced.

Interestingly, this report has no information about mental health status of the elderly. Further demographic projections indicate that the Indian population will exceed 1.4 billion by 2030. The elderly population is likely to reach 198 million by 2030 (Government of India,). India's fertility rate of 2.5 live births may drop further and average life expectancy will rise to 68+ years. This is likely to increase the dependency ratio too. The proportion of people above 80 years is also likely to increase with more women in older age groups (Registrar General of India, 2011). Family continues to be the main source of support for majority of older people.

Health and Psychological Wellbeing in Old Age

People do not age in a vacuum. Socio-cultural context, health care system, political stability, economic development apart from genetic and lifestyle factors will determine how healthy and peaceful old age would be. Health is a major factor that affects wellbeing, life satisfaction and morale in old age. Older Indians report considerable morbidity. Latest survey by National Sample survey organization (GOI, 2015) provides some startling findings of health of average Indians. Survey revealed a higher number of 'Ailing persons' in younger and older age groups. In the 60–69 age group, 259 per 1000 rural and 355 per 1000 urban elderly were found to be having an illness at the time of the survey. Level of living as measured by per capita monthly consumption expenditure (UMPCE) was related to morbidity. Level of morbidity increased with level of living which may also mean that report in morbidity improves with improvement in economic status. Clearly, a higher inclination towards Allopathy treatment was prevalent with 90% of people opting for it. Private doctors were the most important single source of treatment in more than 70% of cases, both urban and rural. On average, a much higher amount was spent for treatment per hospitalized care by people in the private than in the public hospitals. While the rural households primarily depended on their 'household income/savings' (68%) and on 'borrowings' (25%), the urban households relied much more on their 'income/saving' (75%) for financing expenditure on hospitalization. Sadly, as high as 86% of rural population and 82% of urban population were still not covered under any scheme of health expenditure support. Government, however, was able to bring about 12% urban and 13% rural population under health protection coverage through schemes such as Rastriya Swasthya Bima Yojana (RSBY). This compares poorly with the reports that 84% of the citizens in the United States of America are covered with health insurance and the rest are supported by charity organizations and private health care providers through charity programmes (Ridic et al., 2012). SAGE (Study on Global Ageing and

Adult Health) tracks health and health care access in middle and low-income countries. Researchers found evidence of an unusually high burden of health care costs in India. Older Indians had the largest percentage of people receiving out-patient health care (88%) and an extremely large share (94%) paid out-of-pocket for their health care (Population Reference Bureau, 2012a).

A host of psychological factors affect quality of life in old age. Ageing brings with it several physical changes in strength, vigour, attractiveness and looks. These inevitable changes often lead to a sense of anxiety. Loss of older parents, peers and especially of life partners can be a serious threat to wellbeing. India is going through sudden social and cultural changes due to rapid pace of urbanization and modernization. The joint family of the past has gone into oblivion and different types of family units are emerging. Nuclear families, single parent families and more recently surrogacy, adoptions by same sex couples and partners in live-in relationships have changed the dynamics of family bonds. Globalization impacts families and in turn care of elderly and ageing of population also impacts family and social structure. Mass migration and urbanization bring about a 'crisis in care giving'. Changing socio-economic and cultural landscape is paving way for changing "human scape" (Prakash, 2014). Loneliness is a major issue when one of the partners dies reducing the family to a single-person household. Safety of elders is compromised due to crimes against elders, especially in urban areas. Instances of Elder Abuse are on the rise and surveys and studies report shocking figures of older persons being harassed and victimized by family members (Prakash, 2013) Abused elderly suffer from several physical and psychological consequences requiring holistic intervention (Prakash, 2018).

Life satisfaction (LS) is an important component of successful ageing. Successful ageing is not uniform across the different age groups. Level of LS indicates the subjective wellbeing which is associated with the health and mortality status among the elderly. Four factors that directly influences the level of LS among the elderly are: physical health condition, mental health condition, social relationship and environment (WHO, 1997). For improving LS among the elderly, it is necessary to consider factors like satisfaction in residential environment, neighbourhood relationship, economic status, maintaining friendship, family relationship, physical health condition, satisfaction in marital status, job or career and lastly, satisfaction in others aspect of life. LS is influenced by various factors like demographic, socio-economic, health, physical status, mental status, social support, social adjustment and a number of morbidities. Studies indicate that factors such as race, socio-economic status, marital status, education, level of self-esteem, depression, may influence the level of LS. Demographic factors such as rural setting (Banjare et al., 2015), gender (Balachandran et al., 2007), social support network (Marpady et al., 2012), and age (Maheshwaran & Ranjit, 2013) have been linked with LS. LS is a subjective judgement that is part of wellbeing measures (Kirtani & Aminabhavi, 2018). A study on wellbeing of older people in Kerala revealed that nearly half of the subjects interviewed reported low levels of wellbeing (Nair & Anjana, 2017).

As the growing number of elders make their presence felt, quality of their life becomes an important issue. QOL takes into account factors like physical functioning, cognitive functioning, social functioning, emotional functioning, life satisfaction, health perceptions, economic status, recreation, sexual functioning, energy and vitality. The World Health Organization defined quality of life as an individual's perception of their position in life in the context of the culture and value systems in which they live and in relation to their goals, expectations, standards and concerns (WHO, 1997). The WHO definition of QOL has a broad meaning as it includes physical health, mental state, level of independence, social relationships, personal beliefs and their relationship to salient features in the environment. Several studies of QOL of Indian elderly have been carried out in different regions of India such as Karnataka (Barua et al., 2007, Shraddha et al., 2012) Chandigarh (Swami et al., 2002), Delhi (Khokhar & Mehra, 2001), Rural north India (Qadri et al., 2013) Puducherry (Bharathi et al., 2011), Rural Tamil Nadu (Purty et al., 2006), and, Varanasi, UP (Raj et al., 2014). Life satisfaction, a major component of QOL seems to decline with age especially so in case of older females (Priyanka & Misra, 2013; Raj et al., 2014).

Quality of life is affected significantly by health. Physical and psychological well-being are closely related. Physical illness is often associated with and may prove to be an aggravating factor in mental illness. Older Indians suffer from both communicable and non-communicable disorders. This situation is often worsened by age related sensory impairments. Indian elders have transited into a pattern of multi-morbidity (Dey & Nisar, 2014), simultaneous coexistence of more than one chronic condition. This is associated with higher mortality, increased disability and a decline in functional status which lower QOL drastically. According to the Government of India Statistics (2006), the chronic illnesses in the elderly usually include rheumatism, hypertension, coronary heart disease and cancer. Non-communicable diseases (life style related and degenerative) requiring prolonged medical and personal care are common in old age. NCD is found irrespective of socio-economic status in older groups. These NCDs often result in disabilities that compromise the functional ability of elders and affect activities of daily living. The National Sample Surveys of 1986–87, 1995–1996 and 2004 have shown that the burden of morbidity in old age is enormous (Government of India, 2012a, 2012b).

Ageing is not 'non-gendered' or 'gender-neutral. Researchers have documented "feminization of Ageing" and also "feminization of poverty". Many social gerontologists argue that ageing should be looked through 'gender lens' as gender makes a difference to social status, access to resources and wellbeing. It is well established that older women suffer from more chronic disorders and are socially marginalized (Nayar, 2013). Evidence from SAGE studies show that Frailty is higher among female elderly (Chaudhary & Arokiasamy, 2017). Ageing women in India are likely to be more vulnerable in health, economic and social terms. They are likely to be poorer, have more physical complaints and depressive symptoms than men. Their life satisfaction and quality of life are lower than older men. Older women continue to provide care to their elderly spouse but receive less care and support than men (Prakash, 2000). Any type of disability has a much more crippling effect on older women. (Prakash, 2003). Due to poor education and lack of awareness of options, they lack preparation for ageing and future changes (Agarawala & Saikia, 2017). Widowed women still suffer several types of deprivation as reported by surveys conducted in Vrindavan by Guild of Service (2010). Concerned by worldwide discrimination against older women, the UN Convention for Elimination of Discrimination Against Women (CEDAW), took a ground-breaking decision during its 42nd session, to adopt General Recommendations on Older women and protection of their human rights. CEDAW recognized that age is one of the grounds on which women suffer multiple forms of discrimination (Begum, 2008).

Mental Health Issues

Mental health is not merely absence of mental illness. It is a state of wellbeing in which the individual can realize his or her own abilities, can cope with the normal stresses of life, can work productively and is able to contribute to his or her community. While mental illness occurs in all age groups, its manifestation and impact may vary in different age groups. The prevalence of mental disorders among older people is likely to increase as life expectancy increases. Rao (2004) one of the pioneers in Gero-Psychiatry in India stated that psychiatric illness is seldom an 'isolated' event. A minimum of two or three clinical diagnoses in an older person is the rule. The number of symptoms ranging from six to twelve. The nature of modern urbanization may have deleterious consequences for mental health through the influence of increased stressors and adverse events such as overcrowding, pollution, poverty, slums, dependence on cash economy, rising levels of violence, poor social support, etc. (Desai et al., 2004). Psychiatric disorders increase *pari passu* with age. Major disorders in old age are functional disorders followed by organic psychoses, prevalence of neurotic disorders being relatively low. Geriatric depression is the most common diagnosis in older group (Prakash, 2004). There is still considerable stigma attached to accessing mental health care.

A major study conducted by the World Health Organization, the World Bank and Harvard University concluded that mental illnesses account for a substantial portion of the burden of diseases in developing countries (WHO, 2001) mental and behavioural disorders account for 12% of the global burden of disease as an estimated 450 million people in the world suffer from psychological disorders. The psychiatric disorders found in 10% of total population accounts for 5 of 10 leading causes of disability as measured by years lived with a disability. The overall Disability Adjusted Life Years (DALYs) burden for neuropsychiatric disorders is projected to increase to 15% by the year 2020 (Maity & Mukhopadhyay, 2015). Mental health can be considered to be the key to happiness, productivity and harmony. Elderly may be more vulnerable to mental health problems as they experience many losses and stresses. Older adults facing reduced mobility, frailty, chronic pain, bereavement, economic dependence and loneliness experience higher levels of psychological distress (Prakash, 2004). Mental health has impact on physical health and vice versa. Older adults are also vulnerable to abuse, which may increase the likelihood of depression and anxiety. According to a WHO estimate, in India, the burden of mental health problems is of the tune of 2443 DALYs per 100,000 population and the age-adjusted suicide rate per 100,000 population is 21.1. It is estimated that, in India, the economic loss, due to mental health conditions, between 2012 and 2030, is 1.03 trillions dollars. Mental health workforce in India (per 100,000 population) include psychiatrists (0.3), nurses (0.12), psychologists (0.07) and social workers (0.07).

Researchers report that the burden of mental disorders had risen over last few decades in India (Reddy et al., 2013). Exact rates of prevalence are not known as different studies report varied rates of illness depending on the type of study and the condition studied. In a cross-sectional study in South India, 21.7% of total elderly were diagnosed with depressive systems (Barua & Kar, 2010). The number of diagnosed female elderly was almost double that of men and cognitive impairment was higher among the depressed individuals. In 2000, a review of epidemiological studies gave a very high estimate of prevalence of mental disorders in 70.5 per 1000 in rural and 73 per 1000 in the urban population (Ganguli, 2000). A study related to the nature, prevalence and factors health as major risk factors for depression even when good social support was available (Rajkumar et al., 2009). Women, especially rural widowed seem to be at a higher risk for depression (Barua et al., 2007). Singh et al. (2012) report an overall prevalence of 34.2% with mood disorders being most common in geriatric population. Morbidity was higher in females, in the 80+ group and more in community dwelling elderly than residents of old age homes. Maity and Mukhopadhyay (2015) reported rural elderly to be higher on depression and anxiety than their urban counterparts. In 2010, a study conducted in NIMHANS, Bangalore reported that the burden of mental and behavioural disorders ranged from 9.5 to 102 per 1000 population (Math & Srinivasaraju, 2010). Reason behind such wide differences in reported prevalence could be due to wide differences in settings, samples and methods used. National Mental health survey of India was supported by Ministry of Health and family welfare, Government of India was implemented by National Institute of Mental Health and Neurosciences. This study (NIMHANS, 2016) was carried out in 12 states across 6 regions during 2015–16. The overall weighted prevalence for any mental morbidity was 13.7% lifetime and 10.6% current. An estimated 150 million persons are in need of mental health interventions and care (both short term and long term). A GOI report puts the prevalence of psychiatric morbidity in the community to be anywhere from 8.9 to 61.2% (GOI, 2011).

Two psychiatric problems often encountered in older people are depression and dementia. They require immediate attention from health services as they impact quality of life negatively. These two disorders pose a major public health challenge for developing countries. The vulnerability of elderly is due to the multiple medical problems they have along with psychological problems. Cardiovascular diseases, respiratory disorders, hearing and visual impairments, depression and infections such as tuberculosis are common problems in elderly populations. Depression is often associated with suicide in elderly (Jacob, 2012). Depression is under treated in this age group, particularly so because it is not yet perceived as a priority public health problem in developing countries. A meta-analysis of 74 studies (Barua et al.,

2011), including 487,275 elderly individuals found the worldwide prevalence rate of depressive disorders to be between 4.7 to 16%. This study indicates a comparatively higher prevalence of geriatric depression in India (21.9%). Modernization, breakdown in family system, forced retirement leading to inactivity, negative attitude toward elderly, physical illnesses and immobility make elders more prone to depression. Though it is common in old age, it is often underdiagnosed. The social impact of depression is serious as it lowers quality of life, increases chances of other types of morbidity and influences long-term care (Pilania et al., 2013). The goals in treating depression in elderly persons include resolution of symptoms, prevention of relapse and recurrence and improvement of functional capacity. Early diagnosis and treatment are essential as many comorbid conditions exist in elderly. Side effects of anti-depressants are common among elderly and need to be monitored carefully. Psychological interventions along with medical help are required to motivate elderly to continue treatment (NICE, 2009).

Reports of increased cases of dementia indicate that this disease of longevity may be the next silent epidemic in the country. The prevalence of dementia in Indian studies has been shown to vary from 0.84 to 6.7%. The prevalence of dementia was found to be 33.6 per 1000 in a study on urban population of Kerala in 2005. Alzheimer's disease was the most common cause (54%) followed by vascular dementia (39%) (Shaji et al., 2005). Shaji et al. (2010) reviewed articles published in a major Psychiatric journal for 50 years and found very few research reports on dementia. In a ten-year follow up study (Maruthanath et al., 2012), 104 subjects out of 1066 developed dementia, 98 out of them were diagnosed with Alzheimer's. Prevalence for 1000 person years was 11.67 and A.D increased with age. Chandra et al. (1998) report an Indo-US cross national study data from Rural North India. Overall prevalence rate was 1.36% and for AD it was 0.62%. In this population, the prevalence of AD and other dementias was low, increased with age and was not associated with gender or literacy. The early set of data on dementia from LASI project shows lower cognitive function in women even after controlling for socio-economic and health differences (Population Research Bureau, 2012b).

It is estimated that 50 million people worldwide are living with dementia with nearly 60% living in low- and middle-income countries. The total number of people with dementia is projected to increase to 82 million in 2030 and 152 million in 2050. In May 2017, the World Health Assembly endorsed the *Global action plan on the public health response to dementia 2017–2025*. The Plan provides a comprehensive (2018) blueprint for action—for policy-makers, international, regional and national partners and WHO—in areas such as, increasing awareness of dementia and establishing dementia-friendly initiatives; reducing the risk of dementia; diagnosis, treatment and care; research and innovation; and support for dementia carers. It aims to improve the lives of people with dementia, their carers and families while decreasing the impact of dementia on individuals, communities and countries. Depression, psychoses, suicide, epilepsy, dementia and substance use disorders are included in the WHO Mental Health Gap Action Programme (mhGAP) that aims to improve care for mental, neurological and substance use disorders by providing guidance and tools to develop health services in resource-poor areas.

Development of Mental Health Services in India

Before independence, the approach to Mental Health Care consisted largely of building lunatic asylums, which were custodial rather than therapeutic. The first revolution in the care of the mentally ill came with the enactment of the Indian Lunacy Act (1912). In 1947, there were 17 Mental Hospitals with a patient load of 10,000. Since independence, India has been progressively developing basic mental health services infrastructure. The growth has shifted from a vertical approach to a more integrated approach since the 1970s. There was a shift in service delivery with setting up of General hospital Psychiatry units (GHPUs). In the 1980s. non-governmental organizations (NGO) and private sector were increasingly involved in community mental health services. The Indian Mental Health Act was enacted in 1987. The Act came into operation after notification in 1993. The National Mental Health Programme (NMHP) was started in 1982 to provide a framework for mental health services in the country. The main objective was to ensure access to minimum mental health care to all especially to vulnerable groups in society. The District Mental Health Programme (DMHP) was started by the Government of India in 1996–97 on a pilot basis. A detailed account of development of psychiatric services in India and reforms in mental health field is documented in a book edited by Agarwal (2004) titled 'Mental Health: An Indian Perspective: 1946–2003'.

The adoption of National Mental Health Programme (NMHP) by the Government of India in August 1982, was in many ways a landmark event in the history of psychiatry (Wig & Murthy, 2015). In 2014, the revised National Mental Health Policy of India and in 2015, the draft National Health Policy, were released. The new Mental Health Policy, 2014 and the National Health Policy, 2015 both recognize the basic premise of the NMHP (1982), namely, integration of mental health care with the primary care approach. Mental Health Care Act 2017 was passed on 7 April 2017 and came into force on July 7, 2018. The law was described in its opening paragraph as "An Act to provide for mental health care and services for persons with mental illness and to protect, promote and fulfil the rights of such persons during delivery of mental health care and services and for matters connected therewith or incidental thereto." This Act superseded the previously existing the Mental Health Act, 1987 that was passed on 22 May 1987.

Goel et al. (2004) describe the Mental health scene in India as "a bewildering mosaic of immense impoverishment, asymmetrical distribution of scarce resources, islands of relative prosperity intermixed with vast areas of deprivation, conflicting interests and apparent apathy of governments and the governed alike" (p. 24). In a similar pessimistic vein, a WHO-ICMR project on urban Mental health reports uneven availability of mental health services, human resource deficit especially for non-medical mental health professionals and mental health service gap (82% to96%)

(Desai et al., 2004). Obviously, Geriatric mental health was much slower to develop in India. Gopalakrishnan (2014) reports inadequacy of psycho-geriatric services in India and lists several barriers to mental health service in old age. These barriers are due to psychological factors like attitudes, beliefs about mental illness, logistics like access and availability of services and disease related factors. Over use of services, uneven quality of services, budgetary shortages and poor integration with mainstream health and psychiatric services are some other barriers.

Prakash et al. (2013) state that there are four types of resources to address geriatric mental health issues: (1) state funded government psychiatric hospitals and nursing homes; (2) private psychiatric hospitals and nursing homes; (3) non-government organizations; and (4) informal sources- family as caregivers. The country has limited numbers of mental health professionals, around 4000 psychiatrists catering to the 21 million geriatric populations in need of mental health services. Gero-psychiatry is yet to develop as a strong sub-speciality. The ICMR task force project was instituted in 1987 and published in 1990 (Rao, 1990) was perhaps the first important milestone in this field. Other important milestones were creation in 1988 of a separate inpatient ward for elderly by Dr. Natarajan at the Government General Hospital in Madras and an out-patient clinic for the aged in 1996 by Dr. Vinod Kumar at the All India Institute of Medical Sciences, New Delhi. National Policy on Older persons in 1999 mandated establishment of geriatric medicine in all colleges. Post graduate training at Madras Medical College, Chennai; at Amrita Institute of Medical science, Kochi; at Christian Medical College, Vellore; at AIIMS, New Delhi and PG diploma in Geriatric Medicine in IGNOU, are the major training resources in geriatrics available (Dey & Chartterjee, 2014). Geriatric clinics in Hospitals and prime Institutes like NIMHANS and AIIMS are now playing an important role in research, training and service.

Gerontology and Gero-Psychology in India

Gerontology is the study of the ageing process. It includes the study of physical, psychological and social changes in older individuals and the investigation of societal changes resulting from the ageing of the population. This field is also concerned with the application of this knowledge to policies and programmes. Professional Gero-psychology is a speciality in professional psychology that applies the knowledge and methods of psychology to understanding and helping older persons and their families to maintain wellbeing, overcome problems and achieve maximum potential during later life. Professional Gero-psychology appreciates the wide diversity among older adults, the complex ethical issues that can arise in geriatric practice and the importance of inter-disciplinary models of care.

Ramamurti et al. (2015) provide an account of development of Gerontology in India. Research interest in this field began in late 1950s and mostly concentrated on behavioural and social aspects. Since 2009–2010, increased ICMR funding for individual research projects in social and psychological Gerontology has led to an expansion of research areas. New areas of investigation such as senior welfare, economic and demographic aspects emerged. Centre for Research on Ageing at Department of Psychology of Sri Venkateswara University, Tirupati and University departments of Psychology in other states were responsible for the growth of research in Gero-psychology. Over the years, social and demographic aspects have been taken up by Centre for Gerontological Research, Thiruvananthpuram; Tata Institute of Social Sciences, Mumbai; International Institute for Population Studies, Mumbai; and Institute for Socio-economic Change, Bangalore. Gero-psychology is offered as a core subject in very few universities. However, centres such as Centre for Life long learning (TISS), National Institute of Social Defence and several NGOs such as International Longevity Centre offer diploma and certificate courses in Gerontology. Regional Resources and Training Centres sanctioned by Ministry of Social Justice have been offering a wide range of training programmes in collaboration with NISD. In 2000, the Government of India (GOI) recommended that universities and other educational institutions introduce courses in ageing as part of implementing the National Policy on Older Persons (NPOP). Gerontological subjects mostly form part of the curriculum of psychology, sociology and Home science courses in most Universities. In recent years Professional associations have been playing an important role in pushing the frontiers of research by focusing on new and emerging issues. They have also been persistently sending recommendations to the Government to ensure progressive changes.

A major research project titled "building knowledge base on population ageing in India (BKPAI) was launched by UNFPA in collaboration with the Institute of Social and Economic Change, Bangalore and the Institute of Economic Growth, Delhi. The study focuses on social, economic, health and psychological aspects of elderly. Perhaps the first longitudinal study, the LASI or Longitudinal Ageing Study in India was launched in 2009. This is a collaboration between International institute of Population Science of Mumbai, the Harvard school of public health, the School of Medical Sciences, University of California, Los Angeles; and the RAND Corporation. Its objective is to provide reliable information on the health, health care and social and economic aspects of the Indian population, aged 45 and older. Its first phase (2013–2015) covered two waves of data and is made accessible to public (http://www.iipsindia.org/research_lasi.htm). The initiative of the Government to establish National Institute of Ageing in four major regions is likely to give a boost to research and advocacy in this field. Several NGOs like HelpAge India, Alzheimer's and Related Disorders Society of India (ARDSI), are also contributing to research and development. In September 2018, International symposium on Dementia and 22nd National conference of ARDSI was held in Bangalore (Dementia, 2018). It was refreshing to encounter researchers, service providers, informal care givers pooling in information about dementia. Topics ranging from promoting neuroplasticity, framing dementia within a handicapped model, models of care giving, use of technology in dementia care, artificial intelligence, models of integrated care and Dementia-friendly communities were discussed (Personal communication). This trend of academicians, hard core researchers, NGOs and informal carers coming together to address the challenges in geriatric services augurs well for the field.

Interestingly, the progress of Gero-psychology is being fueled by developments in allied fields of study, research and practice. Clinical Psychology is expanding as a profession (Sengar, 2017) and it has moved from a fixation with child and adolescent mental health to attend to later life issues. Diversification of settings and functions of Clinical Psychologists in recent years has led to newer areas of research including clinical gerontology. Cognitive approaches in therapy have started focusing on memory and behaviour disorders in older adults. Behavioural Gerontology is the application of principles of applied Behaviour analysis in elderly patients to address problems of ageing. The Behavioural and Geriatric Neurology studies focus on patients with late-life neurodegenerative disorders, especially those producing dementia. Dementia, as a disorder, has very few curative options and most common approach is to organize long-term care. As a result, the field of psychosocial rehabilitation is expanding in scope. Development in Neuropsychological testing especially cognitive abilities of older patients is emerging as another interesting field of research. Similarly, behavioural methods to manage age related problems and strategies to improve quality of life through non-pharmacological methods are gaining ground. Inputs from these fields are likely to enrich the field of Gero-psychology.

The Challenges Ahead

The writing on the wall is crystal clear. The growing mental health needs of older persons in India are largely unmet. There is human resource crunch, budgetary cuts and lack of integration of services required by the elderly. Most of the policies and programmes of the Government like NPOP and Maintenance Law have not been effectively implemented and monitored. Nayar (2018) concluded during a National Colloquium on the Status of Aged held in 2018 at Thiruvananthapuram that the Government of India has no clear vision on its senior citizens nor has seriously implemented any of its policies and programmes (Personal communication).

Government initiatives such as the Mental Health Policy, the new Mental Health Bill, National Human Rights Commission initiatives and advocacy actions may bring about a change in the mental health scene in the country. Give some hope that the scene may improve. The National Programme for the Health Care of the Elderly (NPHCE), recommends social security provisions for pensions, income tax benefits, provident fund gratuity and strengthening medical assistance. Capacity building is emphasized by expanding infrastructure. Regional Geriatric Centres in district hospitals and opening of community-based geriatric clinics is recommended. Establishing specialized geriatric training programmes and research institutes to improve manpower and utilizing mass media to educate the public are also recommended. The programme also aims to promote strong inter-organizational linkages and referral mechanisms as well as training and support for informal caregivers. Already recommendations have been made to address every possible need of the elderly. Prakash et al. (2012) point to the discrepancy between policies and the ground reality. These policies are not implemented in true sense. The focus is on social benefits in general not specifically on geriatric mental health problems.

The challenge is not about identifying the problems and solutions. It is about implementing what has already been recommended. The NPOP in fact reads like a wish list. It covers everything, every situations, every section of the elderly. Methods to improve economic security, social inclusion, productive ageing, reduction of morbidity, improve community involvement, build intergenerational solidarity- all topics are discussed. Vulnerable groups, women, elderly in disaster situation, rural, widowed- every group is taken into account. Issues of elder abuse, human rights of older people are also touched upon. Ministries involved in implementation and the functions of different directorates are all outlined. What is glaringly missing is the implementation of the policy. Any recommendation made will be a simple reiteration of what is included in the NPOP. However, from the point of specifically addressing psychological issues, the following suggestions are made.

Issue #1: Increased vulnerability of older persons to physical and psychological problems.

Since the problem is a complex result of multiple causative factors, there cannot be a simple or single solution. Vulnerability in old age is a cumulative effect of life cycle experiences, socio-economic conditions and current stresses. Hence, a lifecycle approach to health care is needed. Assuring basic financial security in old age (reduce dependence), Accessible, affordable and appropriate health care (reduce morbidity), social support measures and elder friendly environment (reduce stress) are measures to decrease the chances of multiple morbidities. Screening for age related psychiatric disorders and cognitive impairment could help initiate early remedial measures.

Issue # 2: Inadequacy of existing Geriatric system.

Many recommendations have been made about integrating and mainstreaming elder care are into existing health care delivery system. Adequate budget, availability of generic drugs at low cost increased access to geriatric services have been much discussed. Manpower shortage and lack of trained professionals are major problems needing to be tackled on priority basis. Not only Geriatricians but others serving elderly patients- nurses, paramedics, social workers, family care givers, home health helpers, physiotherapists, to name a few, have to be trained. The initiatives already taken in this direction need to be intensified.

Issue # 3. Need for paradigm shift in Geriatric care.

For a long time, health care had curative approach rather than preventive or health promotive approach. In Geriatrics, prevention of disability and reducing the burden of disease is very important. Rehabilitation services, provision for long-term care, health system geared to 'continuum of care' from out-patient service to end-of-life care have to be developed. Community-based care is a concept that has to be seriously implemented. Strategies to keep old people in their own homes (ageing in place) have to be developed. Suggestions have been already made to involve local governance in health care programmes.

Issue # 4. Lack of involvement from older people, the major stake holders.

This is basically due to cultural factors as well as lack of awareness. Media should be used to spread information about ageing, issues related to ageing, health and well-being in old age and how to keep oneself healthy in old age. Senior citizen clubs and resident associations could be used to educate people about Elder abuse and methods to identify and prevent abuse. Volunteers could be used to create awareness about legal provisions and programmes of the Government. For example, many are still unaware of the Maintenance of parents act. Awareness about rights of elderly is seriously lacking in the community. Seniors do not access many of the benefits that are available either due to ignorance or due to bureaucratic hassles. Non-Governmental organizations working for elderly could play an important role in advocacy and sensitizing elders to their rights. Involving seniors at all levels and in all programmes may improve implementation and monitoring of programmes. As long as older people are perceived as 'beneficiaries" rather than 'participants' in developmental programmes, they will continue to be passive and dependent.

Issue # 5 Not enough focus on Positive Ageing.

The focus is usually on identifying 'problems' of the elderly and try to find solutions for them. For years, Gerontologists have been speaking about 'successful ageing' 'active ageing' and 'productive ageing'. It is time these concepts were translated into action. Successful ageing has three main components- avoidance of disease and disability, maintenance of cognitive capacity and active engagement in life (Rowe & Kahn, 1987). Elder friendly environment and opportunities for social interaction are essential for older people to remain active. Creating new age-appropriate roles to compensate for losses is important for their morale and life satisfaction. People still have many myths about mental illness and stigma is attached to seeking psychological help. Education about mental health, life style modifications and strategies to fight common stress related disorders would help reduce psychological problems. Retirement counselling, grief counselling and support for people suffering from threatening illnesses are ways of reducing psychological distress associated with important life events. Technology could be a boon to elderly in this regard.

In short, there is no dearth of recommendations, policies and legal measures announced by the state time and again. What a senior citizen needs in India today is implementation, evaluation and monitoring of these schemes and policies.

References

Agarawala, N., & Saikia, S. (2017). Trials and tribulations of aged women in Assam. *Indian Journal of Gerontology, 31*(3), 272–288.

Agarwal, S. P. (Ed.) (2004). *Mental health. An Indian perspective 1946–2003.* Directorate General of Health Services, Ministry of Health and Family Welfare.

Balachandran, M., Raakhee, A. S., & Raj, S. S. H. (2007). Life satisfaction and alienation of elderly males and females. *Journal of Indian Academy Applied Psychology., 33*(2), 157–160.

Banjare, P., Dwivedi, R., & Pradhan, J. (2015). Factors associated with the life satisfaction amongst the rural elderly in Odisha, India. *Health Quality of Life Outcomes, 13*, 201. Published online 2015 Dec 21. https://doi.org/10.1186/s12955-015-0398-y

Barua, A., Das, A., Nagaraj, K., Bhat, H. V., & Nair, N. S. (2007). Depression in elderly: A cross-sectional study in rural South India. *Journal of International Medical Sciences Academy, 20*(4), 259–261.

Barua, A., & Kar, N. (2010). Screening for depression in elderly Indian population. *Indian Journal of Psychiatry, 52*(2), 150–153.

Barua, A., Ghosh, M. K., Kar, N., & Basilio, M. A. (2011). Prevalence of depressive disorders in the elderly. *Annals of Saudi Medicine , 31*(6), 620–624.

Begum K. A. (2008). *Ageing, discrimination and older women's rights from the perspective of CEDAW convention.* http://globalageing.org/.ageingwatch/cedaw/cedaw.pdf

Bharati, D. R., Pal, R., Rekha, R., Yamuna, T. R., Kar, S., & Radjou, A.N. (2011). Ageing in Puducherry, South India: An overview of morbidity profile. *Journal of Pharmacology and Bio-allied Sciences, 3*, 537–552.

Chandra, V., Ganguli, M., Pandav, R., Johnston, J., Belle, S., DeKosky, S. T. (1998). Prevalence of Alzheimer's disease and other dementias in rural India—The Indo-US study. *Neurology, 51*, 1000–1008.

Chaudhary, M., & Arokiasamy, P. (2017). Frailty and associated correlates among older adults: Evidence using SAGE states of India HelpAge India. *Research and Development Journal, 23*(1), 18–29.

Dementia 2018. (2018). In *International Symposium on Dementia and 22nd National Conference of ARDSI*, September 14–16, 2018, Bangalore (Personal Communication)

Desai, N. G., Tiwari, S. C., Nambi, S., Shah, B., Singh, R. B., Kumar, D., Trivedi, J. K., Palaniappan, V., Tripathi, A., Pali, C., Pal, N., Maurya, A., & Mathew, M. (2004). Urban mental health services in India: How complete or incomplete? *Indian Journal of Psychiatry, 46*(3), 194–212.

Dey, A. B., & Chatterjee, P. (2014). Development of Geriatric Medicine in India and other parts of the world. In P. Sanchetee (Ed.), *Textbook of geriatric medicine* (pp. 2–5). Paras Medical Publisher.

Dey, A. B., & Nisar, S. (2014). Epidemiological transition and Multi-morbidity. In Sanchetee, P. (Ed.) *Textbook of geriatric medicine* (pp.19–23). Paras Medical Publisher.

Ganguli, H. C. (2000). Epidemiological findings on prevalence of mental disorders in India. *Indian Journal of Psychiatry, 42*(1), 14–20.

Goel, D. S., Agarwal, S. P., Ichhpujani, R. L., & Shrivastava, S. (2004). Mental health 2003: The Indian scene. In S. P. Agarwal (Ed.), *Mental health. An Indian perspective. 1946–2003.* Directorate General of Health Services, Ministry of Health and Family Welfare.

Gopalakrishnan, R. (2014). Management of psychiatric disorders. In P. Sanchetee (Ed.), *Textbook of geriatric medicine* (pp. 559–567). Paras Medical Publisher.

Government of India. (1982). *National Mental Health Programme for India.* Director General of Health Services, Ministry of Health and Family Welfare.

Government of India. (2006). *Morbidity, health care and the condition of the aged.* National Sample Survey Organization 60th Round (January–June 2004)

Government of India. (2011). *Situation analysis of the elderly in India.* Central Statistics Office, Ministry of Statistics & Programme Implementation, Government of India, June 2011.

Government of India. (2012a) *NPHCE. National Programme for the Healthcare of the elderly: an approach towards active and healthy ageing*. http://www.jkhealth.org/notifications/bal456.pdf

Government of India. (2012b). *Operational guidelines (NPHCE)*. Ministry of Health and Family Welfare Government of India. http://www.mohfw.nic.in/showfile.php?lid=1145

Government of India. (2014). *National Mental Health Policy of India: New pathways, New hope*. Ministry of Health.

Government of India. (2015). *National Health Policy 2015 (draft)*. Ministry of Health.

Government of India. (2015). *Key indicators of social consumption in India: Health*. National Sample Survey Office, Ministry of Statistics and Programme Implementation, June 2015.

Government of India Report on Indian Elderly. (2016). *Elderly in India. Profiles and programmes 2016*. Govt. of India. Central Statistics Office Ministry of Statistics and Programme Implementation Government of India. www.mospi.gov.in

Guild of Service. (2010). Dimensions of deprivation. Report on poverty levels of widows of Vrindavan. Survey conducted by the Guild of service, supported by UNIFEM.

Jacob, K. S. (2012). Depression: A major public health problem in need of a multi-sectoral response. *Indian Journal of Medical Researches, 136*(4), 537–539.

Kirtani, S., & Aminabhavi, V. (2018). Impact of membership to groups on Subjective well-being and spiritual intelligence in elderly. *Indian Journal of Gerontology., 32*(3), 231–245.

Khokhar, A., & Mehra, M. (2001). Life style and morbidity profile of geriatric population in an urbans community of Delhi. *Indian Journal of Medical Sciences, 55*, 609–615.

Maheswaran, T., & Ranjit, L. (2013). A study on life satisfaction among elderly people. *Research Journal of Sociology, 1*, 1–8.

Maity, M., & Mukhopadhyay, B. (2015). Is mental health a burning health issue for indian elderly? *Journal of Psychology and Clinical Psychiatry, 3*, 00132. https://doi.org/10.15406/jpcpy.2015.03.00132

Marpady, P., Jyothi, P. S., & Singhe, M. S. (2012). Social support network and life satisfaction among elders in Mangalore Taluk: An implication for social work intervention. *Elixir: Social Science, 48*, 9457–9460.

Maruthanath, P. S., George, A., Ranjith, N., Justus, S., Kumar, M. S., Menon, P. R., Sarma, S., & Verghese, J. (2012). Incidence of Alzheimer's disease in India: A 10 years follow-up study. *Neurology India, 60*(6), 625–630

Math, S. B., & Srinivasaraju, R. (2010). Indian psychiatric epidemiological studies: Learning from the past. *Indian Journal of Psychiatry, 52*, 95–103.

Nair, P. M., & Anjana, A. (2017). Subjective wellbeing of elders in Kerala Helpage India. *Research and Development Journal, 23*(2), 15–23.

National Institute of Clinical Excellence. (NICE) (2009). *National Collaborating Centre for Mental Health Clinical Guidelines 90. Depression. The treatment and management of depression in adults*. London. http://www.nice.org.uk/nicemedia/pdf/CG90NICEguideline.pdf31

National Institute of Health and Family Welfare GOI. (2014). National Mental Health Program.

National Institute of Mental Health and Neurosciences. (2016). *National Mental Health Survey of India, (2015–16)*. Ministry of Health and Family Welfare, Government of India.

Nayar, P. K. B. (2013). Older women: the context, issues and concerns. In P. K. B. Nayar (Ed.), *Older women in India. The context issues and concerns* (pp. 14–34). The Women Press.

Nayar, P. K. B. (2018) Situation of senior citizens in India. An enquiry into their present status problems and needs. In *National Colloquium on the Aged and Ageing in India*, March 14–16, 2018, Thiruvananthpuram (Personal communication).

Pilania, M., Bairwa, M., Kumar, N., Khanna, P., & Kurana, H. (2013). Elderly depression in India: An emerging public health challenge. *Australasian Medical Journal, 6*(3), 107–111.

Population Reference Bureau. (2012a). India's aging population. *Today's Research on Aging, 25*, 1–6.

Population Reference Bureau. (2012). Noncommunicable diseases among older adults in low- and middle-income countries. *Today's Research on Aging, 26*, 1–6.

Prakash, I. J. (2000). Adult women and the ageing process. *Ageing and Society: THe Indian Journal of Gerontology, 10*(3 & 4), 31–42.
Prakash, I. J. (2001). Socio economic security, health and well being of elderly in Karnataka. In A. Bali (Ed.), *Refashioning the new economic order* (pp. 350–363). ICSSR and Rawat Publisher.
Prakash, I. J. (2003). Aging, disability, and disabled older people in India. In P. S. Liebig & I. S Rajan (Eds.), *An aging India. Perspectives, prospects and policies* (pp. 85–108). The Haworth Press Inc.
Prakash, I. J. (2004). Mental health of older people in India. In P.V. Ramamurti & D. Jamuna (Eds.), *Handbook of Indian gerontology* (pp. 176–207). Serials Publications.
Prakash, I. J. (2008). Psychological issues in ageism and its prevention. In M. Rao (Ed.), *Needs and care of the elderly* (pp. 40–49). The Icfai University Press.
Prakash, I. J. (2010). "Agequake"—Managing the impact of population aging in India. In R. Sharma & C. J. Thomas (Eds.), *Ageism: Problems and prospects* (pp. 103–118). Akansha Publishing House.
Prakash, I. J. (2011). Identification, intervention and prevention of elder abuse. In *A manual for professionals and volunteers*. HelpAge India.
Prakash, I. J. (2013) Social well-being of older women in India: Identifying and addressing vulnerabilities. In P. K. B. Nayar (Ed.), *Older women in India. The context, issues and concerns* (pp. 66–92). The Women Press
Prakash, I. J. (2014). Impact of globalization and changing families on older people in India. In P. Sanchetee (Ed.), *Textbook of geriatric medicine* (pp. 58–62). Paras Medical Publisher.
Prakash, I. J. (2018). Psychological impact of Elder Abuse. Some intervention methods to help the victims. HelpAge India. *Research and Development Journal, 24*(2), 6–12.
Prakash, O., & Kukreti, P. (2013). State of geriatric Mental health in India. *Current Transactions in Geriatrics and Gerontology, 2013*(2), 1–6. https://doi.org/10.1007/s13670-012-0034-1
Priyanka & Mishra, S. (2013). Differences in life satisfaction of elderly people in urban and semi urban families of Lucknow (U.P.) *IOSR Journal of Humanities And Social Science (IOSR-JHSS), 16*(6), 28–32
Purty, A. J., Bazroy, J., Kar, M., Vasudevan, K., Veliath, A., & Panda, P. (2006). Morbidity pattern among the elderly population in the rural area of Tamil Nadu, India. *Turkish Journal of Medical Sciences, 36*, 45–50.
Qadri, S. S., Ahluwalia, S., Ganai, A. M., Bali, P. S., Wani, F. A., & Bashir, H. (2013). An epidemiological study on quality of life among rural elderly population of Northern India. *International Journal of Medical Sciences and Public Health., 2*, 514–522.
Raj, D., Swain, P. K., & Pedgaonkar, S. P. (2014). A study on quality of life satisfaction & physical health of elderly people in Varanasi: An urban area of Uttar Pradesh, India. *International Journal of Medical Sciences and Public Health., 3*(5), 616–620.
Rajkumar, A. P., Thangadurai, P., Senthilkumar, P., Gayathri, K., & Prince, M. (2009). Nature, prevalence and factors associated with depression among the elderly in a rural South Indian community. *International Psychogeriatrics, 21*(2), 372–378.
Ramamurti, P. V., Liebig, P., & Jamuna, D. (2015). Gerontology in India. *Gerontologist, 55*(6), 894–900.
Rao, A. V. (1990). *Health care of the rural aged. National task force project*. Indian council of Medical Research.
Rao, A. V. (2004). Psychiatry in old age (gero-psychiatry). In. P. V. Ramamurti & D. Jamuna (Ed.), *Handbook of Indian gerontology* (pp. 117–151). Serials Publications.
Reddy, M. V., & Chandrashekhar, C. R. (1998). Prevalence of mental and behavioural disorders in India: A meta-analysis. *Indian Journal of Psychiatry, 40*, 149–157.
Reddy, B. N., Pallavi, M., Reddy, N. N., Reddy, C. S., Singh, R. K., & Pirabu, R.A. (2012) Psychological morbidity status among the rural geriatric population of Tamil Nadu, India: A cross-sectional study. *Indian Journal of Psychological Medicine. 34*(3), 227–231
Registrar General of India. (2011). *Sample registration system* (p. 47). October 2012

Ridic, G., Gleason, S., & Ridic, O. (2012). Comparisons of health care systems in the United States. *Germany and Canada. Materia Socio Medica, 24*, 112–120.
Roy, S. G. (2004). Demographics of the Indian older population. In P. V. Ramamurti & D. Jamuna (Eds.), *Handbook of Indian gerontology* (pp 1–27). Serials Publications.
Rowe, J. W., & Kahn, R. L. (1987). Human aging: Usual and successful. *Science, 237*, 143–149.
Seby, K., Chaudhury, S., & Chakraborty, R. (2011). Prevalence of psychiatric and physical morbidity in an urban geriatric population. *Indian Journal of Psychiatry, 53*(2), 121–127.
Sengar, K. S. (2017). Clinical Psychology beyond mental hospitals. Changing role of Clinical psychologists. *Indian Journal of Clinical Psychology, 44*(1), 1–5
Shaji, K. S., Bose, S., & Varghese, A. (2005). (2015) Prevalence of dementia in an urban population in Kerala, India. *British Journal of Psychiatry, 186*, 136–140.
Shaji, K. S., Jithu, V. P., & Jyothi, K. S. (2010). Indian research on aging and dementia. *Indian Journal of Psychiatry, 52*(Suppl1), S148–S152.
Shraddha, K., Prashantha, B., & Prakash, B. (2012) Study on morbidity pattern among elderly in urban population of Mysore, Karnataka, India. *International Journal of Medicine and Biomedical Research 1*(3), 215–223.
Singh, P., Kumar, L. K., & Reddy, P. K. C. M. (2012). Psychiatric morbidity in geriatric population in old age homes and community: A comparative study. *The Indian Journal of Psychological Medicine. 34*(1), 39–43.
Swami, H. M., Bhatia, V., Dutt, R., & Bhatia, S. P. S. (2002). A Community Based Study of the Morbidity Profile among the Elderly in Chandigarh, India. *Bahrain Medical Bulletin, 24*(1), 13–16.
UNFPA. (2012). Building knowledge base on population aging in India. In *(BKPAI) Report on the status of elderly in select states of India, 2011*. United Nation Population Fund.
WHO. (1997). WHOQOL. *Measuring quality of life. Division of Health and prevention of substance abuse*. World Health Organization.
WHO. (2001). *The world health report. Mental health: New understanding, new hope*. World Health Organization.
WHO. (2011). *Global health and aging*. World Health Organization and NIH Publication No. 11–7737.
WHO. (2017). *Mental health of older adults, 12 December*. World Health Organization.
WHO. (2018a). *Mental health in India*. WHO, India Country Office for India. Health topic. 2018. Mental health and substance abuse.
WHO. (2018b). *mhGap*. World Health Organization.
Wig, N. N., & Murthy, R. S. (2015). The birth of national mental health program for India. *Indian Journal of Psychiatry, 57*(3), 315–319.

Chapter 5
Gerontological Social Work in India: The Emerging Trends

S. Siva Raju and Vibha Singh

Abstract The ageing discourse has now moved onto acknowledging the greater demand for the ageing-competent practitioners and the dynamic interventions. The review of earlier literature in the field of Gerontological Social Work in India clearly reveals that there exists an inadequate focus of this emerging area. Further, it is noticed that there is a shift in the approach to interventions in elderly care in recent times. The current interventions mainly focus on organizing and empowering older persons for their own development and wellbeing. The focus of the paper is to discuss the context of Gerontological Social Work in India: the role and approaches in Social Work along with the concerns and challenges in the discipline. The paper also discusses the scope for development of interventions in the area of elderly care in India and highlights them with a few selective good practices as adopted and implemented by various agencies in India. The paper concludes with a discussion on the possible solutions for strengthening the competencies of Gerontological Social Work Professionals and the effective interventions that require for facing the challenges of population ageing in developing countries like India.

Keywords Active ageing · Gerontology · Population ageing · Social work

Introduction

Population ageing has emerged as one of the major demographic concerns of recent times. In most parts of the developing countries, the demographic transitions are negatively affecting the social fabric and local community arrangements. While the ageing population is a sign of successful development in medical sciences and technology, living standards and education, it also brought distinct social, economic and clinical challenges such as growing demand for increasingly complex health care services (Evans et al., 2011). India is still considered a youth nation and probably this is why population ageing is not seen as an immediate threat. However, the projection

S. Siva Raju (✉) · V. Singh
Tata Institute of Social Science, Mumbai, India

M. K. Shankardass (ed.), *Gerontological Concerns and Responses in India*,
https://doi.org/10.1007/978-981-16-4764-2_5

of population growth of elderly is faster in developing countries than many developed countries. The demographic structure of India is expected to shift dramatically from a young to an ageing population with 316 million elderly persons by 2050 (James, 2011). These are absolute demographic propositions where proportion of elderly is increasing with social and health care needs. This is a call for social work educators and practitioners to integrate gerontology into formal academic training programmes.

Elderly in India face multiple vulnerabilities due to various reasons. The structural inequalities, inadequate place of elder care in policies and insignificant attention from the Non-Profit sector are a few to name. The discipline of Gerontology is still in infancy stage in the country. The population ageing has been discussed widely in the Ageing allied disciplines like rehabilitation, nursing, disability, public health, social work and demography. Social work professionals come to front because they facilitate the needs of elderly and enable help from different service providers. Considering the increasing population of elderly people, more social work professionals will be needed to deal with the issues related to population ageing, followed by adequate training for developing the competencies. There is a greater demand for ageing-competent practitioners who can understand the social, environmental and personal needs, as people age.

As the major service providers to older adults and families, Social work professionals require to have varied skills and competencies to meet the need. Social work professionals, regardless of their current area of specialization, cannot underestimate the potential impact that ageing population will have on all their future professional roles (Wheeler & Guinta, 2009). The field of ageing is multifaceted and involves meeting needs through a variety of roles. Social work is one of important fields that cater to the needs of elderly. In large measure, social work practice "is always shaped by the needs of the times, the problems they present, the fears they generate, the solutions that appeal and the knowledge and skill available" (Reynolds (1935) as cited in Greene & Cohen, 2005). Social work professionals work closely with the elderly and their families and social welfare and health organizations. These roles will be discussed further in the paper.

Evolution of Gerontological Social Work in India

The early foundation of social work practice was recognized in 1601 with The Elizabethan poor law which had shifted the responsibility of relief of the poor from the traditional agencies to the government authorities. However, the roots of social work education can be traced back in the nineteenth century in Britain and other European countries and later in the United states, Asia, Africa and South America. The first recognized University to teach Social Work in Asia was Yenching University in 1922 but it was suspended because of some political reasons. That's why the credit of starting the first School of Social work in Asia goes to Tata Institute of Social Sciences in 1936. By 1950, India had developed many universities and institutes offering the education of social work like Kashi Vidyapeeth, Varanasi and College of Social Service, Gujarat Vidyapeeth, Delhi School of Social Work, University of Baroda and University of Lucknow. The initial focus of majority of these institutes was poverty, education and health. But gradually they expanded their area of interventions and targeted the population group like children, women, elderly and other vulnerable groups in the society. These institutes, later on, started providing specialization papers at the master's level, e.g. social work with elderly.

However, the initial development in the education of Gerontology was in the field of psychology and medicine. The Department of Psychology, S.V University, introduced the first graduate course in Gerontology in 1976, followed by a master's specialized course, with the support of University Grant Commission and the first research centre on Ageing in India called 'The centre for research on Ageing' in 1983. In 1980, the medical institutes expanded their wings to geriatrics and started offering specialized programmes, e.g. doctoral programmes by the Centre for Molecular Biology of Ageing at Banaras Hindu University and post graduate courses in geriatric by Madras Medical College in 1996.

National policy for Older persons (1999) recommended universities and institutes to introduce courses on Ageing. As a result, several institutes now offer courses on Ageing at various levels in different disciplines like Social Work, Psychology, anthropology, occupational therapy and rehabilitation, etc. Albeit, there are some challenges and concerns in social work education which need to be addressed to improve the efficiency of the profession. Some of the concerns and challenges are the quality of services provided by the social work professionals, competencies of the professionals, inadequate formal training to social work students, unattractive job prospects, lack of scholarships to pursue research on Ageing and other financial constraints, inadequate number of faculty to supervise students in gerontology and in-service training to the professionals and ageism in general. This paper attempts to touch upon some of these concerns and discuss the recent developments in the field of Ageing and the status of Gerontogical practices in India and their further scope of development.

Evolution of 'New Gerontology'

The new gerontology is built on a successful-ageing paradigm. This new and positive gerontology is based on the philosophy of wellness where active ageing, successful ageing and productive ageing are the commonly referred words. For Atchley (1999), maintaining thinking patterns, activities, living arrangements and social relationships despite changes in health constitutes the idea of continuity (Greene & Cohen, 2005). A subtle transition in the paradigm was observed in 1980s where Rowe and Kahn and other authors made significant arguments about Positive ageing. The philosophy of 'life continuity' replaced the perspective that growing old is a time of loss and decline. Rowe and Kahn (1998) as cited in Greene & Cohen, 2005 suggested that leading a salutary life involves minimizing risk and disability, maximizing physical and mental abilities and engagement in an active life. Rowe and Kahn emphasized that the effects of ageing are not equivalent to disease as seen previously.

These philosophies are in line with the theory of Salutogenesis proposed by Antonovsky in 1998. It posits that people use their resources naturally to strive for health. The focus here is on the factors that optimize the health rather than the treatments or prevention of the diseases. Therefore, in the new gerontology, the focus of the interventions should be more on facilitating the individuals in mobilizing the resources for development, health and wellbeing. The successful-ageing paradigm also envisions confident ageing older adults to be financially secured, productive and educated about their health care (Corman & Kingson, (1996) as cited in Greene & Cohen, 2005)).

Majority of work in research and practice based on the philosophies on new gerontology. Recent researches in the country Focus on active ageing, volunteerism, social participation, age-friendliness. (Kaushik, 2011; Singh, 2016; Vasi, 2016). The Journal of Madras School of Social Work brought out a special edition (Guest Editor: Siva Raju, 2016) to highlight the studies and practices on 'Positive Ageing'.

Understanding Older Adult Population from the Social Work Perspective

A social work professional understands that the culture, gender, ethnic group membership, sexual orientation and life experiences add to the uniqueness of the ageing experience for each older adult. Elderly population can be grouped as 'young-old', 'middle-old' and 'oldest-old'. Each group has different concerns and requires distinct interventions. Young-old is a group of age between 60 to 70 years. This group doesn't really associate themselves with the old population. They might still be working or newly retired, comparatively still be socially engaged and with less health problems. On the other hand, people aged between 70 to 80 years and till 85 years in some regions are called middle-old group. This group has their own characteristics and they experience more health problems, restrictions in mobility, with growing needs for supportive services. Most of these older adults are out of the labour force. People in this age group also experience loss of spousal company and shrinking social networks. The group which needs the assistance the most is oldest-old. These are people with age 80 years and plus. The needs of this group are different from the other groups. They are more likely to experience some serious health issues and require assistance with the activities of daily living. Each group need specific social, health and mental services to maintain the functioning of optimum health and independence. Early life experiences also affect the socio-economic well-being of individuals in old age. Therefore, there are several factors that determine the experiences of elderly which need to be considered for designing the diagnosis and interventions.

The elderly in India are a heterogeneous population with variations in morbidity across several dimensions, gender, location and socio-economic status in particular, as well as great diversity in cultures, religions and languages (Evans et al., 2011). Therefore, the intervention should be individualistic, based on the principle of self-determination. Social Work professionals also understand that there are even more marginalized groups within the ageing population which requires interventions based on distinct and right based approaches. From the perspective of social inclusion, elderly from rural areas, transgender, disabled, women, single elderly, poor elderly and migrants are some of the vulnerable sections within the ageing population which needs special attention.

Main Concerns Affecting the Elderly in India

Population ageing is inevitable and should be seen as an achievement, as it is a result of better living opportunities and further advancement in health care system. There is a need to have a holistic view of ageing in the country. In the era of new gerontology, Ageing India report (UNFPA, 2017) identified four main concerns of elderly population in India, namely, Participation and contribution, Income security, health and enabling and supporting environment.

Participation and contribution: In order to prepare the people to live a hundred-year life, there is a need to support them in continue participating in social, economic, political systems. Wishing ageing to be successful, active and healthy necessarily entails considering social participation as a key concept of social policy (Raymond et al., 2013). Some activities help older adults develop knowledge and skills that boost their self-image and mental outlook (Harlow-Rosentraub et al., (2006) as cited in Zedlewsk & Butricai, 2007). Engagement provides the sense of purpose to older adults. Therefore, in this era of new and positive gerontology, researches and programmes should be initiated to promote social and productive engagement of elderly.

Income security: For a country like India, one of the major concerns for elderly is the financial security. Only small proportion of people retire from organized sector receives pension and other retirement benefits. But for others, actual struggles start when they stop working and become dependent on their family for economic needs. Government of India and state governments provide a small pension which has very nominal coverage. The needs of elderly women are more critical, as some of them never worked in formal employment and have always been dependent on their family members for their needs. Social inequalities and processes make the economic disparity even greater for some elderly like migrants, disabled and transgenders. Therefore, suitable measures should be initiated by both government and non-government sectors to secure financial needs of elderly.

Health of elderly: Health is such important component in old age that healthy ageing and active ageing are used interchangeably. Health issues of elderly are not restricted to a set of diseases but also include functional incapacitation due to senescent changes in body. Chronically ill patients suffer from diseases like diabetes, heart ailments, cancer and they face various complex medical and psychosocial problems which require special interventions from social work professionals. The role of social workers for this section of elderly is to enable them access and utilize social and health care services effectively. As social workers use life cycle approach to make intervention, there is an urgent need to advocate the long-term care policy in India. Social workers also need to focus on End-of-Life patients to make life less miserable at that stage of life.

Supportive environment: Ageing occurs primarily in the community and familial context. People in old age may find it difficult in adjusting to the fast changing social and physical environment. Various studies have confirmed the influence of social and physical environment on the quality of life of elderly and conclude that small modifications in the physical environment may help in maintaining the independent functioning among elderly (Singh, 2016). Therefore, adequate attention should be given to creating a suitable environment for elderly to embrace the changes. The role of social workers is very crucial in this context. Social workers with the necessary knowledge and skills are needed to work with elderly and families.

Role of Social Work in Care of Elderly

Social work professionals have a very important role to play to deal with the issues related to ageing, ranging from direct services to elderly and families to macro-level interventions. Social Workers are the important actors of the inter-disciplinary team aiming at contributing to the wellbeing of the elderly. They are the mediators which connect different service providers to the clients in various forms. In a way, we can say they connect the dots. Social workers play the role of an advocate, manager, educator, facilitator, organizer, enabler, mediator, coordinator, analyst, initiator and researcher. The role consists of connecting the elderly and families with the right resources and services in the community. The varied services range from counselling to consultation with family members to plan the long-term care for the elderly and to resource mobilization. Their role is not limited to working with elderly who are coping with physical and mental problems but also enables the elderly to lead active and productive lives. With a sound understanding of the social processes, social work professionals don't underestimate the influence of the environment on the clients. Social work practices the principle of Person-in-Environment approach which holds the belief that environment is one of the most influential factors. Direct services to elderly involve community social service settings, geriatric case management, independent and assisted-living communities, home health care agencies, adult day health settings, hospitals and nursing homes. Macro-level roles include planning at local, state and regional levels; legislative and political advocacy; creating awareness and research and education and consultancy in business and industry. The role of social work professionals is basically discussed under the three main types; Action, Advocacy and Research.

Action: Social Work professionals can take various actions to empower older adults. They can assist older adults with preparing the advanced care plans especially for end-of-life patients, employment opportunities for young older adults, strengthening the role of families by family therapies, younger generation & community, intergenerational solidarity, enabling older adults to make best use of technology to make their lives easier. Social Work professionals also help elderly people in times of natural calamities by providing relief and rehabilitation.

Advocacy: The advocacy is a powerful tool for social workers to empower older adults. They can educate elderly for financial preparedness, health promotion and for active ageing. They can advocate the rights and concerns of elderly population like universal pension, policies on long-term care plans, opportunities for social participation, housing for elderly and other inequalities and opportunities. Social workers can also initiate public campaigns for creating age-friendly societies and educating public to accept the population ageing positively. Social workers can also Strengthen the civil society for the cause of elderly people, promote innovation in elder care.

Gerontological Research: The robustness of gerontological education's trajectory has been less than gerontological research development. Social and behavioural gerontology covers more than half of ageing research (Ramamurti et al., 2015). The researches are mainly in: markers of successful ageing; assessment of disability and coping, characteristics among the centenarians; and developing conceptual model of ageing (Ramamurti & Jamuna, 2010a, b), gender, mental health, empowerment and ageing (Prakash, 2003, 2004); health and ageing of urban elders (Siva Raju, 2002), advocacy and rights of the elderly population (Nayar, 2003), elder abuse and sociological perspectives (Shankardas, 2003), rural ageing and loneliness (Prafulla, 2009), anthropometry of the elderly population, female ageing and health (Bagga, 1994, 2013), old age homes and security, pensions and coping with disasters (Anupama & Sonali, 2012), social security and the demographics of ageing and social security (Ramamurti et al., 2015).

Indian Gerontological Society's Indian Journal of Gerontology, HelpAge India's Research and Development Journal, Calcutta Metropolitan Institute of Gerontology's Ageing and Society: The Journal of Gerontology and the Indian Journal of Geriatrics, besides some of the international journals like Ageing and Society, The Gerontological Society of America's The Journals of Gerontology, Journal of Ageing and Health covered major researches in ageing. There is also an effort in the country to create a large database about the ageing population by the academic institutes through the large scale surveys like Building knowledge base on Population Ageing in India (BKPAI) and Longitudinal Ageing Study in India (LASI).

Competencies and Skills Required Among the Social Work Professionals

In order to improve the efficiency of the social work professionals, following are the keys points that the academic institutions need to consider training young social work students.

Knowledge about the health and emerging trends: Social work professionals must continuously update their knowledge of basic mechanisms of health care and prevention and interventions for the impact created by the illnesses. The understanding of the working of health care system, financial structures and related management process is essential for health social workers.

Practice skills in ageing: The social work professionals need to develop new skills and strengthen the foundation skills in order to keep pace with the societal changes with regards to ageing. bio-psychosocial assessment, counselling and case management over the continuum of care. Family practice and advocacy for the needs of individuals and their families will remain the essential practice skills of social workers in health care and ageing (Berkman et al., 2006).

Cultural competency and skills for ethical practices: Given the heterogeneity among the elderly, it is very essential for social workers to remain sensitive towards each case and must practice competently and creatively with older adults and their families from a variety of cultural backgrounds. At times, social work professionals may have to serve as the family therapist, counsellors, mediators in addressing the ethical dimensions of medical decisions, for example, for end-of-life patients. This, along with other family interventions, requires high skill level of ethical practice.

Social work profession specific competencies: The knowledge and practice of conducting Case work and group work will be very helpful for Social workers to understand the clients properly and bring out the suitable interventions specific to their context.

Existing Intervention Models: Changing Approaches

Social work interventions in India are not limited to social work professionals. There are various actors who are contributing their bit for the wellbeing of the elderly. Traditionally, the interventions were limitedly from the Social work institutions, government and non-governmental agencies. There are new emerging social models of care. A special report on good practices of elder care in India by UNPFA mentioned five such good practices. These are ESHG by HelpAge India, Kudumbshree in Kerala, palliative care model in Kerala by, dementia and active ageing initiatives and food security initiative in Tamil Nadu. A thorough analysis of the approaches of these good practices shows that the philosophy behind these programmes is to make elderly self-sustained groups of empowered elderly. There is shift in the approach from welfare to empowerment of the people. For example, ESHG helps elderly in managing finances in order to lead a risk-free life. Similarly, Kudumbashree works with volunteers at various levels. It is more of a participatory programme than working for the elderly. Let's discuss some of the good practices from recent times.

ESHG is Self-help group for elderly and the philosophy considers that elderly group is heterogeneous in nature. It creates the foundation of 'Elder for Elder' spirit where they can help each other instead of relying on the younger generation. It doesn't only ensure economic wellbeing but also provides an opportunity to engage in different financial and social activities like maintaining the records, attend meetings and additional bank related work. This enhances their capabilities and enables them in leading an active life. It also strengthens their social participation which is an important pillar of active ageing. On similar lines, Kudumbashree pilot project for elderly in Kerala targets social development activities like social security, health care, social protection and livelihood support, etc. Kudumbashree community organizations functions at three levels: Neighbourhood group, area development society and community development society. This ensures the sustainability of elder care through livelihood support. The next best practice targets end-of-life patients, i.e. the palliative care. Every state in India should have a palliative care policy like Kerala. What makes it different and successful is the collaborative efforts of community, NGOs and states involving the home-care teams. The Malapurram model of palliative care is a successful example which can be followed in other parts of the country. It functions with the help of state and community participation where medical professionals, volunteers and family members are trained to provide care to elderly people.

Another best practice targets 3.7 million people who are going to be affected by dementia (The dementia report 2010). The Bengaluru based Nightingales Centre for Ageing and Alzheimer's (NCAA) provides the largest comprehensive care facility for dementia with 88 inpatient beds. The services range from memory clinics, assessment of challenging behaviours, a multi-disciplinary team to take care of all aspects of dementia and non-pharmacological interventions like art, music, dance therapies along with professional counselling. The day care centres also emphasize wellness to ensure active ageing. Other activities like physical activities, cognitive activities and social cognitive activities are done at The Bagchi centre for active ageing.

Noon Meal Programme (NMP), Amma canteen aim to reduce malnutrition among the elderly and alleviate nutritional insecurity among the poor elderly. NMP is successful because it is working with the existing resources of Integrated Child Development Services (ICDS) and Public Distribution System (PDS). Amma canteen usually serves 55,000 people every day in various branches across Tamil Nadu. Not only it serves the nutritional needs of elderly, but also provide livelihood opportunities to women by working in the canteens. PDS, being a poverty alleviation programme, promotes social welfare by supplying essential commodities like rice, sugar, wheat, kerosene, etc. to elderly people. The combined benefits of these food security programmes might be useful in other parts of the country.

Another example of community-based practice is by The Family Welfare Agency (FWA), Mumbai which developed from working with general community-based issues to providing specialized services in the field of Ageing and Mental Health. The FWA has worked at three levels preventive, promotive and curative within the community and nearby areas. The agency has, thus progressed from 'remedial' to 'therapeutic' and has now broadened its approach with a 'social development' perspective, emphasis on integrating approaches. Various need based services are provided through the MSC to cater to the health care and management (physical and mental), educational, recreational, social security, rights and facilities for senior citizens, Community outreach, counselling—personal and family issues of and related to senior citizens.

The concept of Mobile Medical Units (MMU) by HelpAge India programme also takes health care to the doorstep of the needy in the community. The MMUs address the problems of unaffordability, inaccessibility and non-availability of basic essential health care to poor elderly. This programme has immediate short-term impact towards improvement in the quality of life of marginalized elderly beneficiaries. The MMU provides basic diagnostics, free treatment, free medicines, home visits by doctor, counselling for patients, elders, family members and caretakers, community awareness on the rights of the elderly, referral linkage with local health providers, linkage with Govt. schemes and programmes.

Elderly Care Through Corporate Social Responsibility (CSR)

CSR has been a longstanding phenomenon in India and has a great potential for improving the quality of life of elderly. Its beginnings were in the concept of corporate philanthropy where business houses made occasional charitable donations. The CSR practices in India have evolved from the notions of pure charity to its practice as part of social development, to the multi-stakeholder approach that is the current global trend. Most recent and welcome change in India has been the specification by the Government through an amendment in the Companies Act- 2013, of the amount that a corporate company has to 'spend mandatorily' for the 'specified activities' they may undertake to fulfil their CSR obligation for social development.

The Government's (revised) notification with the amendments to Schedule VII (10 items of social development for which CSR expenditure is mandatory) of the Companies Act, 2013 was issued on 27 February 2014, after substituting the 10 items with items that were inclusive of the elderly and declared it effective from 1st April 2014. Pertaining to the elderly, it broadly stipulated activities such as enhancing vocational skills, initiating livelihood enhancement projects, setting up old age homes, day care centres and such other facilities and benefits for armed forces veterans and war widows. Due to the amendment to the 10 items of Schedule VII in the Companies Act, 2013, elderly can now hope for some reprieve due to the initiatives by the corporate sector and look forward to a dignified old age. This mandate will also mean that the corporate companies have to undergo the Government audit and provide evidence of their accountability in working with the elderly. Non-Governmental agencies, senior citizens and individuals working on elderly issues have since begun to take financial assistance from corporates to improve the quality of life of elderly through various activities.

Challenges in Gerontological Social Work Profession

In 2002, Rosen & Zlotnik brought attention to the disconnection between social work and gerontology. He emphasized that Social work must find its unique way to address the disconnect between demographic reality and a contemporary educational environment that does not prepare most social workers for a growing ageing population (Rosen & Zlotnik, 2002). He further emphasized that the social work profession is well suited to work with older adults and their families and that there are a variety of opportunities to strengthen ageing and gerontology education for social work. A lack of current curriculum, encouragement among the social work students and limited gerontological expertise are the main concerns about Social Work and Gerontology.

He conducted research to study the course curriculum, interests and competencies of the professional. Similar studies should be initiated in India so that the understanding could be used to promote the discipline accordingly. Crewe (2005) endorsed Ethnogerontology in order to cater the issues of the heterogeneity among the elderly. India is lagging behind to even consider these concerns. Gerontology hasn't really attracted young professionals yet. Moreover, there is shortage in faculty as well, who can promote the field among the young graduates. Job opportunities for interested candidates are very few and often not very lucrative. Due to lack of interest and availability of scholarships in the field of Ageing, there are very few early career researchers working in the field of Ageing. These are some other academic and professional challenges Social work Gerontology need to tackle for its development in the country like Ageism and social attitude, Counter transference, Independence, Self-awareness and faculty development.

Way Forward

Clearly, there is a need to promote healthy and productive ageing in the country. It is better to be done at earliest; otherwise, there would be a greater concern like in China, Japan and other western countries. The transition from a 'youth' country to a 'silver' county will be faster than anticipated. Wheeler and Guinta (2009) suggested four areas in gerontological social work to promote productive ageing. These are: (1) employment and retirement; (2) volunteerism and civic engagement; (3) informal caregiving; and (4) investment in local, cross-sector planning and collaborative community development.

India's elders make an important contribution to society. As per Krishnaswamy et al. (2008), these include contribution through the formal workforce, household contribution such as raising grandchildren, caring for the sick, resolving the conflict, maintain and transferring culture and religious heritage and volunteerism in society. Therefore, there is need to look beyond the 'ageing as burden' and replace it with the perspective of 'celebrate age', which focus on opportunities than the problems. Traditionally, the focus of gerontological social work in India has been on the issues related to destitution, pension, migration, care giving aspects, activities of daily living, social needs and other family and community-based interventions. The second wave shifted the focus to mental health, strengthening intergenerational solidarity and elder abuse. Now the issues that require attention and promotion are age: friendliness, lifelong learning, third age career, volunteerism, ageism, productive engagement, housing, technology and innovations, social entrepreneurship. Given the dramatic growth in the numbers and proportion of older adults in our society and in the financing, delivery and technological advances of bio-medical health care, it is time to bring the concept of ageing and health care together in the social work educational programmes, practice, policy and research (Berkman et al., 2006). A standard curriculum of gerontology, with local context, should be included in Social Work institutes. There is need to have more 'Centres of excellence on Ageing' in universities in India to attract and encourage scholars to study ageing issues in India.

For many elderly persons, remaining in the labour pool is not a choice; but the necessity while some choose to remain in employment. Social work interventions embedded in the framework of productive ageing suggest capitalizing the strengths and resources of elderly. Enhancing Social participation and adopting the Active ageing policies in the interventions is the need of the hour. There is a need to encourage social entrepreneurship/ social business in elder care among young social work professionals. State and CSR ventures need to encourage social innovations for elder care. Adequate funding opportunities are required so that under-represented communities and their issues could be focussed. Other important areas to be focussed are: Palliative care as the part of health care system, End-of-life and long-term care.

Acknowledgements The authors would like to acknowledge with thanks the contribution of Mr. Gandharva Pednekar for highlighting the issues related to Ageing and Corporate Social Responsibility.

References

Anupama, D., & Sonali, S. (2012). Elder abuse in India. New Delhi, India: HelpAge India.

Bagga, A. (1994). Health status of women in old age homes. *Ageing and Society: The Indian Journal of Gerontology, 4*, 11–21.

Bagga, A. (2013). Women, aging, and mental health. New Delhi, India: Mittal Publications.

Berkman, B., Gardner, D., Zodikoff, B., & Harootyan, L. (2006). Social work and aging in the emerging health care world. *Journal of Gerontological Social Work, 48*(1–2), 203–217.

Caring for Our Elders: Early responses—India ageing report (2017) UNFPA.

Crewe, S. E. (2005). Ethnogerontology: Preparing culturally competent social workers for the diverse facing of aging. *Journal of Gerontological Social Work, 43*(4), 45–58.

Evans, J. M., Kiran, P. R., & Bhattacharyya, O. K. (2011). Activating the knowledge-to-action cycle for geriatric care in India. *Health Research Policy and Systems, 9*(1), 42.

Greene, R. R., & Cohen, H. L. (2005). Social work with older adults and their families: Changing practice paradigms. *Families in Society, 86*(3), 367–373.

James, K. S. (2011). India's demographic change: Opportunities and challenges. *Science, 333*(6042), 576–580.

Kaushik, A. (2011). *Active ageing: A study of elderly contributing in urban.* VDM Verlag Dr. Mullar Publication.

Krishnaswamy, B., Sein, U. T., Munodawafa, D., Varghese, C., Venkataraman, K., & Anand, L. (2008). Ageing in India. *Ageing International, 32*(4), 258–268.

Nayar, P. K. B. (2003). Senior grassroot organizations in India. In: Liebig, P. S., & Irudaya Rajan, S. (Eds.) An aging India: Perspectives, prospects, and policies (pp. 193–212). Binghamton, NY: Haworth Press.

Prafulla, C. (2009). The sunset years. Calcutta, India: Abhiyan Publishers Pvt. Ltd.

Prakash, I. J. (2003). Home alone: Older people coping with loneliness. In: Prakash, I. J. (Ed.) Aging: Emerging issues (pp. 31–36). Bangalore, India: Bangalore University.

Prakash, I. J. (2004). Mental health of older people in India. In: Ramamurti, P. V., & Jamuna, D. (Eds.) Handbook on Indian gerontology (pp. 176–208). Delhi, India: Serials Publications.

Ramamurti, P. V., Liebig, P. S., & Duvvuru, J. (2015). Gerontology in India. *The Gerontologist, 55*(6), 894–900.

Raymond, E., Sevigny, S., Tourigny, A., Vezina, A., Verreault, R., & Guilbert, A. (2013). On the track of evaluated programmes targeting the social participation of seniors: A typology proposal. *Ageing and Society, 33(2),* 267–296. https://doi.org/10.1017/S01447686X11001152.

Ramamurti, P. V., & Jamuna, D. (2010a). Geropsychology in India.

Ramamurti, P. V., & Jamuna, D. (2010b). Developments and research on aging in India. In: Palmore, E. B., Whittington, F., & Kunkel, S. (Eds.). The International handbook on aging: Current research and developments (pp. 260–269). Santa Barbara, CA: Praeger.

Rosen, A. L., & Zlotnik, J. L. (2002). Demographics and reality: The "disconnect" in social work education. *Journal of Gerontological Social Work, 36*(3–4), 81–97.

Shankardas, M. K. (2003). Combating elder abuse in India-An emerging social, legal, and public health concern-A status report. In: Proceedings of 7th Asia Oceania Regional Congress of Gerontology, Tokyo, Japan.

Singh, V. (2016). Environmental factors influencing active ageing amongst elderly women. *The Journal of the Madras School of Social Work, 10*(1 & 2), 113–128.

Siva Raju, S. (2016). Need for promoting positive ageing: Some empirical evidences. *The Journal of the Madras School of Social Work, 10*(1&2), 1–8.

Siva Raju, S. (2002). Health Status of the Urban Elderly: a medico-social study. B.R. Publishing Company, Delhi.

United Nations Population Fund . (2017). *'Caring for our elders: Early responses'—India ageing report—2017*. UNFPA.

Vasi, S. (2016). Active ageing through volunteerism: A review. *The Journal of the Madras School of Social Work, 10*(1 & 2), 61–89.

Wheeler, D. P., & Giunta, N. (2009). Promoting productive aging. *Health & Social Work, 34*(3), 237.

Zedlewski, S. R., & Butrica, B. A. (2007). Are we taking full advantage of Older Adults' full potential?, *Perspectives on Productive Ageing, 7.* The Urban Institute. http://citeseerx.ist.psu.edu/viewdoc/download;jsessionid=550AFB8671E6906F239D8A78CE179D23?doi=10.1.1.508.6520&rep=rep1&type=pdf

Chapter 6
Demographic Dimensions and Gerontological Issues in India

S. Irudaya Rajan and S. Sunitha

Abstract Ageing is a natural process and none can stop or avoid it. But any being, community or nation can face it bravely if there is good governance and pragmatism about the future. The government, which represents the people, is responsible for delivering a minimum standard of living for the welfare of the citizens of the nation. India now deals with the aged population through different social security schemes with minimal compatibility among them. Everywhere, the older persons are the major beneficiaries of social security and their needs include food, clothing, shelter, health care and emotional support. All these needs barring emotional support can be met through an income. Therefore, need for income security is the pioneer requirement for older persons. Though India is a welfare nation, social security given to the citizens is inadequate for their daily life. In India, majority of the workforce earns through unorganized labour markets. The issues which generally happen among the aged are increasing number of aged women due to widowhood, health and financial problems that lead to elder abuse and neglect. Most often, the abusers are the caregivers who are particularly family members. Another important problem among the aged is the migration of their children which induces increasing risk to managing elderly life owing to physical absence of their children. This chapter confronts the current demographic situation in India, living arrangements, marital status, working status and places of residence based on various Censuses. Migration impact is examined using data collected through the Kerala Ageing Survey 2013 conducted by the Centre for Development Studies, Kerala and funded by the Government of Kerala.

Keywords Welfare of the citizens · Social security · Emotional support · Aged women · Migration · Demographics · Living arrangements · Marital status and working status

S. I. Rajan (✉) · S. Sunitha
The International Institute of Migration and Development, Kerala Thiruvananthapuram, India

M. K. Shankardass (ed.), *Gerontological Concerns and Responses in India*,
https://doi.org/10.1007/978-981-16-4764-2_6

Introduction

Population ageing is increasing globally faster than all other age groups. According to United Nations (2017), 962 million older people over the world comprising 13% of the total population which is nearly 7.6 billion in mid-2017. Europe has the highest proportion of elderly (25%). Countries like India and China are frontrunners in terms of world's highest total population as well as elderly population. The process of ageing has been taking place at a much faster rate in Asia than in European countries. An ageing world in India is increasing at an average rate of 2.9% per annum. Thus, as population ageing is an emerging concept in the perspective of demographic transition, India is voyaging through population ageing since 2001 with 77 billion elderly population. In 2011, this number of older adults was increased to104.2 million. The proportion of elderly to the total population was increased from 5.6% in 1961 to 8.6% in 2011 (Rajan & Mishra, 2020). There is significant disparity between the states in terms of growth and levels of the elderly population (UNFPA, 2017). While considering the state-wise proportion of older persons, Kerala has the highest proportion with 12.6% followed by Goa (11.2%) and Tamil Nadu (10.4%) (Table 6.1). In 2001, 16 out of 29 states of India had elderly population of more than 7% of the total population (Rajan et al., 2014) while in 2011, 24 out of 29 states crosses this percent.

In northern part of India, Punjab (10.3%) and Himachal Pradesh (10.2%) had the highest proportion of older persons. This uneven distribution of older persons may be due to the socio-economic, cultural and political variations across the states. Still, there are some most remote areas with no access to immediate attention even for their emergency situation. It is very much a concern that even India is emerging as greying and need more attention to become elderly friendly. Free to communicate with society, free to move anywhere, free to access the infrastructure facilities may be the future concerns.

Current Demographic Situation in India

India is now passing through the third stage of demographic transition with a reduction in birth and death rates (Rajan & Sunitha, 2018a). Total fertility rate (TFR) determines the growth of younger population while life expectancy determines the growth of older population (Rajan & Sunitha, 2015). Based on the census 2011, Total Fertility Rate was estimated at 2.7 for India (Guilmoto & Rajan, 2002; 2013). According to the study, fertility has gone below the replacement level of 2.1 children per woman in less than 12 states and union territories in India. Of the 621 districts, 174 have fertility levels below 2.1 and the lowest fertility level is estimated in Kolkata (1.2). Thus the pace of demographic transition varies across the states.

The increase in life expectancy changed the age structure. In Table 6.2, the average age of a male person who is aged 60 is expected to live 16 more years. That is, a

Table 6.1 Proportion of Older persons by states and union territories, 2011

States and union territories	Proportion of older persons	States and union territories	Proportion of older persons
India	8.6	Assam	6.7
Jammu and Kashmir	7.4	West Bengal	8.5
Himachal Pradesh	10.2	Jharkhand	7.1
Punjab	10.3	Odisha	9.5
Chandigarh	6.4	Chhattisgarh	7.8
Uttarakhand	8.9	Madhya Pradesh	7.9
Haryana	8.7	Gujarat	7.9
NCT of Delhi	6.8	Daman & Diu	4.7
Rajasthan	7.5	Dadra & Nagar Haveli	4.0
Uttar Pradesh	7.7	Maharashtra	9.9
Bihar	7.4	Andhra Pradesh	9.8
Sikkim	6.7	Karnataka	9.5
Arunachal Pradesh	4.6	Goa	11.2
Nagaland	5.2	Lakshadweep	8.2
Manipur	7.0	Kerala	12.6
Mizoram	6.3	Tamil Nadu	10.4
Tripura	7.9	Puducherry	9.7
Meghalaya	4.7	Andaman & Nicobar Islands	6.7

Table 6.2 Expectation of life at ages 60 and 70 for India (in years)

Year	Male		Female	
	e60	**e70**	**e60**	**e70**
1971	13.80	8.57	14.75	9.10
1981	14.25	8.83	15.31	9.42
1991	15.01	9.27	16.23	9.97
2001	15.74	9.70	17.05	10.45
2011	16.29	10.03	17.75	10.87

male person born in 40 s, would live up to age 76 years and females up to 78 years. The older persons at the age of 60 years are more likely to live 6 more years than the older persons at the age of 70 years. Even though the levels of life expectancy are similar, different populations can have varying levels of inequality in length of life (Smits & Monden, 2009). Comparison of the state level life expectancies reveals that although life expectancy has shown drastic improvement in past decades in India, not much has changed in inequality regarding length of life.

Living Arrangements

As per the 2011 Census, the average size of Indian households is 4.5 and average size of elderly in the household is 2.4. In other words, an average Indian family has more than two older adults to look after. The households with more than one older adult increased during the inter-census period, 2001–2011. Of the 248.8 million households in India, 31.3% have at least one older person which is higher in rural areas (32.5%) compared to urban areas (29%). About 4.1% are elderly alone or all elderly households. About 27.2% households have elderly living with adult members. The remaining 68.7% households have no older members. Elderly households are seen more in rural areas than urban areas. The households with more than one elderly increased during the inter-census period (Table 6.3).

In India, joint familial system of living is followed in comparison to the western countries, where nuclear family system is dominated. It is often seen that older persons who earn money will be considered as an asset to the family and those who depend on family are considered a burden (Rajan et al., 2017). On the other hand, co-residence of older parents can provide child care for their grand children and at the same time children can take care of their parents (Sudha et al., 2006).

It is clear from Table 6.4 that, about 7% females and 3% males are living alone. As per Census 2011, 10.3 million households had only one member and among this

Table 6.3 No of aged persons in HH, India, 2001 and 2011

No. of Older persons	2001			2011		
	Total	Rural	Urban	Total	Rural	Urban
None	69.8	68.4	73.4	68.7	67.5	71.2
One	21.3	22.0	19.4	21.6	22.1	20.5
Two	8.4	9.1	6.8	9.3	9.9	7.9
Three or more	0.4	0.4	0.3	0.5	0.5	0.4

Source Registrar general of India, census 2001 and 2011

Table 6.4 Living arrangements of older persons in India, 2011

	Male	Female
Living Alone	2.7	6.9
Living with one person	16.0	13.6
Two	10.0	8.3
Three	10.9	10.6
Four	13.5	16.3
Five	14.7	15.2
Six or More	32.2	29.2
Total	100.0	100.0

Source Compiled from census 2011, registrar general of India

48.3% are elderly households. Among these, 72.8% are older women. More women than men lived alone. In about 13% households, elderly are living with one person. In reality, about one fifth of the older women is living in households that have only older persons and no other adults. As per the 2011 Census, the average size of Indian households is 4.5 and average size of the household with older adults is 2.4. In other words, an average Indian family has more than two older persons to look after.

Living arrangement of the elderly plays a vital role in empowering older persons by giving dignity. According to Rajan and Sunitha (2018b), older people who experience life satisfaction have dignity when they are living with their family. One can enjoy their life at the later stages of life if they would get proper care and love (Rajan & Sunitha, 2018b). Table 6.5 shows most of the older persons are living with spouse only or living with spouse and adult children and their percentage is increasing over the years. But the older people who are living with children only are decreasing over the years. Most probably, spouse themselves are the caregivers. If there is a serious health problem, then they need support of children and other immediate relatives as caregivers.

Table 6.5 Living arrangements among the older persons in India, 1995–96 to 2014 (NSSO)

Living arrangements	Period	Rural	Urban
Alone	1995–1996	4.3	6.0
	2004	5.3	4.3
	2014	4.4	3.5
With spouse only	1995–1996	10.7	5.7
	2004	12.5	10.4
	2014	14.7	15.1
With spouse and adult children	1995–1996	46.2	29.7
	2004	44.2	46.8
	2014	46.4	48.1
With adult children	1995–1996	33.1	51.2
	2004	32.0	32.2
	2014	31.7	30.5
With other relations and non-relations	1995–1996	5.9	6.5
	2004	5.6	4.9
	2014	2.9	2.9
Not recorded	1995–1996	1.0	0.9
	2004	1.9	1.1
	2014	–	–
Total	1995–1996	100.0	100.0
	2004	100.0	100.0
	2014	100.0	100.0

Source Compiled from National Sample Survey, 1995–1996, 2004 and 2014

Table 6.6 Marital Status of the Older persons in India, 1961–2011

	60 +				70 +			
	Married		Widowed		Married		Widowed	
	Male	Female	Male	Female	Male	Female	Male	Female
1961	69.1	23.7	27.5	75.4	60.5	24.8	36.1	84.4
1971	74.7	30.0	22.4	69.2	66.6	19.0	30.4	80.3
1981	78.2	34.9	19.4	64.3	70.5	21.7	27.2	77.6
1991	80.7	44.2	15.5	54.0	72.2	29.9	21.4	67.2
2001	82.1	47.3	15.0	50.7	74.8	32.6	21.4	64.9
2011	82.1	49.6	14.6	47.8	73.8	33.9	22.1	63.2

Source Compiled from various censuses, registrar general of India

Marital Status

Older people are mainly associated with widowed group than the married group. Particularly among women, ageing problems started with widowhood since most of them are unemployed, dependent on others for their financial needs and less educated compared to men. Table 6.6 shows a marked variation in the marital status by gender. There is a marked disparity between men and women in widowhood mainly because of long life span of women, remarriage among men and gap in marital age. Majority of men will receive care at right time from their wives while most of the widows would depend on adult children or other relatives for their immediate needs (Rajan & Balagopal, 2017). Table 6.6 shows that though the frequency of widowhood is favourable to females, it is decreasing over the years. The frequency of widowhood among females has been increasing according to their age. But there was a decline of 27.6 points from 1961 to 2011 in widowhood of older women while it was 21.2 for the adult aged 70 and above. The trend in widowhood among older adults is decreasing maybe because of the universality of remarriage system in society than in earlier times. Remarriage is not just a marital union but to care for each other at their later ages as they live longer and children are less or none to live with them. Gender difference in marital status shapes the living arrangements of the older persons (Rajan & Sunitha, 2015).

Working Status

A significant percentage of older persons are working at their later ages for their livelihood. The work participation rate of older women is increasing over the period compared to their male counterparts. About 40% of the older persons are working and among this 58% are older men. About 22% of elderly are working even at their oldest age, 80 years and above (Table 6.8). The overall work participation among the

Table 6.7 Work participation rate of older persons in India, 1961–2011

Year	Total	Male	Female
1961	49.5	76.6	22.4
1971	43.2	73.8	10.5
1981	40.1	65.1	14.0
1991	39.1	60.5	16.1
2001	40.3	60.3	20.9
2011	39.8	57.6	22.5

Source Compiled from various censuses from 1961 to 2011, Registrar General of India

Table 6.8 Workers and non-workers in India, 2011

	Workers			Non-Workers		
	Persons	Males	Females	Persons	Males	Females
60 +	39.8	57.6	22.5	60.2	42.4	77.5
70 +	28.7	43.7	14.2	71.3	56.3	85.8
80 +	21.6	33.9	10.7	78.4	66.1	89.3

elderly are continuing in a constant proportion (Table 6.7). Most of the older workers are involved in informal sectors such as agricultural or non-agricultural sectors or engaged in small scale businesses.

The older person who is working in informal sector has increased in rural areas over the years for both males and females (Dhar, 2014). The incidence of financial insecurity has been found to be greater among the older persons in rural areas, older widows, the aged residing in nuclear families or alone and the aged afflicted with health problems (Rajan et al., 2003).

While analysing the Census figures, over the years, child dependency ratio has declined and aged dependency ratio has increased. The index of ageing (ratio of older persons to the child population) takes into consideration both ends of the age distribution and captures the effect of fertility decline on ageing population. According to this measure, the ageing process was slow in India during 1961–2001but gathered pace between 2001 and 2011 (Rajan & Balagopal, 2017).

Table 6.9 explains the level of economic dependency among older persons in India by using NSSO data. The older persons in urban areas are economically more independent and are continued over the years for both males and females compared to their rural counterparts. Elderly males in rural areas are more dependent on their families compared to those in urban areas. On the other hand, older women in the urban areas are more dependent than that in the rural areas.

This economic dependency enhanced the migration of their children for a better living conditions to what they faced at their younger ages. Though the economic needs may fulfil through the migration of their children, need for physical care and attention from their children may not be there because it is not a priority for them

Table 6.9 Level of economic independence among the older persons in India, from 1995–96 to 2014 (NSSO, various years)

Level of economic independence	Period	Rural			Urban		
		Male	Female	Person	Male	Female	Person
Economically independent	1995–1996	48.5	12.1	30.1	51.5	11.5	31.1
	2004	51.3	13.9	32.7	55.5	17.0	35.9
	2014	42.6	11.2	26.6	51.5	12.9	31.9
Partially dependent	1995–1996	18.0	14.6	16.3	16.9	11.0	13.9
	2004	15.2	12.4	13.8	13.4	9.5	11.4
	2014	23.9	19.1	21.5	18.5	15.3	16.9
Fully dependent	1995–1996	31.3	70.6	51.1	29.7	75.7	53.2
	2004	32.0	72.0	51.9	30.1	72.1	51.6
	2014	33.5	69.6	51.9	30.0	71.8	51.2
Not recorded	1995–1996	2.2	2.6	2.4	1.9	1.8	1.9
	2004	0.2	0.2	0.2	1.0	1.3	1.2
	2014	–	–	–	–	–	–

as most of them lead a nuclear familial system. Next section describes some impact of migration on elderly with special analysis of Kerala Ageing Survey conducted in 2013 by the Centre for Development Studies, Thiruvananthapuram.

Impact of Migration on Elderly—Special Analysis of Kerala Ageing Survey 2013

Kerala is pioneering in human development as a model for many states in India. Low fertility and long longevity are the peculiar achievements of Kerala for years. But the increasing longevity keeps the elderly population as the highest proportion to the total population in India. As child population decreases and elderly population increases, there will not be anyone in the family to take care of these elderly. Also, the impact of migration reduced the population growth and sex ratio favourable to females. Thus, as the living arrangement of the older persons is changing from joint to nuclear family system, the older adults tend to live alone or live with their spouse only. Number of old age homes are increasing in Kerala as there are fewer children in the family and there is increase trend in migration of the children loneliness, physical dependence, insecurity, abuse, etc.

Table 6.10 established that the family system of both migrant and non-migrant families has changed. Most of the households have two adults only. One out of 10 elderly households has no adults. In most of the migrant households, older persons are living with one adult person mostly female adults. Thus, the number of children

Table 6.10 Elderly HH with adult members (20–59 years) and Migration Status, 2013

	Migrant	Non-migrant	Total
No Adult	9.3	11.9	10.9
One	24.1	14.4	18.2
Two	31.8	41.1	37.5
Three	18.6	19.3	19.0
Four	9.1	8.3	8.6
Five	3.8	2.9	3.2
Above Five	3.3	2.1	2.5
Total	100.0	100.0	100.0

Source Kerala ageing survey, 2013, conducted by centre for development studies, Thiruvananthapuram and sponsored by Government of Kerala

is limited and these children are away, so they are living alone or living with spouses or others.

In Table 6.11 the older persons are divided into two categories. The first category is those who are residing with children or could get an immediate attention of their children physically (Type 2). The second category is those who are living alone or living with spouse or others and whose children are outside the district (Type 1). These children have migrated to other states or other countries and no one will be available for their immediate needs. The older persons whose children are away had a good or fair perception of health compared to the older persons whose children are near to them. This may be because, if they are residing alone they may be more conscious about their health and mentally they will prepare that they are alone and should be alert of any health problems. But the health perception had no relation with their disease pattern. Irrespective of their type about 30% older persons have no disease. Among the older persons who have two or more chronic diseases, older persons in type 1 are slightly high. The older persons in type 1 are more independent compared to the older persons in type 2. The older persons who need special care fall in type 2 category. The depression scale is categorized into three levels, high, medium and low. While analysing their depression index, older persons in type 2 have a medium level.

Older persons in type 1 category have the best living standard compared to those in type 2 category. On the other hand, older persons with low living standards have a higher percentage in type 2 category compared to that of type 1 category. Thus it can be concluded that older people who live alone, live with spouse or others have a better economic background compared to those who are living near to/with their children. However, they have some diseases or mental depression due to the absence of attention from their children. Parents are always keen in mind that their children should be with them and look after the mat their later life. If something happened contrary to their mindset they would suffer from mental dilemmas.

Table 6.11 Profile of older persons by residence of children, 2013

	Type 1—children residing outside	Type 2—children residing near or With them
Health Perception	Percent	
Poor	29.0	34.5
Fair	36.3	31.2
Good	34.7	34.2
Financial Status		
Fully Dependent on Others/ Spouse	49.8	56.3
Partially Dependent	15.3	21.6
Fully Independent	35.0	22.1
Need Special Care		
Yes	23.5	30.9
No	76.5	69.1
Depression Index		
High	18.4	17.2
Medium	63.2	67.6
Low	18.4	15.2
Chronic Diseases		
2 or More Diseases	35.6	34.8
One Disease	34.4	35.2
No Disease	29.9	30.0
Standard of Living Index		
Low	22.5	26.9
Average	21.6	29.4
Better	24.3	23.2
Best	31.6	20.6
Total	100.0	100.0

Source Same as Table 6.10

Conclusion

Migration is a major factor in the financial security of older persons. It keeps social security and health care but does not keep up care from their children that they deserve most in their later life. But the situation of older persons in non-migrant households is different. Most of them have no financial security, social security and other caring. One solution for this problem is to empower them financially or give care. For this, the children irrespective of their gender, who are not looking after their parents, should be given a fixed amount every month for their wellbeing (if the parents shared their property with their children). The maintenance shall be payable by children in the proportion in which they would inherit his/her property. The child who is looking after them need not be given the fixed amount because he/she already spent time and money for them. This will encourage people to look after their parents or otherwise older persons will be financially secured.

References

Dhar, A. (2014). Work force participation among elderly in India struggling for economic security. *The Indian Journal of Labour Economics, 57*(3), 221–245.

Guilmoto, C. Z., & Irudaya Rajan, S. (2002). District level estimates of fertility from India's 2001 census. *Economic and Political Weekly, 37*(7), 665–672.

Guilmoto, C. Z., & Rajan, I. (2013). Fertility at the district level in India: Lessons from the 2011 census. *Economic and Political Weekly, 48*(23), 59–70.

Irudaya Rajan, S., Kurusu, V., & Sunitha, S. (2014). 'Demography of ageing in India' Chapter 2 in Section 1: Introduction pp. 6–18, in P. Sanchetee (Ed.)—Text book of geriatric medicine, Under the Aegis of Indian Academy of Geriatrics published by Paras Medical Publisher.

Irudaya Rajan, S., & Sunitha, S. (2018a). 'Demographic changes in Kerala', in the book, B.A. Prakash & Jerry Alwin (Eds.). Kerala's Economy Since 2000: Emerging Issues. Sage Publishers.

Irudaya Rajan, S., Sunitha, S. (2018b). Empowering the Elderly by giving dignity in the book H. Çakmur (Ed.) *2018 Geriatrics Health*, IntechOpen, ISBN: 978-1-78923-761-0.

Irudaya Rajan, S., & Sunitha, S. (May 2015). Demography of ageing in India—2011–2101. *Helpage India, Research and Development Journal 21*(2).

Irudaya Rajan, S., Sunitha, S., & Arya, U. R. (2017). Elder care and living arrangement in Kerala, in S. IrudayaRajan, & G. Balagopal (Eds.) *Elderly care in India: Societal and state responses*, Springer.

Irudaya Rajan, S., & Balagopal, G. (2017). Caring India: An introduction. Chapter 1 in the book, S. IrudayaRajan & G. Balagopal (Eds.). *Elderly care in India: Societal and state responses.* Springer Nature. pp. 1–36.

IrudayaRajan, S., Sarma, P. S., & Mishra, U. S. (2003). Demography of Indian ageing, 2001–2051. *Journal of Ageing and Social Policy, 15*(2–3), 11–30.

Rajan, S. I., & Mishra, U. S. (2020). *Senior citizens of India: Emerging challenges and concerns*, Springer.

Smits, J., & Monden, C. (2009). Length of life inequality around the globe. *Social Science and Medicine, 68*(6), 1114–1123.

Sudha, S., Suchindran, C., Mutran, E. J., Rajan, S. I., & Sarma, P. S. (2006). Marital status, family ties, and self—rated health among elders in South India. *Journal of Cross-Cultural Gerontology, 21*(3–4), 103–120.

United Nations, Department of Economic and Social Affairs, Population Division. (2017). World population prospects: The 2017 revision, key findings and advance tables. Working Paper No. ESA/P/WP/248.

Chapter 7
Health and Social Concerns in Elderly Men

Prabhat Gautam Roy, Rakshit Bhardwaj, and Ashish Goel

Abstract India, the world's second most populous country, has seen a rapid increase in its share of older people in the last decade. Elderly population, (defined as age $\geq$ 60 years) made up for 5.6 percent population in 2001 which increased to 8.6 percent in 2011. This number is expected to increase further in the coming years. In view of the above, it is imperative for the society to recognize problems faced by the elderly and try to address them so as to provide them a good quality of life. This chapter addresses health and social concerns of older men. The present chapter discusses not only the health issues but also the social concerns of elderly men and deals with the basic concepts of disease, prevention and rehabilitation with an aim to demystify the concepts surrounding illness. Common health issues covered include–strokes, heart diseases, chronic airway disease, incontinence, diabetes, hypertension, dental issues, hearing or visual impairment, anemia, asthenia, unintentional weight loss, constipation, arthritis, impotence, addictions, falls, cancers, cognitive impairment, rigidity, insomnia and depression. Social issues specific to elderly men like loneliness, economic dependence, living wills and advanced directives are also discussed.

Keywords Elderly population · Older men · Quality of life · Health issues · Social concerns

Introduction

India, the world's second most populous country, has seen a rapid increase in its share of older people in the last decade. Elderly population, (defined as age $\geq$ 60 years) made up for 5.6% population in 2001 which increased to 8.6% in 2011. This number is expected to increase further in the coming years.

Geriatric medicine is an upcoming sub speciality in medicine that focuses on health issues of older population. Need for specialized care for the elderly was long desired and due. With the advent of formal courses in geriatric medicine, this demand

P. Gautam Roy · R. Bhardwaj · A. Goel (✉)
University College of Medical Sciences and Guru Teg Bahadur Hospital, Delhi, India

M. K. Shankardass (ed.), *Gerontological Concerns and Responses in India*,
https://doi.org/10.1007/978-981-16-4764-2_7

has started being met and the course has gathered momentum with increasing number of doctors opting to practice geriatric medicine.

There are health issues that are specific to older men which need to be addressed. These include stroke, heart diseases, chronic airway disease, incontinence, diabetes, hypertension, dental issues, hearing or visual impairment, anemia, asthenia, unintentional weight loss, constipation, arthritis, impotence, addictions, falls, cancers, cognitive impairment, rigidity, insomnia and depression.

This chapter deals with these medical problems covering salient features of each disease with a focus on epidemiology, pathophysiology, clinical features, management and prevention. It also deals with social issues faced by older men like malnutrition, loneliness, economic dependence. Finally, it also touches upon the controversial topic of living wills and advanced directives.

Stroke

Stroke is defined as a sudden onset neurological deficit of vascular origin lasting more than 24 h. Stroke is a term used for a condition wherein the patient develops a deficit in terms of motor or/and sensory function of limbs, speech, vision, higher mental functions like intelligent thinking and understanding of complex tasks and consciousness.

The underlying mechanism which leads to stroke is inadequate blood supply to the brain which leads to damage to that part of the brain which controls the above-mentioned functions. Two prominent causes of inadequate blood supply to brain are rupture of the vessel supplying the brain (Hemorrhagic Stroke) and occlusion of the vessel supplying the brain (Ischemic Stroke).

Risk factors leading to stroke include modifiable factors high blood pressure, diabetes, obesity, smoking and tobacco consumption. There are a few non-modifiable factors too, like Type A personality, positive family history and certain genetic mutations.

Stroke generally presents as weakness of one half side of the body. It may be sudden (within minutes) or gradual (few hours) in onset. It can be associated with loss of sensations like pain and temperature over the affected area. Another common presentation of stroke is deviation of angle of mouth. It leads to loss of facial symmetry, drooling of saliva from the affected site, inability to close eyes forcefully and weakness in blowing air from the mouth/whistling. Stroke can also present as an inability to speak (Aphasia), personality disturbances and decreased consciousness.

In case of occurrence of any of the above-mentioned symptoms, the patient must be immediately taken to the hospital. It must be understood that time taken from onset of symptoms to appropriate medical intervention can have lasting effects on the quality of life the patient leads after having a stroke. In case of Ischemic stroke, the standard treatment involves thrombolysing (re-opening) the blocked vessel, provided the patient presents within 3 h of onset of symptoms. If there is a longer delay in presentation or if thrombolysis cannot be administered due to certain reasons, the treatment involves lifelong therapy with oral medications. In case of Hemorrhagic stroke, the standard treatment is controlling the blood pressure to ideal levels and relieving raised intracranial pressure (caused by hematoma) using medical or surgical techniques.

The quality of life after stroke depends on residual neurological deficit after the event which is directly related to the area of brain damaged and time taken from onset of symptoms to receiving appropriate medical care. Most patients who receive timely medical care and are lucky enough to get away with little cerebral damage recover significantly and are able to carry out most activities. Patients with greater deficit usually take longer time. The role of physiotherapy is of great importance for these patients to help them achieve certain level of recovery.

Coronary Artery Disease

CAD is defined as a condition where the oxygen consumption of the myocardium exceeds its supply. On account of suboptimal blood and oxygen supply, there is damage to the myocardium at risk which leads to symptoms. The underlying mechanism behind CAD is obstruction of the arterial supply of the heart, most commonly due to deposition of atherosclerotic plaques on the vessel wall. Other causes of CAD are occlusion of artery by a thrombus, dissection of coronary artery and increase in oxygen demand of myocardium due to cardiac muscle hypertrophy.

Risk factors leading to CAD can be broadly classified as modifiable and non modifiable. Modifiable risk factors include smoking, tobacco consumption, obesity, hypertension, diabetes and hyperlipidemia. Non-modifiable risk factors include family history, Type A personality and genetic causes of accelerated atherosclerosis and CAD.

CAD commonly presents as chest pain (angina), however many angina equivalents have also been described as presenting symptoms of CAD. Classically, chest pain is described as retrosternal/central in location and constricting in character. It usually occurs on physical exertion, however, it may also occur at rest. The pain may radiate to left arm or anywhere from jaw to umbilicus. Rarely, the pain may only occur in left arm, therefore left arm pain in an elderly man should not be taken lightly. Other symptoms which may be harbingers of CAD are shortness of breath, anxiety, palpitations, unexplained sweating, or fainting spells (syncopal attacks).

In case of occurence of any of the above-mentioned symptoms, the patient must be taken to nearest hospital. It must be understood that time taken from onset of symptoms to appropriate medical care can have an impact on final outcome. In case of an acute event of angina, the first investigation is a 12 lead ECG. Further investigations include cardiac biomarkers and Echocardiography. In case patient has an Acute Coronary Syndrome, the standard of care is Coronary Angiography followed by Percutaneous Coronary Intervention. Other procedures like thrombolysis, although very effective are slightly inferior to PCI in terms of long-term outcome. However, they continue to be widely used in developing areas. Following acute intervention, the patient requires to take lifelong antiplatelet medicines (Aspirin and clopidogrel) and antihyperlipidaemic drugs (Atorvastatin).

Life after CAD/ACS depends on the duration of time taken to receive appropriate medical care after onset of symptoms. In case of timely care, there is virtually no damage to myocardium and the patient can lead a normal life, however, he may need to take lifelong medications. On the contrary, if there is delay in seeking medical care, the patient has to live with residual myocardial damage and may suffer shortness of breath, palpitations and sudden cardiac arrhythmias.

Cognitive Impairment and Forgetfulness

Dementia is a disorder characterized by a decline in cognition involving one or more cognitive domains. The deficits must represent a decline from previous level of function and must be severe enough to interfere with daily function and independence. Mild cognitive impairment is defined as presence of difficulty in remembering things but preserved ability to do activities of daily life.

Impaired cognition is a common problem in elderly men, as is evident by the fact that as many as 5–7% of elderly men exhibit symptoms. Most patients with dementia do not present with a complaint of memory loss, it is often the family member who brings the patient for medical attention. However, even family members are often delayed in bringing the patient for medical attention as they inaccurately ascribe the forgetfulness to ageing. Symptoms at onset of cognitive impairment include problems in retaining new information and rate of processing information. (1).

Major dementia syndromes include.

Alzheimer's disease- a disorder in which.

Vascular dementia- a disorder that happens when brain cells do not get enough blood supply and the patient has recurrent CVAs.

Other causes: Dementia with Lewy bodies, Fronto-temporal dementia.

Most elderly patients have Alzheimer's disease (around 60–80%) (2).

Evaluation of dementia involves history taking by family members, administering objective scales to document cognitive impairment like Mini Mental State Examination (MMSE), Montreal Cognitive Assessment (MCoA) and Clinical dementia rating. A thorough physical examination and investigatory workup must always be done to rule out atypical presentation of a curable medical illness before labeling any patient as a case of dementia.

Treatment of dementia depends on type of dementia. There are drugs used to treat Alzheimer's disease like donepezil, rivastigmine, galantamine and memantine. Treatment for vascular dementia includes controlling blood pressure and cholesterol. There are no proven ways to prevent dementia, however indulging in physical activity, healthy balanced diet and social interaction help keep the brain healthy.

Malignancies and Cancer

Cancer is a latin word for crab- since it adheres to any part that it seizes in an obstinate manner, similar to a crab's behaviour. In medical terms, the term used for cancer is malignant neoplasm. Malignancies carry with them great social stigmata and most people associate a diagnosis of malignancy with end of life. However, with the advent of modern technology thrust in research related to oncology, this scenario is changing fast, so much so that there is a cure available for many cancers. Common cancers affecting elderly men include (in order of prevalence) Ca Prostate, Ca Lung and bronchus, Ca Colon and Rectum, Ca urinary bladder and Melanomas.(3).

Risk factors for developing these cancers include smoking and tobacco consumption (Ca Lung, Bronchus and Urinary bladder), increasing age (Ca Prostate), family history and inflammatory bowel disease (Colorectal Ca), occupational exposure to nitro dye and chronic cystitis (Ca Urinary bladder) and excessive exposure to sunlight (Melanoma).

Presenting symptoms common to all cancers include constitutional symptoms like low grade fever, lethargy, malaise. Apart from this anorexia and weight loss is present in most cancers. Lung and bronchial malignancies present as cough with sputum- which may contain blood (hemoptysis), progressive shortness of breath and dull aching pain chest in initial stages when the malignancy is restricted to lungs. Common site of spread of Ca Lung and bronchus is brain, where metastasis can present as seizures or focal neurological deficits. Prostate cancer is usually asymptomatic till late in natural history of disease. Symptoms usually occur after metastasis to bones and include severe bony pains and pathological fractures. Other presenting complaints include progressive weakness, exertional shortness of breath and decreased exercise tolerance with or without passage of blood in stools. These symptoms are due to anemia secondary to chronic blood loss via faeces in patients with Colorectal carcinoma. Bladder malignancies also present with symptoms of anemia secondary to blood loss in urine. Melanomas are easy to recognize for the patient as it is a rapidly increasing dark colored patch over skin in areas exposed to sun.

In case of any of these symptoms, one must visit a general physician who usually does the basic workup of the patient before referring him to an oncologist. Investigations are specific for each type of cancer but they broadly involve imaging of the involved part and microscopic evaluation of the part involved (biopsy). Newer modalities of imaging like PET-CT involve scanning of complete body using a radioactive substance and findings of the extent of spread of cancer.

As discussed earlier, these days there is a therapy available for most cancers. With the advent of biologically targeted molecular therapy, prognosis of most cancers has improved. However, early detection and timely intervention remain the cornerstone in prognosis of cancer patients.

Hearing Impairment

Age related hearing loss which is also called Presbycusis is one of the common reasons for auditory impairment in adults. The prevalence of hearing loss increases with age. Presbycusis affects more than fifty percent adult males by the age of 75 years and nearly all adults above 90 years of age. (4–6).

Risk factors for presbycusis include male gender (probably because of more exposure to noise), low socio-economic status, ototoxic drugs like aminoglycosides and chemotherapeutic agents, hypertension, diabetes, immunological disorders and vascular diseases. (7).

Four pathological types of presbycusis have been described.

Sensory: this is characterized by degeneration of organ of corti (an organ in internal ear which is a very important component of auditory pathway)

Neural: this involves degeneration of cells of spiral ganglion.

Strial/ Metabolic: this is characterized by atrophy of stria vascularis in all turns of cochlea.

Cochlear conductive: this occurs due to stiffening of basilar membrane of internal ear.

Classically, presbycusis presents as gradually progressive and bilaterally symmetrical loss of hearing which begins in high frequency range. It is the high frequency sounds which carry consonants, thereby making for majority of heard information. Low and mid frequency sounds consisting of vowels are well heard. As a result of this pattern of hearing loss, patients can hear that someone is talking to them (from the low frequency vowels) but they are not able to comprehend what is being said (due to loss of information carried by consonants). Apart from hearing loss, it can also be accompanied by ringing like sensations in ear (tinnitus), vertigo and dysequillibrium.

Diagnostic evaluation of an elderly man with hearing loss is usually done on the basis of classical history of disease, simple tuning fork tests and audiometry. Advanced imaging techniques like CT and MRI, although of some help in excluding neural or central pathology, are rarely used for diagnosis.

Despite widespread prevalence of Presbycisus, a complete 'cure' to this disease is not available. However, supportive measures are quite effective and routinely used. Hearing aids can improve hearing function in most cases leading to improvement in quality of life. In patients with severe presbycusis which is unaffected by conventional hearing aids, cochlear implantation provides a ray of hope. Great majority of patients undergoing cochlear implantation achieve significant functional improvement. Other supportive measures for managing hearing impairment include use of assistive listening devices and auditory rehabilitation techniques like active listening training, speech reading and use of sign language for communication. There is also active research going on to develop genetic and cellular interventions which induce regeneration of hair cells and prove to be 'cure' for presbycusis.

Undernutrition and Anorexia

Malnutrition, mistakenly taken as synonymous with undernutrition, is a state of disturbed calorie intake. It can either be excessive calorie intake- overnutrition; or decreased calorie intake- undernutrition. Diagnosing undernutrition, even though widely prevalent, is a difficult task. The following criteria have been recommended by the American Society for Parenteral and Enteral Nutrition (ASPEN):

Insufficient energy intake.
Weight Loss.
Loss of muscle mass.
Loss of subcutaneous fat.
Localized or generalized fluid accumulation that may mask weight loss.
Diminished functional status as measured by handgrip strength.
Presence of two or more of these six criteria signifies undernutrition. (8).

Increased ageing is commonly associated with undernutrition. The causes for poor nutrition are multifactorial in elderly males-disease related organ system compromise, depression, inadequate finances, loneliness and stringent food preferences being prominent among them.

Social life of older people plays a significant part in nutrition. In one study it was found that older individuals who have food in presence of others eat more than those who have food alone. (9) Another factor of significance is that in our country, most elderly people depend on pensions or on money given by children for their survival. In the backdrop of illnesses associated with older age, they tend to use money previously spent on food for medications and other needed items.

Several physiologic factors like delayed gastric emptying and prolonged antral distension, early satiety, impairment in regulation of food intake and alteration and taste and smell physiology also play their part in poor nutrition. (10)Threshold for odor detection and taste perception also increases with age which leads to increased tendency of tasteless in food, thereby affecting amount of food consumed. (11).

Two syndromes associated with undernutrition are Cachexia and Sarcopenia. Cachexia is defined as "A syndrome associated with underlying illness and characterized by loss of muscle with or without loss of fat mass"(12). Sarcopenia is characterized by a low muscle mass, loss of muscle strength and performance(13). The major difference between sarcopenia and cachexia is that the former need not be associated with an underlying disease.

Once the underlying cause for undernutrition has been identified, such as depression or a medical illness, the primary aim is correction of that cause. Apart from addressing the underlying cause, treatment of undernutrition is mainly based on replenishing calories and proteins, providing nutritional supplements and use of appetite stimulants.

Calorie requirement for elderly men is calculated by the formula:

$661.9–(9.53 \times \text{age}) + \text{PAC x} [(15.91 \times \text{weight in kg}) + (539.6 \times \text{height in meters})]$.

Appetite stimulants are a new class of drugs used for undernutrition. Commonly used among them are Megestrol acetate, Mirtazipine and Ghrelin mimetics. Mirtazipine is a drug from the antidepressant group which leads to weight gain, hence is an ideal drug for elderly with depression and weight loss.

Visual Problems

Visual problems are a common health issue faced by the elderly. A common misconception in our society is that most visual impairment is due to refractive errors, which leads the patient to an optometrist rather than consulting an ophthalmologist. However, evidence shows that leading cause of visual impairment among elderly people is Age Related Macular Degeneration (ARMD; 36.2%), followed by refractive errors (31.6%), cataract (24.5), glaucoma (11.6%) and Diabetic eye disease(2.3%).(14).

Age Related macular degeneration is a disease of central vision. Early symptoms include blurring of central vision, requirement of bright lights or magnifying glasses to read. Smoking is commonly associated with ARMD and its cessation can help delay the onset of disease.

Refractive errors include myopia, hypermetropia, astigmatism and presbyopia. Myopia (nearsightedness) is the most commonly seen refractive error seen in elderly males. It is a disorder of the lens where the image is formed in front of retina as a result of axial elongation of the eyeball or increased refractive power of the eye. This results in blurred distant vision and relatively normal near vision (hence the term nearsightedness). Hypermetropia (farsightedness) leads to a normal distant vision but a defective near vision. Astigmatism (Greek: lack of pinpoint) is a condition where an uneven corneal surface causes light rays to focus unevenly onto the retina. This causes distorted images at all viewing distances. Presbyopia is a term used to signify 'ageing sight'. It is a phenomenon that usually begins after the age of 40 when the lens loses its normal accommodating power.

Cataract (meaning waterfall) is a disorder in which there is opacification of the lens. It presents as a painless disease with insidious onset and gradually diminishing visual acuity. Patients usually complain about problems with night driving, reading road signs and fine prints, change in visual acuity, or paradoxically improving vision which ameliorates the need for using glasses.

Glaucoma is characterized by elevated intraocular pressure and damage to optic nerve. It is painful if acute in onset, however, chronic forms are painless. Visual loss in glaucoma is peripheral, to begin with and central vision is spared till late in course of this disease.

Since ophthalmic diseases can have so many varied etiologies, one must always consult an ophthalmologist and have himself evaluated thoroughly before attributing visual problems to increasing age and refractive errors.

Treatment of ARMD is by taking a special combination of vitamins and minerals, called the "AREDS Formula"(15). Besides dietary considerations, cessation of smoking is also a part of the treatment. Refractive errors are treated using techniques that augment the refractory powers of the human lens. Common methods include spectacles, contact lenses and refractive surgeries. Cataract is treated by removing the defective opaque lens and replacing it with a synthetic intraocular lens. Glaucoma is managed using techniques that reduce intraocular pressure. Common techniques to do this involve eye drop medicines (Prostaglandins and Beta Blockers), Laser therapy and Ocular surgery (to relieve intraocular pressure by promoting drainage of aqueous humor).

Sexual Dysfunction

Ageing brings with it many health issues and sexual problems constitutes a very important but seldom discussed health issue among elderly men. With increasing age, most men report having less interest in sex (decreased libido), requiring more stimulation to achieve erection (erectile dysfunction), having trouble in reaching orgasm and having orgasms that are less satisfying than they were at a younger age (ejaculatory disorders).

Decreased libido is estimated to be present in around 5–15% of men. (16) It increases with age and is commonly associated with other sexual disorders. Causes of decreased libido include Antidepressants (SSRI), Depression, Fatigue, Underlying systemic illnesses and Alcoholism. Treating the underlying cause usually leads to restoration of libido. Erectile dysfunction(ED) is the most common sexual problem faced by elderly men. It is defined as consistent or recurrent inability to acquire or sustain an erection of sufficient rigidity and duration for sexual intercourse. Risk factors associated with erectile dysfunction are obesity, chronic medical diseases like diabetes mellitus and cardiovascular disorders, smoking and watching television for long duration. Physical activity, weight loss and healthy lifestyle confer protection against ED.(17) Treatment of ED includes correction of the underlying causes and use of phosphodiesterase-5 inhibitors like sildenafil.

Ejaculatory disorders include Premature, Delayed and Retrograde ejaculation. Premature ejaculation(PE) is defined as ejaculation which occurs prior to vaginal penetration or within one minute of penetration.(18) Penile hypersensitivity, depression and performance anxiety are etiological factors associated with PE. SSRI's forms the mainstay of treatment in candidates with PE. Ejaculatory disorders also include other disorders associated with delayed ejaculation and absence of ejaculation (Anejaculation). Psychotherapy, use of vacuum assisted devices and testosterone supplements have been used in treatment of these disorders.

Falls

Incidence of falls increases with age and accounts for major morbidity among elderly individuals. Falls often go without much attention from the family members and the clinician, reason being that since all falls do not result in significant injury, the patient doesn't inform the clinician. Falls, being associated with low self esteem are often masked by the patient. The patient, family members and clinician might erroneously believe that falls are an inevitable part of ageing thereby not giving it due importance.

Around 30–40% individuals above the age of 65 falls each year(19). This number rises to about 50% among octogenarians(20). Risk factors for falls can be extrinsic (uneven terrain, poor quality walking aids, etc.) or intrinsic. Intrinsic causes include increasing age, balance problems, visual problems, weakness, arthritis, stroke, dizziness and chronic illness.

Diagnostic evaluation of falls must be done for elderly with history of 2 or more falls in last year. Besides history taking which helps in characterizing the cause of falls, physical examination of musculoskeletal function forms an integral part of patient evaluation. Performance Oriented Mobility Assessment (POMA) tool(21), Get up and Go test(22) and Functional Reach Test(23) are a few methods of assessing musculoskeletal function. Apart from these routine investigations must also be done to exclude other comorbidities.

While addressing the underlying health condition makes up for a large part in prevention of falls, the final responsibility lies with the individual himself. To avoid falling, one can make their home safer by getting rid of things like loose rugs, slippery flooring and cords which might make them trip. Having a well lighted home also helps. Wearing sturdy footwear at home, using good quality walking aids and staying mentally alert are other measures that help in preventing falls.

Urinary Incontinence

Urinary Incontinence is defined as involuntary leakage of urine due to loss of control over urinary bladder. Prevalence of incontinence increases with age such that it is approximately 5% in 19–44 years, 11% in 45–64 years and about 21% in elderly men aged above 65 years. (24).

Risk factors associated with incontinence are advanced age (leading to weak pelvic floor muscles), Prostatomegaly, UTIs', Diabetes and Neurological diseases like stroke. There are various types of urinary incontinence found in elderly males, common among them are:

Stress Incontinence- leakage of urine on laughing, sneezing, or coughing (anything which increases intrabdominal pressure)

Urgency Incontinence- this is related to a sudden urge to urinate which is so strong that the person passes urine before he can reach the toilet.

Mixed incontinence- this has features of both stress and urgency incontinence.

Incomplete bladder evacuation- this is related to partial bladder evacuation on account of some obstruction to urine outflow. It is commonly seen in patients with prostatomegaly.

Diagnostic evaluation of urinary incontinence revolves around laboratory investigation and imaging. Urine analysis and urine cultures are done in almost all patients. Prostate Specific Antigen (PSA) testing is considered in men with high suspicion of prostatomegaly to rule out coexistence of carcinoma. Imaging techniques involve an ultrasound of the kidneys and urinary bladder. It can detect local pathologies and also give information about type of incontinence in the patient.

Since etiologies of urinary incontinence are multifactorial, a multicomponent approach is required to tackle this problem. Non-pharmacological steps include reducing the amount of water and liquids consumed per day, strict control of diabetes, bladder training and pelvic muscle exercises. Pharmacological interventions are aimed at relaxing the bladder (antimuscarinics and beta-3 agonists) and improving urinary flow (alpha blockers-tamsulosin). Unresponsive cases require surgical intervention to improve the flow of urine by removing a part of enlarged prostate gland, repairing tissues that hold urinary bladder in its anatomical location and repairing muscles that control urinary flow.

Frailty

Frailty is basically age related physiological decline characterized by susceptibility to adverse health outcomes. There is a common misconception that increased age is synonymous with frailty. Some old men have a very active and vigorous lifestyle while others who are relatively young have a decline in physiological functioning. Incidence of frailty in adult men over 65 years is estimated to be around 8.4%. (25).

Factors associated with increased frailty include:

Increasing age.
Unmarried/ Single men.
Smoking.
Low Education.
Intellectual disability.
Depression.

Since frailty captures the essence of age related physiological decline, there can't be a single criteria or a laboratory test to define or diagnose frailty. There are two scales used to diagnose frailty: Hopkins Frailty Phenotype and FRAIL Scale.

Hopkins Frailty Phenotype is one universally accepted scale to diagnose frailty. It defines frailty as meeting three or more of following five criteria:

Weight loss $\geq$ 5% in last one year.
Exhaustion.
Weakness (decreased grip strength).

Slow walking speed (>7 s to walk 15 feet).
Decreased physical activity (Males spending < 383 kcal per week)(26).

FRAIL Scale is a quicker and easier way to diagnose frailty:

Fatigue.
Resistance to climb one flight of stairs.
Ambulation (Can you walk one block).
Illnesses (more than 5).
Loss of weight (more than 5%).

The answer Yes to three or more of these indicates frailty. (27).

Management of frailty involves a multipronged approach. The following graphic provides an outline of interventions carried out at various stages of frailty.

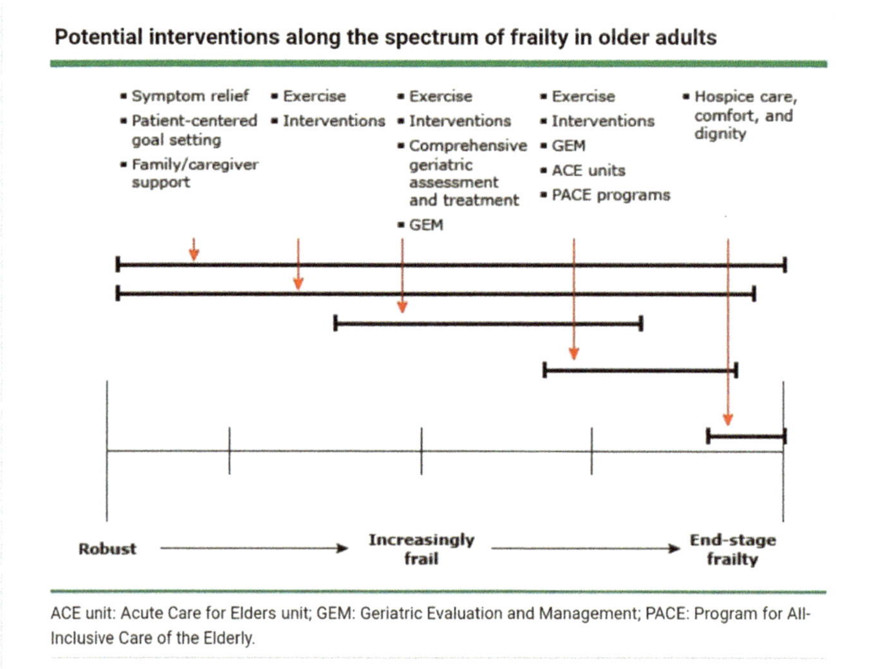

Source Walston JD, Fried LP. Frailty and its Implications for Care. Chapter 9. *In: Geriatric Palliative Care, Morrison RS, Meire DE. Oxford University Press, New York 2003. p.93. Copyright ©2003 Oxford University Press.*

Exercise forms the cornerstone of managing frailty. It is associated with improvement in carrying out activities of daily living, improved bone mineral density, decreased falls and increased general wellbeing.(28).

Comprehensive Geriatric Assessment (CGA) comprises an inter-disciplinary care team, consisting of geriatrician and other specialists, that coordinate management of frail individuals and develops a plan for integrated care.

Programme of All inclusive Care for the Elderly (PACE) is also a similar setup where geriatricians, nurses, occupational therapists and social workers work together to provide comprehensive care to frail individuals.

Emotional Support and Economic Dependence

India, world's second most populous country has seen an alarming boom in population over the last 50 years. Demographers have placed India in phase 4 of demographic cycle over the last 4–5 decades, implying persistence of high fertility rate and a rapidly declining mortality rate. This translated into rapid population expansion and current situation of population overload. Elderly people comprise around 5.5% of total population. Working population of India (aged 15–64 years) is believed to be only 46% of the total. This means that age dependency ratio is 8.4%. Put in simpler words, it means that less than half of India's population has to earn and cater to the remaining more than half.

Old age is faced with many challenges. While retiring from a job leads to free time and greater independence, dwindling social circles, health issues and changing social roles lead to emotional vulnerability. While parents take responsibility for their children and ensure that all their needs are met, this role often reverses in old age. Many a time old people have to lean on their children for meeting very basic needs. They may feel uncomfortable asking for help and even avoid it on many occasions, dependence on children causes decreased self esteem and adds to emotional vulnerability. Post retirement people may feel a void in their daily schedule where there is nothing much to be done. Boredom and depression can creep in due to this and it is a significant cause of morbidity in the elderly.

With old age, declining physical activity, decreased self sufficiency, health problems and passing away of people in social circles takes a huge toll on mental aspect of an individual. Since emotional wellbeing is as important as physical health, depression and feeling of social disconnection can lead to unwillingness to live any longer. Besides lack of emotional support, dwindling finances is also a major concern of old age. Source of income is very limited and finances can be a huge problem if the person hasn't planned for retirement in advance. Changing social roles and dynamics with family members means that all elderly people can't openly ask for money from their children or younger relatives. To add to this, dwindling health also leads to expenditure. With a limited income, expenses for health, food and daily routine can make for a very gloom and vulnerable old age.

Advanced Directives

Advanced directives are legal documents that allow a person to decide what kind of medical care should be given if ever he reaches a stage where he can't decide for himself. These documents, besides upholding the person's choices and preferences, also make things easier for the caregivers.

Following are different kinds of advanced directives:

Health Care Proxy (Durable power of attorney for health care): This is a system wherein the person chooses someone to make medical decisions for him in situations where the person is unable to decide for himself.

Living Will: A living will is a written document that tells the health care providers what type of care the person wants if he is unable to decide for himself.

Do Not Resuscitate orders: These are orders given to the health care team by the person that he doesn't want them to try and restart his heart if it stops beating once.

Advanced directives have been shown to decrease rate of hospitalization, chances of dying in hospital and duration of palliative care received by the patient. (29) There are many legal issues associated with advanced directives. Religious myths and social pressure make exercising advanced directives a challenging task. Fear of litigation may also prompt caregivers to extend complete life support to the patient with virtually no chances of recovery. Therefore understanding the legal aspects of end of life care and discussing it openly with a lawyer and trusted caregivers can go a long way in providing the kind of medical attention as desired by the patient himself in grave situations.

Ethical issues also arise with advanced directives because of concerns about how much care makes sense for a patient who is terminally ill or is expected not to come out of a vegetative state. It may also lead to a conflict between caregivers who have different opinions about end of life care. Therefore, it is in best interest of the patient to plan ahead and give clear instructions about the extent to which he wants to be medically pursued should he land in a situation with potentially no chances of complete recovery.

Chronic Obstructive Pulmonary Disease

COPD or chronic obstructive pulmonary disease is a lung condition in which the lung airways become narrowed, thus limiting the airflow into the lungs. These airways are also inflamed and there is destruction of the air sacs (alveoli) of the lungs. As the lung destruction progresses, there is progressive increase in difficulty of breathing, decreased oxygenation of blood and decreased ability of the lung to get rid of carbon dioxide. The term COPD includes chronic bronchitis (inflammation of the lung airways and associated with chronic cough and phlegm) and emphysema (destruction of alveoli).

Smoking is the most common cause of this disease. Harmful gases and microscopic particles which are inhaled while smoking or breathing smoke filled air (secondhand smoke) or from air pollution irritate and injure the airways and lungs and cause inflammation. Over time, this inflammation becomes chronic and irreversibly damages the lung tissue and may cause scarring or fibrosis. Most people with COPD have components of chronic bronchitis and emphysema. Some also have features of asthma. In a minority of people with asthma, chronic inflammation permanently restricts airflow. When this airway narrowing cannot be completely reversed with treatment, the person is said to have COPD.

Smoking cigarettes and beedi are the most common risk factors. However, 15–20% of those who have never smoked, also develop COPD. Other factors contributing to development of COPD include exposure to second hand smoke, environmental dust and organic materials, air pollution and hyperactive airways. Genetic factors also contribute. Deficiency of alpha 1 anti-trypsin, a protein that protects alveoli from oxidative harm can cause emphysema. The most common symptoms include:

Coughing with sputum production.

Wheezing (a squeaking noise on breathing).

Shortness of breath at first with activity and later even at rest as disease progresses.

Fatigue.

The tests used in diagnosing COPD(30) are Pulmonary function test—Spirometry. During spirometry, a deep breath is taken in and then blown out with maximal force into a tube connected to a machine called a spirometer. The spirometer measures the velocity and the volume of air one can blow. If the measurement is abnormal, the test is repeated after using a bronchodilator. In people with asthma, there is demonstrable bronchodilator reversibility with the test measurements returning to normal after bronchodilator use. However, in people with COPD, the test measurements may only partially improve. Chest X-ray shows changes only when the disease is advanced and severe. It helps to exclude other diseases. CT scan is helpful in diagnosing emphysema.

The most important part of treatment for COPD is cessation of smoking. The disease progression is slowed, irrespective of the severity of the disease post smoking cessation. Unfortunately, there is no cure for COPD; however, many treatments are available for the symptoms and complications of this disorder, which include:

Bronchodilators—in form of metered dose inhalers (MDI) which include anti-cholinergic agents and beta agonists.

Oral or IV steroids in severe exacerbations.

Theophylline.

Antibiotics in exacerbations.

Supplemental oxygen therapy—only therapy proven to reduce mortality.

Non-pharmacological treatment.

Pulmonary rehabilitation.

Lung volume reduction surgery.

Lung transplantation.

Weight Loss

Unintentional or involuntary weight loss occurs in 15 to 20% of older adults. It is frequently insidious and often may be a harbinger of a serious underlying medical disorder. It is associated with increased mortality and morbidity. Clinically important is defined as the loss of > 4.5 kg or > 5% of one's body weight over a period of 6–12 months. It leads to various deleterious effects such as decline in activities of daily living, hip fractures, impaired immunity, pressure ulcers and increased risk of other diseases(31).

Body composition changes as the person ages. Lean body mass begins to decline by up to 0.3 kg per year in the third decade. This loss is countered by increase in fat mass that continues until 65 to 70 years of age. Total body weight usually peaks at 60 years of age. Thereafter, there are small decreases of 0.1 to 0.2 kg per year after 70 years of age. Mean energy intake is reduced in the elderly reflecting the reduced physical activity and loss of mean body weight. Many hormones and peptides involved in hunger are altered in their levels and lead to reduced appetite and early satiety, which collectively contribute to 'anorexia of ageing'. Substantial weight changes should not be attributed to anorexia of ageing.

Causes of involuntary weight loss can be divided into 4 categories.

(1) Malignant neoplasms
(2) Chronic inflammatory or infectious diseases,
(3) Metabolic disorders (e.g. hyperthyroidism and diabetes)
(4) Psychiatric disorders.

A quarter of the weight loss patients is caused by malignant disease. Organic diseases are responsible for one-third of the cases. Remainder is due to psychiatric disease, medications, etc. There is no identifiable cause in up to one-quarter of patients despite extensive investigation. The most common cancers responsible for involuntary weight loss are gastrointestinal, hepatobiliary, lung, breast, genitourinary, ovarian and prostate. The prognoses with those cancers which present with weight loss are very poor.

Oral and dental factors such as poor dental hygiene, dry mouth, inability to chew, edentulousness (loss of tooth), pain due to temporomandibular joint syndrome, caries, etc. can lead to weight loss too.

Chronic inflammatory diseases such as malabsorption, peptic ulcer, inflammatory bowel disease, celiac disease, chronic pancreatitis, obstruction/constipation, pernicious anemia in gastrointestinal system; congestive cardiac failure, chronic obstructive pulmonary disease, renal insufficiency are responsible for weight loss. Hyperthyroidism, diabetes mellitus, pheochromocytoma and adrenal insufficiency are a few metabolic and endocrinal disease causing weight loss.

Neurological diseases such as stroke, quadriplegia, parkinson's disease and dementia predispose to weight loss. Infections such as HIV, tuberculosis, parasitic infections, subacute bacterial endocarditis and certain medications like sedatives, antibiotics, pain-killers, antidepressants, metformin, levodopa, anti-hypertensive (ACE inhibitors) can lead to weight loss.

Psychiatric diseases like depression, anxiety, paranoia, bereavement, alcoholism, eating disorders lead to malnutrition and weight loss. Social causes such as poverty, isolation need special mention as they may be the important cause for weight loss and related comorbidities.

Diagnosis of the cause of weight loss can be done by thorough evaluation such as complete blood counts, Liver function test, erythrocyte sedimentation rate, renal function tests, thyroid profile, chest radiograph, abdominal ultrasound, age, sex and risk factor–specific cancer screening tests, such as mammography and colonoscopy. Patients at risk should have HIV testing. All elderly patients with weight loss should also undergo screening for dementia and depression. Treatment is aimed at correcting the underlying cause. An early contact with health care can avert the serious consequences of some grave diseases associated with this symptom of weight loss.

Constipation

Constipation is a very common symptom encountered in daily clinical practice. It usually has different meanings. Stools may be too hard or too small, difficult to pass, or infrequent (less than three times per week). Many patients may have a normal frequency of defecation but complain of excessive straining, hard stools, lower abdominal fullness, or a sense of incomplete evacuation. Constipation is more frequent as one gets older(32).

Causes of constipation may be for convenience divided into recent onset or chronic. Colon obstruction due to cancer or stricture, anal sphincter spasm due to anal fissures, or painful hemorrhoids and certain medications are the causes of constipation of recent onset. Whereas, the causes of chronic constipation are many. It generally results from inadequate fiber or fluid intake or from disordered colonic transit or anorectal function. Irritable bowel syndrome, pelvic floor muscle dysfunction, endocrine disorders such as hypothyroidism, hypercalcemia, pregnancy, depression, neurologic diseases such as parkinsonism, multiple sclerosis, spinal cord injury, prolonged immobilization and certain drugs (calcium channel blockers, antidepressants) are important causes of chronic constipation(33).

Constipation can be diagnosed from symptoms and physical examination. Rectal examination may be needed. Further testing may be done in some situations like a recent change in bowel habits, blood in the stool, weight loss, or a family history of colon cancer which includes blood tests, x-rays, sigmoidoscopy, colonoscopy, or more specialized testing if needed.

Treatment for constipation includes eating foods high in fiber (20 to 35 g of fiber per day) and using laxatives or enemas if needed. Behaviour changes include paying attention to bowel movements and not ignoring them. Many fruits and vegetables can be particularly helpful in preventing and treating constipation.

Patients with constipation are treated with laxatives (bulk, osmotic, prokinetic, secretory and stimulant) including fiber, psyllium, milk of magnesia, lactulose, polyethylene glycol, bisacodyl and some newer drugs like lubiprostone, linaclotide and prucalopride. If the constipation is not responding to above medications along with pelvic floor training, psychological counseling and dietary modifications, surgery in the form of colectomy with ileorectostomy may be considered.

Prostate

The prostate is a small gland situated just below the urinary bladder. It is a part of the male reproductive system. It is about a size of a walnut. Prostate gland surrounds the urethra (the tube that carries urine from bladder). It is made of 2 lobes.

There are mainly 2 major concerns regarding the prostate gland in elderly males.

(1) Benign Prostatic Hypertrophy (BPH).
(2) Prostate cancer.

Benign Prostatic Hypertrophy (BPH): The prostate normally enlarges to some degree in all men with advancing age. But not everyone develops the symptoms of BPH or lower urinary tract symptoms. The symptoms usually begin after the age of 50 years.

The most common symptoms of BPH are:

1. Increase frequency of micturition, especially at night.
2. Urinary hesitancy interrupted or weak stream of urine.
3. Leaking or dribbling of urine
4. Inability to completely empty bladder

Some men have significant symptoms with slightly enlarged prostate whereas other men with very enlarged prostate can have only minor urinary symptoms. In some, the symptoms gradually worsen over years and in few symptoms eventually stabilize and improve over time.

The symptoms of BPH can also be caused by.

- UTI
- Prostate or bladder cancer
- Kidney stones
- Narrowing of urethra
- Problems with the nerves controlling bladder (overactive bladder)

Diagnosis

(1) Rectal examination—To feel the size and shape of the prostate gland. It also helps to determine some signs of prostate cancer.
(2) Urinalysis
(3) Blood Test-Serum PSA (prostate specific antigen) levels- It is a protein produced by prostate cells. It can be elevated both in BPH and prostate cancer
(4) Urodynamic studies

(5) Ultrasound studies

Treatment

Options include medical and surgical procedures. Mild BPH usually does not require treatment. Moderate to severe symptoms usually require treatment. Medical treatment involves 2 types of drugs, Alpha blockers (tamsulosin, alfuzosin, doxazosin), Alpha reductase inhibitors (finasteride, dutasteride), or combination of both.

Surgical—

(1) Trans Urethral Resection of Prostate(TURP)
(2) Prostate ablation by laser or radio frequency
(3) Removal of prostate (prostatectomy)
(4) Suprapubic catheterization—as a temporary measure or in few cases, permanently

Prostate Cancer

Prostate cancer symptoms are usually similar to the enlarged prostate gland as seen in BPH. Other much less common symptoms include blood in the urine or semen and erectile dysfunction. The screening of prostate cancer is usually done by serum PSA levels and digital rectal examination. Further, biopsy of the gland may be required to confirm and for staging of cancer. Treatment options vary according to the stage of cancer. Available treatment options include radical prostatectomy (removal of prostate), radiation therapy sometimes along with androgen deprivation therapy (drugs like leuprolide, flutamide and procedures like orchidectomy) and chemotherapy.

Parkinson's Disease

Parkinson's disease is the second most common neurodegenerative disorder after Alzheimer's. It is because of damage to nerve cells that produce dopamine—'a chemical messenger'. Parkinson's disease affects people of both sexes, of all races and countries. The mean age of onset is about 60 and the condition worsens as the age advances.

There is no exact cause of Parkinson's disease, but observed risk factors for Parkinson's include: Genes - It is identified that specific genetic mutations can cause Parkinson's disease, especially in younger patients. However, it is uncommon. Environmental Factors - Exposure to certain toxins or environmental agents have been proposed to increase the risk of Parkinson's disease. Age -Even though it is usually seen in the elderly, few cases especially involving genetic mutations are seen in young patients at 20 years of age or even less. The symptoms tend to worsen gradually as age advances.

The dopaminergic neurons in the basal ganglia are affected and the denervation of these causes the loss of facilitatory action basal ganglia on the cortex of brain leading to the parkinsonian features.

It can be broadly divided into motor or non-motor features. The 3 cardinal motor features of Parkinson's include

(1) Akinesia or bradykinesia: Inabilityor slowness in initiating movements
(2) Rigidity of movements
(3) Resting tremors in extremities

The patients often show a lack of associated movements like swaying of hands while walking, reduced blinking of eyes and may have masked face, i.e. patient doesn't show any associated expressions with respect to the subject of speech (the person does not show a smile on his face even though he is happy). Pill rolling tremors, i.e. as the name suggests the person shows finger movements as if he is rolling them over a pill is seen in affected patients. Gait of the patients with Parkinson's is described as festinating gait where the patient involuntarily moves with short, accelerating steps, often on tip toe as if he is trying to catch the centre of gravity of his body. Patients often have freezing episodes that are, he/she may stay as it is with difficulty initiating further movement. Some of the non-motor features include mood disorders like depression, sleep disturbances, dementia, features of autonomic involvement like orthostatic hypotension, gastrointestinal, genitourinary and sexual dysfunction.

Drugs are the mainstay of Parkinson's treatment. There are many classes of drugs used.

1. Levodopa in combination with carbidopa—mainstay of treatment
2. Dopamine agonists like ropinirole, pramipexole
3. MAO-B inhibitors like Rasagiline and selegiline
4. COMT inhibitors like entacapone, tolcapone
5. Surgical treatment includes deep brain stimulation (DBS)

Type 2 Diabetes

Worldwide prevalence of DM (diabetes mellitus) has risen dramatically over the past 2 decades. India being called the "diabetic capital of the world" has as many as 50 million people suffering from this condition. Most of the individuals with diabetes are between the age group of 40 s and 60 s, however, it is being seen now in younger individuals, maybe because of changing diet habits, lack of activity and obesity.

Diabetes is gaining much importance now-a-days as it affects a person's health in many ways. It has implications not only from a financial point of view, but also increases the morbidity and mortality. Diabetes when uncontrolled, causes an immunocompromised state with increased susceptibility to infections, delayed wound healing, accelerates atherosclerosis leading to cardiac and cerebrovascular diseases. The long-term complications of Type 2 DM like neuropathy, retinopathy and nephropathy are often disabling and lead to a significant decrease in quality of life. It is for all these reasons that early recognition, life style modifications, proper treatment and adherence to the drugs are of utmost importance to control this disabling, multi system involving ailment.

Risk factors can be classified as.

1. Unavoidable risk factors
2. Avoidable risk factors

Unavoidable risk factors.

- Family history—type 2 DM has a strong genetic component
- Age
- History of gestational diabetes
- Race

Avoidable risk factors.

- Obesity or being overweight
- Hypertension
- Little or no exercise
- High levels of HDL or triglycerides
- Smoking
- Stress and lack of minimal sleep

Type 2 DM is a condition that hampers the way body handles the level of glucose in blood. This condition is associated with insulin resistance (insulin helps in entry of glucose from blood into other cells of the body) and/or decreased body insulin levels because of under secretion of insulin from pancreas. Other mechanisms involved include increased production of glucose from liver and impaired fat metabolism in the body.

The criteria for diagnosis of diabetes is mentioned below:

- Symptoms of diabetes plus random blood glucose level $\geq$ 200 mg/dL or
- Fasting plasma glucose $\geq$ 126 mg/dLor
- Hemoglobin A1c $\geq$ 6.5% or
- 2-h plasma glucose $\geq$ 200 mg/dL during an oral glucose tolerance test

Persons with (1) fasting glucose of 100–125 mg/dL, [called as impaired fasting glucose (IFG)]; (2) plasma glucose levels between 140 and 199 mg/dL following an oral glucose challenge [called as which is termed impaired glucose tolerance (IGT)]; or (3) HbA1c of 5.7–6.4% - are called as prediabetics and are at increased risk of developing overt diabetes and cardiovascular complications.

The management of diabetes involves a multi-disciplinary approach. The salient features of each are described below:

1. Diabetes education—It involves sensitizing the patients regarding the adequate control of blood glucose, dietary and lifestyle modifications, right way of taking drugs or insulin, prevention and management of hypoglycemia.
2. Nutrition—Low carbohydrate, low fat diet, using low glycemic index diet, consuming less sucrose, increasing consumption of dietary fibers, vegetables, fruits, whole grains, low sodium intake and use of non-nutrient sweeteners.
3. Regular exercise, for a minimum of 20 min, at least five days a week, encouraging weight loss.
4. Oral hypoglycemic agents—various classes of drugs are now used for treating diabetes. Some of these include-

   - Biguanides - Metformin
   - Sulphonylureas - Glimepride, gliclazide, glipizide, glyburide
   - DPP4 inhibitors—Sitagliptin, vildagliptin, linagliptin, teneligliptin
   - Glinides - Repaglinide, nateglinide
   - SGLT2 inhibitors - Canagliflozin, dapagliflozin, empagliflozin
   - Thiazolidinediones - Rosiglitazone, pioglitazone
   - GLP-1 receptor agonists - Exenatide, liraglutide, dulaglutide

5. Insulin—Insulin is now considered as the preferred initial therapy in type 2 DM, particularly in lean individuals and with severe weight loss, those with underlying renal or hepatic disease, or in individuals who are hospitalized or acutely ill.

The use of oral drugs or insulin is often individualized according to the requirements.

6. Treatment of associated conditions like dyslipidemia, hypertension, obesity, coronary heart disease.
7. Frequent follow-up for screening of or management of complications of diabetes such as retinopathy (yearly eye-checkup), cardiovascular disease, nephropathy and neuropathy.

Depression in Elderly

Geriatric depression is a mental and emotional disorder affecting older adults. Feelings of occasional sadness and low mood are normal, however, depression lasting longer is not. Older adults are often misdiagnosed because their symptoms of depression mimic normal age related issues or may be attributed to a concurrent illness. Hence, depression should not be considered a normal part of ageing and an early medical consult should be sought, as it is a treatable condition.

Several factors or a combination of factors may contribute to depression.

- Genetic: Persons with family history of depression are at increased risk of developing depression
- A past history of depression also increases risk at elderly age

- Female sex
- Stress in the form of loss of loved one, divorce, widowhood, loneliness
- Lack of social supportive network
- Financial hardships
- Prolonged substance abuse
- Many diseases co-occur with depression. Major ones include
  - Cardiac illness (20–30% patients)
  - Cancer (25% patients)
  - Neurologic disorders (cerebrovascular diseases, Parkinson's, dementia
  - Diabetes mellitus
  - Hypothyroidism, also hyperthyroidism
  - HIV, chronic hepatitis C infection
  - Chronic fatigue syndrome, fibromyalgia
  - Chronic severe pain due to any cause
- Medications (steroids, anti-hypertensive, antibiotics, anti-arrhythmic agents, etc.)

There are several symptoms of depression, but it varies individually. Few symptoms are listed below and persistence of these symptoms for $\geq$ 2 weeks may indicate depression.

- Persistent sadness or 'empty' mood
- Feeling of worthlessness, helplessness, hopelessness
- Loss of interest in life—not enjoying what one usually used to
- Frequent crying spells
- Decreased energy, fatigue
- Feeling irritable, restless
- Lack of concentration
- Difficulty in concentrating, remembering
- Sleeplessness
- Eating more or less than usual
- Suicidal thoughts, attempts
- Aches and pains, digestive problems without a physical cause, or not responding to treatment
- Withdrawal from social activities

Treatment choices vary from person to person. Most common forms of treatment are psychotherapy and medications. Psychotherapy helps to see how depression may be connected with what has happened in the past. Cognitive Behavioural Therapy helps to see how some of the ways one thinks or behaves may be causing depression. Also, it helps one think more realistically. Antidepressants are the drugs used to treat depression. With the advent of newer drugs, better options are now available to treat depression with relatively lesser side effects. They usually take 2–4 weeks to work. Some of the classes of medications used to treat depression include:

Selective serotonin reuptake inhibitors (SSRIs).

Selective serotonin-norepinephrine reuptake inhibitors (SNRIs).
Tricyclic antidepressants.
Monoamine oxidase inhibitors (MAOIs).

Some of the changes in life style such as regular exercise, healthy balanced diet, being prepared for major life changes, more social interaction and sharing of feelings with family and friends, good sleep can help prevent and also treat depression.

Insomnia in Elderly

Insomnia is a very frequent problem encountered in late life. Despite its large prevalence, it is often underdiagnosed and untreated. Insomnia is difficulty in falling asleep or staying asleep, despite adequate opportunity to sleep. Sleep is reported as insufficient and non-freshening. It should not be attributed to normal part of ageing. The prevalence of insomnia ranges from 30–60%(34).

The average adult needs about 7.5 to 8 h of sleep per day. There are two basic states of sleep. (1) rapid eye movement (REM) sleep and (2) non–rapid eye movement (NREM) sleep. NREM sleep is further subdivided into three stages: N1, N2 and N3. NREM stage N3 sleep is also known as slow-wave sleep (SWS) and is believed to be the most restorative part of sleep. After the onset of sleep, it usually progresses through NREM stages N1–N3 sleep within 45–60 min. The first REM sleep episode usually occurs in the second hour of sleep. NREM and REM sleep alternate through the night with an average period of 90–110 min.

As the age progresses, the sleep architecture also changes. Sleep initiation is more difficult. The N3 sleep (SWS) duration gradually decreases and may be completely absent in old individuals. The NREM sleep becomes more fragmented with more frequent awakenings. There are also changes in the natural circadian rhythm, causing many elderly people to go to bed earlier and to wake up earlier. Also, they find more difficulty in staying awake during the day. They tend to take more frequent daytime naps.

Insomnia is classified as transient (few nights), acute (less than 3–4 weeks) and chronic (more than 3–4 weeks).

Transient or acute insomnia usually occurs in people with no history of sleep disturbances and a cause for the same is often identifiable. Usual causes include acute medical illness, stressful or bad news, jet lag, changes in sleeping environment, medications. Chronic or long-term insomnia may be associated with a variety of underlying disorders such as medical (sleep apnea, restless leg syndrome, musculoskeletal pain, heart failure, COPD, peptic ulcer disease, constipation, diarrhea, urinary incontinence, nocturia, Parkinson's, Alzheimer's, etc.), psychiatric (anxiety, depression, delirium), behavioural (excessive daytime sleeping, early retirement to bed), medications (caffeine, nicotine, antidepressants, levodopa, diuretics, beta blockers, laxatives, etc.) and substance abuse.

Timely diagnosis and treatment of insomnia are very essential as it is associated it increased morbidity and mortality. It causes chronic fatigue, decreased memory, impaired concentration and impaired functional performance of daily activities, increases risk of falls and accidents. It can also lead to glucose intolerance and diabetes, obesity, metabolic syndrome, accelerated atherosclerosis, increased risk of coronary artery disease and stroke and impaired immunity.

Treatment options include(35).

Non-pharmacological—Improvement of sleep hygiene, cognitive behavioural therapy. Various sleep hygiene recommendations that may be helpful in elderly patients are:

- Avoid caffeine, alcohol and nicotine
- Develop a consistent sleep routine
- Perform regular exercise (preferably in the morning or early afternoon);
- Using the bed only for sleep and sex
- Avoid heavy meals within 2–3 h of bedtime
- Avoid large amounts of fluids 2–3 h before bedtime
- Restful sleep environment
- Avoid napping especially after 3 pm
- Avoid solving problems, thinking about life issues, reviewing events of the day when trying to fall asleep
- Prepare for sleep with 20–30 min of relaxation (e.g. soft music, meditation, yoga, pleasant reading)

Pharmacological—

Bezodiazepenes(alprazolam, clonazepam, temazepam).
Non-benzodiazepenes (zolpidem, zaleplon, zopiclone).
Antidepressants (trazodone, amitriptyline, doxepin).
Antihistamines (diphenhydramine).
Melatonin related drugs (ramelteon).

Osteoarthritis

Osteoarthritis (OA) is the most common form of arthritis. In OA, the cartilage in the joints (which normally protects bones from rubbing together) wears down gradually and bony spurs occur. Although OA can affect almost any joint, it most often affects the hands, knees, hips, feet and spine; and usually, wrist, elbow and ankle are spared(36). The prevalence of OA rises strikingly with age—it is uncommon in adults under age 40 and highly prevalent in those over age 60 years. Risk factors include:

- Age — Advancing age is one of the strongest risk factors for OA.
- Gender—Women are 2–3 times more likely to develop OA than men.
- Heredity—OA is a highly heritable disease
- Obesity — People who are obese are at high risk of developing OA.

- Occupation — OA of the knee has been linked to certain occupations that require frequent squatting, kneeling, lifting heavy loads.
- Previous injury or surgery to knee also increases risk of OA
- Sports — The risk of OA is increased in those who participate in wrestling, boxing, cycling, gymnastics, football; by contrast, sports like running do not have increased risk of OA.

Osteoarthritis symptoms often develop slowly and worsen over time. Signs and symptoms of osteoarthritis include:

- Pain — Joint pain in OA is worse with activity and relieved by rest. In severe cases, the pain may also occur at rest or at night.
- Stiffness — Joint stiffness may be most noticeable on waking up in the morning or after a period of inactivity.
- Loss of flexibility—Inability to move joint through its full range of motion
- Swelling (effusion) — OA may cause a type of joint swelling called an effusion, which results from the accumulation of excess fluid in the joint.
- Crackling or grating sensation (crepitus) — Movement of a joint may cause a crackling or grating sensation called crepitus.
- Bony outgrowths (osteophytes) — These extra bits of bone, which feel like hard lumps, may form around the affected joint.

Diagnosis of OA can be made by the history and clinical symptoms and imaging in the form of X-ray are helpful(37) to rule out other causes of joint pain and also to know the severity of the disease.

Osteoarthritis (OA) is a progressive disease which generally worsens slowly over time, although it may stabilize in some people(38).

Treatment options include(39):

Non-pharmacological—Weight loss, avoiding activities that overload the joint, exercises to improve strength of muscles that bridge joint, redistributing load within the joint using a brace, or a splint or by unloading the joint during weight bearing with assistive devices such as a cane or a crutch.

Pharmacological—

- Topical nonsteroidal anti-inflammatory drugs (NSAIDs), Capsaicin
- Oral nonsteroidal anti-inflammatory drugs (NSAIDs)
- Paracetamol (Acetaminophen)
- Joint injections such as steroids or hyaluronans

Surgical—Surgery is usually reserved for severe osteoarthritis (OA) that significantly limits daily activities and that did not respond to other arthritis treatments. Surgical options include joint realignment, fusion and joint replacement.

Anemia in Elderly

Anemia is a very common, underdiagnosed disease in elderly. Though its prevalence increases with age, it should not be considered an inevitable consequence of ageing. The WHO definition of anemia can also be applied to the elderly, which is, hemoglobin < 13 g/dl in men and < 12 mg/dl in women. In elderly, any degree of anemia contributes to increased morbidity and mortality and significantly affects the quality of life. Anemia may be harbinger of a serious underlying illness.

Symptoms of anemia may be non-specific such as fatigue, breathlessness on exertion, generalized weakness, dizziness. It may also manifest as cognitive impairment or exacerbation of an underlying illness such as cardiac failure.

Anemia in the elderly is particularly relevant as it has a number of serious consequences. Anemia is associated with a higher incidence of cardiovascular disease, cognitive decline, decreased physical performance and quality of life, increased risk of falls and fractures and increased duration of hospital stay(40).

Anemia in elderly can be broadly divided into the following subgroups.

- Anemia due to nutritional deficiency—Among this group, iron deficiency is the most common cause of anemia. Other causes include vitamin B12 and folic acid deficiency.
- Anemia of chronic disease—It is the most common cause of anemia in elderly. This group of diseases can be summarized as having a functional iron deficiency due to an underlying disease. In other words, there is inefficient utilization and recycling of iron due to the inflammatory mediators associated with various diseases.
- Malignancy—An underlying malignancy like myelodysplastic syndrome, chronic leukemia or lymphoma, gastrointestinal cancers can present like anemia.
- Other causes—Diseases like chronic kidney disease, hypothyroidism, hypersplenism, hemolytic anemias can cause anemia. However, in about 15–25% of the patients, no underlying cause of anemia is found.

Blood investigations in the form of complete hemogram with RBC indices, peripheral smear, reticulocyte count help in the identification of type and probable cause of anemia. Further investigations include serum iron studies, vitamin B12, folate levels, renal function tests, thyroid hormone levels and stool for occult blood(41). When malignancy is suspected, bone marrow examination and other additional investigations are required to arrive at a diagnosis. The diagnostic workup does not end when the diagnosis of iron deficiency anemia is made. Further workup for chronic blood loss from gastrointestinal tracts like endoscopy or colonoscopy is necessary. When anemia of chronic disease is suspected, investigations directed towards the identification of the underlying disease are done.

Treatment is aimed at correcting a specific cause. Iron supplementation in iron deficiency anemia, vitamin B12 and folate supplementation when their deficiencies are found. Malignancies are treated according to the current protocols. Chronic kidney disease and some anemias of chronic disease respond to erythropoietin supplementation, whereas the main treatment of anemia of chronic disease is treating the underlying chronic disease(42).

Conclusion

Having covered individual topics in great detail, before concluding we would like to emphasize a few things again. Lifestyle changes contribute significantly to most age related problems like stroke, coronary artery disease, hypertension, diabetes and malignancies. It is therefore of utmost importance to adopt a healthy lifestyle, quit smoking and recreational drugs, eat a balanced diet and exercise regularly. Early recognition and prompt action in setting of alarming clinical symptoms can go a long way in deciding the prognosis of an individual. It is, therefore, reiterated that professional medical help must be sought at the earliest in the event of red flag symptoms. These should not be ignored and attributed to other things. Other than physical wellbeing, mental and social health also comprise of holistic wellbeing concept propagated by the WHO. Therefore, due importance must be given to treating oneself with kindness, avoiding self criticism, indulging in hobbies, planning for old age well in advance with regards to finances and keeping negative thoughts away. One must also take good care of his relations, surround himself with good people, remain happy and try and spread positivity.

References

Althof, S. E., McMahon, C. G., Waldinger, M. D., Serefoglu, E. C., Shindel, A. W., Adaikan, P. G., et al. (2014). An update of the International Society of Sexual Medicine's guidelines for the diagnosis and treatment of premature ejaculation (PE). *The Journal of Sexual Medicine, 11*(6), 1392–1422.

Bacon, C. G., Mittleman, M. A., Kawachi, I., Giovannucci, E., Glasser, D. B., & Rimm, E. B. (2003). Sexual function in men older than 50 years of age: Results from the health professionals follow-up study. *Annals of Internal Medicine, 139*(3), 161–168.

Bergen, G., Stevens, M. R., & Burns, E. R. (2016). Falls and Fall Injuries Among Adults Aged >/=65 Years - United States, 2014. *MMWR. Morbidity and Mortality Weekly Report, 65*(37), 993–998.

Brinkman-Stoppelenburg, A., Rietjens, J. A., & van der Heide, A. (2014). The effects of advance care planning on end-of-life care: A systematic review. *Palliative Medicine, 28*(8), 1000–1025.

Bennell KL, Hunter DJ, Hinman RS. Management of osteoarthritis of the knee. BMJ. 2012;345:e4934.

Bharucha, A. E., Pemberton, J. H., & Locke, G. R., 3rd. (2013). American Gastroenterological Association technical review on constipation. *Gastroenterology, 144*(1), 218–238.

Bross, M. H., Soch, K., & Smith-Knuppel, T. (2010). Anemia in older persons. *American Family Physician, 82*(5), 480–487.

Buta, B. J., Walston, J. D., Godino, J. G., Park, M., Kalyani, R. R., Xue, Q. L., et al. (2016). Frailty assessment instruments: Systematic characterization of the uses and contexts of highly-cited instruments. *Ageing Research Reviews, 26*, 53–61.

Chew, E. Y., Clemons, T. E., Agron, E., Launer, L. J., Grodstein, F., Bernstein, P. S., et al. (2015). Effect of Omega-3 Fatty Acids, Lutein/Zeaxanthin, or Other Nutrient Supplementation on Cognitive Function: The AREDS2 Randomized Clinical Trial. *JAMA, 314*(8), 791–801.

Cruz-Jentoft, A. J., Baeyens, J. P., Bauer, J. M., Boirie, Y., Cederholm, T., Landi, F., et al. (2010). Sarcopenia: European consensus on definition and diagnosis: Report of the European Working Group on Sarcopenia in Older People. *Age and Ageing, 39*(4), 412–423.

Duncan, P. W., Studenski, S., Chandler, J., & Prescott, B. (1992). Functional reach: Predictive validity in a sample of elderly male veterans. *Journal of Gerontology, 47*(3), M93–M98.

Evans, W. J., Morley, J. E., Argiles, J., Bales, C., Baracos, V., Guttridge, D., et al. (2008). Cachexia: A new definition. *Clinical Nutrition, 27*(6), 793–799.

Evans, J. R., Fletcher, A. E., Wormald, R. P. (2004). Assessment MRCTo, management of older people in the C. Causes of visual impairment in people aged 75 years and older in Britain: An add-on study to the MRC trial of assessment and management of older people in the community. Br J Ophthalmol. 88(3), 365–70.

Gaddey, H. L., & Holder, K. (2014). Unintentional weight loss in older adults. *American Family Physician, 89*(9), 718–722.

Gates, G. A., & Cooper, J. C. (1991). Incidence of hearing decline in the elderly. *Acta Oto-Laryngologica, 111*(2), 240–248.

Goodnough, L. T., & Schrier, S. L. (2014). Evaluation and management of anemia in the elderly. *American Journal of Hematology, 89*(1), 88–96.

Gopinath, B., Rochtchina, E., Wang, J. J., Schneider, J., Leeder, S. R., & Mitchell, P. (2009). Prevalence of age-related hearing loss in older adults: Blue Mountains Study. *Archives of Internal Medicine, 169*(4), 415–416.

Gorina Y, Schappert S, Bercovitz A, Elgaddal N, Kramarow E. Prevalence of incontinence among older americans. Vital Health Stat 3. 2014(36):1–33.

Guidelines for the initial evaluation of the adult patient with acute musculoskeletal symptoms. (1996). American College of Rheumatology Ad Hoc Committee on Clinical Guidelines. Arthritis Rheum, 39(1):1–8.

Hochberg, M. C. (1996). Prognosis of osteoarthritis. *Annals of the Rheumatic Diseases, 55*(9), 685–688.

Horowitz, M., Maddern, G. J., Chatterton, B. E., Collins, P. J., Harding, P. E., & Shearman, D. J. (1984). Changes in gastric emptying rates with age. *Clinical Science (london, England), 67*(2), 213–218.

Huang, Q., & Tang, J. (2010). Age-related hearing loss or presbycusis. *European Archives of Oto-Rhino-Laryngology, 267*(8), 1179–1191.

Hunter, D. J. (2011). Osteoarthritis. *Best Practice & Research Clinical Rheumatology, 25*(6), 801–814.

Jemal, A., Siegel, R., Xu, J., & Ward, E. (2010). Cancer statistics, 2010. *CA: A Cancer Journal for Clinicians, 60*(5), 277–300.

Kamel, N. S., & Gammack, J. K. (2006). Insomnia in the elderly: Cause, approach, and treatment. *American Journal of Medicine, 119*(6), 463–469.

Keysor, J. J. (2003). Does late-life physical activity or exercise prevent or minimize disablement? A critical review of the scientific evidence. *American Journal of Preventive Medicine, 25*(3 Suppl 2), 129–136.

Laumann, E. O., Paik, A., & Rosen, R. C. (1999). Sexual dysfunction in the United States: Prevalence and predictors. *JAMA, 281*(6), 537–544.

Locher, J. L., Robinson, C. O., Roth, D. L., Ritchie, C. S., & Burgio, K. L. (2005). The effect of the presence of others on caloric intake in homebound older adults. *Journals of Gerontology. Series a, Biological Sciences and Medical Sciences, 60*(11), 1475–1478.

Mathias, S., Nayak, U. S., & Isaacs, B. (1986). Balance in elderly patients: The "get-up and go" test. *Archives of Physical Medicine and Rehabilitation, 67*(6), 387–389.

McCall, W. V. (2004). Sleep in the Elderly: Burden, Diagnosis, and Treatment. *Prim Care Companion J Clin Psychiatry., 6*(1), 9–20.

Muller-Lissner, S. A., Kamm, M. A., Scarpignato, C., & Wald, A. (2005). Myths and misconceptions about chronic constipation. *American Journal of Gastroenterology, 100*(1), 232–242.

Petersen, R. C., Smith, G., Kokmen, E., Ivnik, R. J., & Tangalos, E. G. (1992). Memory function in normal aging. *Neurology, 42*(2), 396–401.

Qaseem, A., Wilt, T. J., Weinberger, S. E., Hanania, N. A., Criner, G., van der Molen, T., et al. (2011). Diagnosis and management of stable chronic obstructive pulmonary disease: A clinical practice guideline update from the American College of Physicians, American College of Chest Physicians, American Thoracic Society, and European Respiratory Society. *Annals of Internal Medicine, 155*(3), 179–191.

Rahkonen, T., Eloniemi-Sulkava, U., Rissanen, S., Vatanen, A., Viramo, P., & Sulkava, R. (2003). Dementia with Lewy bodies according to the consensus criteria in a general population aged 75 years or older. *Journal of Neurology, Neurosurgery and Psychiatry, 74*(6), 720–724.

Rolls, B. J. (1999). Do chemosensory changes influence food intake in the elderly? *Physiology & Behavior, 66*(2), 193–197.

Rosenhall, U., Moller, C., & Hederstierna, C. (2013). Hearing of 75-year old persons over three decades: Has hearing changed? *International Journal of Audiology, 52*(11), 731–739.

Shikany, J. M., Barrett-Connor, E., Ensrud, K. E., Cawthon, P. M., Lewis, C. E., Dam, T. T., et al. (2014). Macronutrients, diet quality, and frailty in older men. *Journals of Gerontology. Series a, Biological Sciences and Medical Sciences, 69*(6), 695–701.

Stauder, R., & Thein, S. L. (2014). Anemia in the elderly: Clinical implications and new therapeutic concepts. *Haematologica, 99*(7), 1127–1130.

Tinetti, M. E. (1986). Performance-oriented assessment of mobility problems in elderly patients. *Journal of the American Geriatrics Society, 34*(2), 119–126.

Tinetti, M. E., Speechley, M., & Ginter, S. F. (1988). Risk factors for falls among elderly persons living in the community. *New England Journal of Medicine, 319*(26), 1701–1707.

White JV, Guenter P, Jensen G, Malone A, Schofield M, Academy Malnutrition Work G, et al. Consensus statement: Academy of Nutrition and Dietetics and American Society for Parenteral and Enteral Nutrition: characteristics recommended for the identification and documentation of adult malnutrition (undernutrition). JPEN J Parenter Enteral Nutr. 2012;36(3):275–83.

Woo, J., Yu, R., Wong, M., Yeung, F., Wong, M., & Lum, C. (2015). Frailty Screening in the Community Using the FRAIL Scale. *Journal of the American Medical Directors Association, 16*(5), 412–419.

Chapter 8
Health Issues and Services for Women in Old Age

Jasbir Kaur

Abstract Older women are usually seen engaged in social and economic roles responsibilities that are most frequently governed by their family or society. There are specific issues concerning uniquely older women in context of gender influences, health risks and health outcomes. Further, it also undermines their access to health care system and response of the health system catering to their needs. Ageing is an evolving process that occurs differently among various individuals or societal groups. It is often evident that socially and economically privileged remain free from health concerns till their 70s and 80s. But in contrast poor and disadvantaged women start showing ageing changes as early as even in their forties. Ageing can also be seen on a continuum, where on one extreme there are women who are socially and economically independent and living active ageing to those who are completely dependent on their family or society for their survival needs. This chapter illustrates health issues and concerns of the old women and also suggest an age responsive framework for action.

Introduction

> "Old age is not a disease-it is strength and survivorship, triumph over all kinds of vicissitudes and disappointments, trials and illnesses."
>
> Maggie Kuhn.

India, the largest democracy in the world and second most populous country is now also emerging as the 6th largest economy in the world. In terms of the population, India harbours 16% of the world's population. There are varying rates of Literacy, employment, health and morbidity among different regions. Quality of life at any age is also strikingly different in urban and rural counterparts (Prakash, 1999).

At the time of independence, life expectancy was only 32 years, since then there is a gradual improvement in public health and medical services. Further, this has led to significant control of specific infectious diseases and hence decline in

J. Kaur (✉)
MM College of Nursing, Solan, Himachal Pradesh, India

M. K. Shankardass (ed.), *Gerontological Concerns and Responses in India*,
https://doi.org/10.1007/978-981-16-4764-2_8

mortality rates. By 1990, life expectancy at birth reached 60 years. There was reduction in infant mortality too due to improved sanitation, increased attention towards maternal health and better child care facilities. Demographic projections reveal that in upcoming years, the shape of the population pyramid will gradually change from a wide base/narrow top to a barrel-shaped form.

Most often, age above 60 Years is regarded as 'old age' and people are called with the nomenclature as 'senior citizens. Ancient culture of India documents total human life span as hundred years. Dharmasastra, written by Manu, the ancient law giver, has divided the human life span into four 'ashramas' of life stages, brahmacarya', 'grihsta' 'vanaprastha' and 'samnyasa' or asceticism. The last two stages present a mature and ageing man who would gradually give up his worldly pursuits, move away from the mundane routine of the householder and turn inward in search of spiritual growth. Through this scheme of a man's life did not have any mention of a women's life, it was assumed that a wife would follow her husband faithfully in his move through different stages. In the societal context, old age is connotated with marriage of one's children irrespective of the person's chronological age and for women menopause and arrival of grandchildren is seen as transition from adulthood to elder.

Currently, age 58 is fixed as retirement age for most of the government officials in our country. Usually, ageing is correlated on the continuum of chronological age with a cut off age of 60 or 65 years. This definition is partly due to the fact that retirement age is also similar to this cut off age. But, chronological age has got little significance in many developing countries including India as elderly people in these countries continue to work in informal sector as no specific age of retirement is fixed for such instances. Therefore, under such circumstances, socially constructed meaning of age is more relevant as the new roles are assigned or loss of certain roles is primarily determined by physical decline with old age.

India has around 104 million elderly persons (8.6%, Census, 2011) and this number is expected to increase to 296.6 million making 19% of the total population by 2050, as depicted in Fig. 8.1 (United Nations, 2017). By the end of the century, the elderly will constitute nearly 35% of the total population in the country. The data also suggest that a significant proportion of elderly live in rural areas with large number of old-oldest age and well documented phenomenon of feminization of ageing. The increasing trend of population of elderly women in upper age groups is also quite evident. At the age of 65, 70, 75 & 80 there are 1310, 1590, 1758 & 1980 elderly women respectively per 1000 elderly men (Fig. 8.2). The sex ratio of the elderly has increased from 938 women to 1000 men in 1971 to 1033 in 2011 and is projected to increase to 1060 by 2026. With feminization of ageing, there are other related consequences as discrimination and neglect, often exacerbated by widowhood and complete dependence on others. Loss of spouse in old age adds significant vulnerability in later years. The data also suggest that three out of five single older women are very poor and about two-thirds of them are completely economically dependent upon their families.

The issues concerning women didn't get much attention earlier, but now due to increased life expectancy, feminization in ageing, their issues can't be neglected. It is

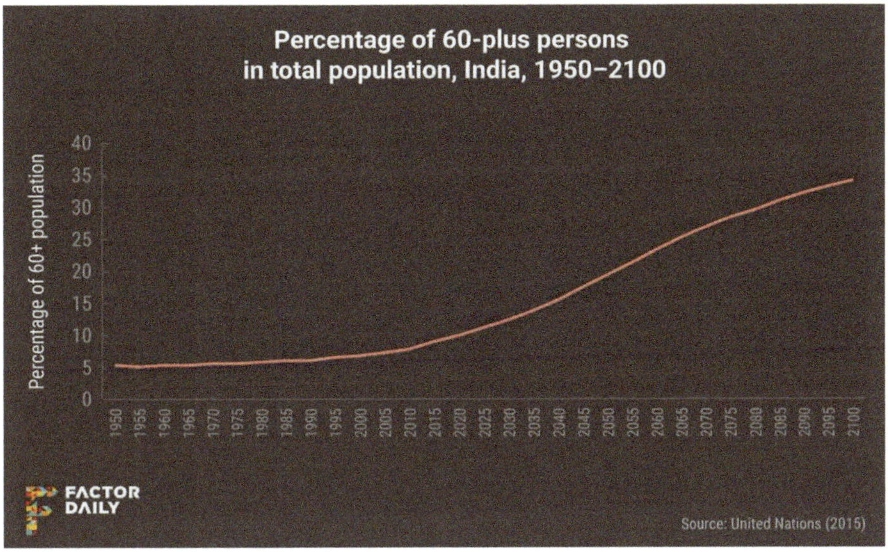

Fig. 8.1 Percentage of elderly (60 and above) persons in total population, India, 1950–2100. *Source* United Nations (2015)

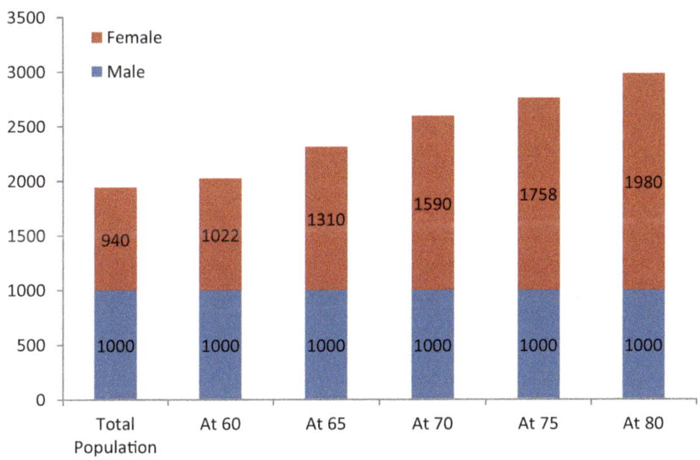

Fig. 8.2 Male female ratio: total population and above 60 years in India. *Source* Agewell Research & Advocacy Centre analysis based on census of India's data

an appropriate time and context to discuss issues related to old women to effectively overcome major social and developmental challenges.

Major Concerns of Old Women

Age well foundation has delineated following major concerns of old women in India.

Destitution/Alienation/Isolation: As our overall socio-economic environment is changing very rapidly, life style has turned fast paced and so called modern where young ones in the family hardly get time to interact with their elderly members of the family. Further with popularity of nuclear family structure, intergenerational bond has weakened. Grandchildren are not able to cherish the love and warmth of their grandparents. Therefore, elderly are left on their own and feel isolated.

Social insecurity: Due to rapid urbanization and dissolution of joint family structures, older women who live in cities have became more vulnerable to alienation/marginalization as compared to rural older women. Further, lack of any social security adds to their distress. As they remain neglected by their own family, they don't expect any kind of social security from others.

Financial Insecurity: As the life expectancy of women has increased, so are their financial needs. Even, if they have property or money, they are not allowed to take decision about utilizing these assets. Societal rules and traditions don't allow them to make use of their ancestral property or money for their own welfare. They remain financially dependent upon others for their day to day needs.

Medical Problems: Older women often suffer from acute problems due to negligence, lack of awareness, financial support and religious mindset of women. As they are bound to live within four walls of their house, very rarely they will come to open places, their health problems remain unnoticed. Their family usually ignore their health problems believing these as a consequence of old age. Under such circumstances, they are not able to ventilate their health concerns. Symptoms of disease are often ignored due to lack of health awareness leading to delayed diagnosis and inappropriate treatment.

Health Concerns of Old Woman

Salagre (2013) has conceptualized the term Geriatric Syndrome, which depicts physiological decline brought by ageing (Fig. 8.3). After infants and children, old people are most vulnerable to morbidity and mortality as health. While the debilitating effects of old age cannot be avoided, risks can be minimized through careful planning and prevention beginning from middle age (Patwardhan, 2003). Advances in medical technology over the past years have promoted longevity but not good health. Advancing age add to their vulnerability and prolongation of life is not sufficient unless the extended period of life is made liveable.

The illness pattern of the old is quite different from that of the young and so the basic philosophical approach and mode of treatment to the illness of the old also need to be different. The National opinion Research Centre defined illness as "any condition, i.e. any disease, impairment, symptom or a group of related symptom,

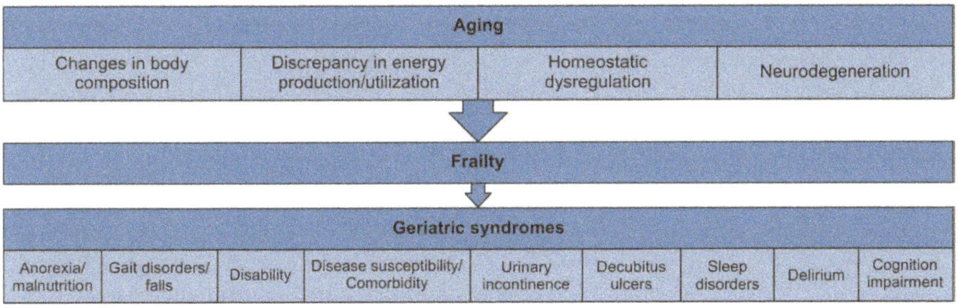

Fig. 8.3 Pathophysiology of health issues in geriatrics

which was reported by the aged as having bothered them" (Soodan, 1975). The aged have different health problems. Generally, they have complaints towards muscular, pain, eye and hearing impairment and respiratory problem. Some major diseases like blood pressure, arthritis, asthma are seen to be more pronounced during old age. The National Sample Survey data shows that 7.4% in rural and 7.9% in urban areas were suffering from one of the other chronic diseases (Chaturbhuj, 1998).

A variety of data on health problems of elderly is available. In 1996, there were nearly nine million hypertensives among the elderly population. Urban elderly had three times more prevalence of coronary heart disease as compared to their rural counterparts. (Shah and Prabhakar, 1997). An estimated five million were diabetic and the prevalence rates were about 177 for urban and 35 per 1000 for rural elderly people. Crude prevalence rate of strokes is estimated to be about 200 per 100,000 persons. Older persons surviving through peak years of stroke (55–65 years) with varying degrees of disability are already a major medical Problem (Dalal, 1997).

Geriatric medicines have made rapid strides in the west but the concept is hardly popular even among professionals in India. There are many similarities in western and Indian societies regarding old age diseases though not on the causes of death. It is widely known that old patients suffer from multiple pathologies. Ramachandran and Radhika (2006) in their comparative study on elderly women in India and Japan found that elderly women in India face different types of health-related issues due to various socio-economic factors. Lack of health awareness among the elderly and financial constraints are the major contributory factors for the poor health of the elderly in India.

The health profile of elderly women is more compromised as compared to elderly males. The differences could lie in biological, social and cultural factors. Various studies based on primary and secondary data have analysed various health and health-related issues faced by elderly people especially elderly women. Singh and Yesudian (2007) in their analysis using NSSO 2004 and Census 2001 suggest that the physical mobility is high among elderly men than elderly women in both urban and rural areas. The health condition and physical mobility are poorer for urban elderly women than rural elderly women. Rural elderly women perceive that they are in poor health condition than their urban counterparts.

Hiremath (2012) studied the health status of elderly women in rural Karnataka. The findings revealed that nearly three fourth of the elderly suffer from Hypertension (78.65%), Osteoarthritis (73.03%), Diabetes (66.29%) and Bronchial Asthma (77.52%). Other health problems included Cataracts (65.16%), Anemia and Skin problems (61.79%). The findings also revealed that most of the elderly women suffered from more than one health problem. The author concluded that the older women as they age, often reflect the cumulative impact of poor diets, lack of good food and safe drinking water, a gender-based division of domestic tasks; environmental hazards, etc.

In another study on elderly by Audinarayana et al. (2002) in Tamil Nadu, reported marked gender-wise differentials in health status of the elderly. Chronic morbidity due to poor vision, cataract, blood pressure, back pain/slipped disc was significantly higher among women as compared to elderly men. Similarly perceived health status of elderly men was significantly better ($p < 0.001$) 'healthy' than those of elderly women.

Lena et al. (2009) in their study on health and social problems of the elderly in Karnataka depicted that 60.3% of the elderly women were hypertensive, 57.9% had osteoarthritis, more pronounced as compared to men. More than half, 55.8% of the women felt that they are burden on their family, unhappiness with their life was also reported by more of the women as compared to elderly men. Women also had poor perceptions regarding economic and social security as compared to men.

Kaur et al. (2004) in their study on physique of rural and urban Jat Sikh women studied the change in weight with ageing. The study findings revealed that there was a decrease in mean weight of Jat Sikh women from 66.94 kg at age 61–65 years to 49.68 kg at 81+ years. Another interesting finding of the study was in relation to change in weight as depicted by comparison with another study conducted by Singal and Sidhu (1981). The results depicted that mean weight has increased significantly in all age groups as mean weight of Jat Sikh women was 51.37 kg in 1981 and 66.94 kg in 2004. The results conclude that such an increase in weight due to rapid change in life style increases their vulnerability to chronic diseases.

In a study on 150 aged widows in rural areas of Hissar district, Haryana, Sushma and Darshan (2004) noticed that most of them were suffering from multiple ailments. Around 45% widows had asthma, 90% had general weakness, problems of eyesight, teeth and forgetfulness, 31% had mental anxiety, 21% reported to have heart diseases and various other chronic illnesses. The findings also reveal that only three- fourth cases consulted a physician for serious conditions, 16% always consulted the doctor while others never consulted a doctor.

Functional impairments like malnutrition, depression, impaired physical performance and urinary incontinence were documented to be present more significantly among female elderly as compared to their male counterparts (Shan etal., 2003). Marital status and economic dependence play a significant role in determining morbidity among elderly women (Dilip, 2003). The authors concluded that with increasing age, diseases are more likely to increase with widowhood, divorce and economic dependence. Similarly, in another study of elderly rural females in Rajasthan, Sharma (2003) found that widowhood, economic dependency, lack of proper food and clothing, fear of the future, lack of caring and progressive decline in health made coping with health problems difficult. Elderly widows from poor socio-economic families had very poor health status. Adequate financial status, good physical and mental health, active participation in leisure activities, continuation of hobbies, maintenance of daily schedule, retaining social networks and assuming social roles influenced healthy ageing positively.

Joshi, Kumar and Avasthi (2003) studied morbidity profile and its relationship with disability and psychological distress among elderly people in Northern India. The findings of the study reveal that was more (94.1%) as compared to 81.3% of the males. Similar trend was noticed in both rural and urban areas. The physician diagnosed morbidities (7–9 in number) were observed among 26.4% of the women. The most common observed morbidities among women were Anaemia, Dental problems, Hypertension, Cataracts and Osteoarthritis. Psychological distress was reported by 66.6% of the urban and 82.3% of the rural women. Fractures after falls were also reported more frequently among females (26.4%) compared with males (16%).

In a study to elicit morbidity and health care utilization by elderly women in an urban slum in Chennai, Balagopal (2009) revealed that 40.5% of ailments of the elderly women were medically untreated. The most important reasons for not seeking care were financial problems, the perception of ailments as not serious. This information is indicative of inaccessible health care which increases financial burden on elderly women and absence of social security and health insurance. The author concludes social policy of developing countries like India underplays the health care requirements of elderly women.

Mental health of the elderly is another important area in understanding their overall health situation. Sharma (2009) in his study on mental health issues of elderly depicted that elderly women are affected more frequently by dementia, depression and psychosomatic disorders than the male elderly.

Kaur et al. (2004) studied psychosocial stresses in Rural and Urban Jat Sikh Women with special reference to senescence. The researchers revealed that the stress score of rural married women was more than urban. The stress score of whole life was the highest for rural widows.

Roy and Chaudhari (2008) reported influence of socio-economic status, wealth and financial empowerment on gender differences in health and health care utilization in later life among nationally representative 34,086 older men and women. The results indicated that older women report worse self-rated health, higher prevalence of disabilities, marginally lower chronic conditions and lower health care utilization than men. Further statistical analysis revealed that by controlling for economic independence, gender differentials disappear or are reversed, with older women having equal or better health than otherwise similar to men. The study findings conclude that financial empowerment might confer older women the health advantage reflected in developed societies by enhancing a woman's ability to undertake primary and secondary prevention during the life course.

Rastogi et al. (2014) carried out a cross-sectional study on major health problems of the geriatric in Ahmadabad. The study findings revealed that among females memory disturbance (42.8%) and depression (28.6%) is more as compared to males.

Beyond physical, mental and social problems unique to elderly women, another challenge in today's scenario is elder abuse. Here, also vulnerability of women is more owing to significant financial, social dependency of women upon their families. Chokkanathan and Lee (2006) examined the extent and correlates of elder mistreatment among 400 community dwelling older adults in Chennai. Mistreatment was reported by 14% of the elderly. Most frequent form of mistreatment was chronic verbal abuse followed by financial abuse and the rate of physical abuse and neglect was similar. Half of the elderly reported more than one type of mistreatment (multifaceted-mistreatment). With the exception of financial abuse, verbal and physical abuse, as well as neglect, was significantly higher among women as compared to men. Adult children, daughters-in-law, spouses and sons-in-law were the prominent perpetrators. Depression and lesser satisfaction with life were reported more frequently by mistreated older adults as compared to not mistreated. Gender, social support and subjective rating of physical health were reported as significant factors associated with abuse on logistic regression.

Another unique problem faced by elderly women is related to their sexual health which is considered taboo in many cultures. The research has brought to light several serious problems. For example, older women are at increased risk of being victims of sexual violence because of their socio-economic dependency and, in some settings, because of gender-based inequities. It is quite evident that sexual harassment and violence often take place within the home. Women who become dependent on their families, especially widows, are particularly vulnerable to these forms of abuse. Sexual abuse among older people not only put them at greater risk of exposure to STIs; they are also physiologically more vulnerable to these infections, as there are marked changes to the lining of the vagina among post-menopausal, which further reduces innate protective mechanisms against infection. There is also a gradual decline in immune function with advancing age. Older women who already suffer from chronic or acute pelvic infections have increased vulnerability to additional infectious diseases.

It is clear from the above review of above studies regarding multifaceted issues faced by elderly in general and elderly women in particular. Health and well-being of the elderly are affected by many closely knit aspects of their social and physical environment. Although, the socio-economic and health needs of the elderly are huge and manyfold but, the financial resources, policies and programmatic capacity available to meet these needs are highly scarce and challenging.

Services for Older Women in India

In view of the multifaceted problems experienced by elderly women, very little attention has been paid in India towards developing a model of health and social care for elderly, which is in tune with the changing need and times of society. The developed countries have evolved many models for elderly care, e.g., nursing home care, health insurance, etc. In our country, the major focus regarding implementation of health policies and programmes has remained on control of population, reproductive health and disease prevention. But the increasing number of elderly people in our country has added another dimension to existing health care services. Trends in ageing like demographic transition and feminization of ageing have brought along a new range of medical, social and economic problems which require a timely intervention by our programme managers and policy makers.

There are no separate programmes for elder women in India. The policies and programmes for the welfare of elderly are neither exclusively for elderly men nor for elderly women. Their discretions and directions are common to both sexes. The privileges and services for elderly in general are being discussed here:

Article 41 of the Constitution: Article 41 of Directive Principles of State Policy has particular relevance to Old Age Social Security. According to Article 41 of the constitution of India, "the state shall, within the limits of its economic capacity and development, make effective provision for securing the right to work, to education and to public assistance in cases of unemployment, old age, sickness and disablement and in other cases of undeserved want."

Article 47 of the Constitution: Article 47 of the constitution of India provides that the state shall regard the raising of the level of nutrition and the standard of living of its people and improvement of public health as among its primary duties.

Maintenance and Welfare of Parents and Senior Citizens Act, 2007 The Maintenance and Welfare of Parents and Senior Citizens Act, 2007 was enacted in December 2007, to ensure need based maintenance for parents and senior citizens and their welfare. Section 19 of the Maintenance and Welfare of Parents and Senior Citizens Act, 2007 envisages provision of at least one old age home for indigent senior citizens with a capacity of 150 persons in every district of the country. The objectives of the Act are:

- Revocation of transfer of property by senior citizens in case of negligence by relatives.
- Maintenance of Parents/senior citizens by children/ relatives made obligatory and justifiable through Tribunals.
- Pension provision for abandoned senior citizens.
- Adequate medical facilities and security for senior citizens.
- Establishment of Old Age Homes for indigent Senior Citizens.

The Act was enacted on 31st December 2007. It accords prime responsibility for the maintenance of parents on their children, grandchildren or even relatives who may possibly inherit the property of a senior citizen. It also calls upon the state to provide facilities for poor and destitute older persons. The Act has to be brought into force by individual State Government. Himachal Pradesh is the first state and Punjab is the fifth state where old parents can legally stake claim to financial aid from their grown-up children for their survival and denial would invite a prison term. As on 3 February 2010, the Act had been notified by 22 states and all UTs.

The National Policy for Older People (NPOP) 1999 announced by the government of India in 1999 acknowledges the problems faced by elderly and also addresses the concerns of older women in India. It states that there is need for developing and elaborating social and community services for older persons, especially for women. It also emphasizes increasing accessibility and use of welfare services by removing socio-cultural, economic and physical barriers and making the services client oriented and user friendly.

National Policy on Senior Citizens 2011 This revised policy document advocates issues related to senior citizens living in urban and rural areas, special needs of the 'oldest old' and older women. It will endeavour to strengthen integration between generations, facilitate interaction between the old and the young as well as strengthen bonds between different age groups. It believes in the development of a formal and informal social support system so that the capacity of the family to take care of senior citizens is strengthened and they continue to live in the family. The policy seeks to reach out in particular to the bulk of senior citizens living in rural areas who are dependent on family bonds and intergenerational understanding and support.

The focus of the new policy:

- Promote the concept of 'Ageing in Place' or ageing in own home, housing, income security and homecare services, old age pension and access to health care insurance schemes and other programmes and services to facilitate and sustain dignity in old age. The thrust of the policy would be preventive rather than cure.
- Mainstream senior citizens, especially older women and bring their concerns into the national development debate with priority to implement mechanisms already set by governments and supported by civil society and senior citizens' associations. Support promotion and establishment of senior citizens' association, especially among women.
- The policy will consider institutional care as the last resort. It recognizes that care of senior citizens institutional care as the last resort. It recognizes that care of senior citizens has to remain vested in the family which would partner the community, government and the private sector.
- long-term savings instruments and credit activities will be promoted to reach both rural and urban areas.
- Recognize the senior citizens are a valuable resource for the country and create an environment that provides them with equal opportunities, protects their rights and enables their full participation in society.
- Employment in income generating activities after superannuation will be encouraged.
- States will be advised to implement the Maintenance and Welfare of Parents and Senior Citizens Act, 2007 and set up Tribunals so that elderly parents unable to maintain themselves are not abandoned and neglected.
- Support and assist organizations that provide counselling, career guidance and training services.
- States will set up homes with assisted living facilities for abandoned senior citizens in every district of the country and there will be adequate budgetary support.

National Council for Older Persons (NCOP) A National Council for Older Persons (NCOP) was constituted in 1999 under the chairpersonship of the Ministry of Social Justice and Empowerment to operationalize the National Policy on Older

Persons. The NCOP is the highest body to advise the Government in the formulation and implementation of policy and programmes for the elderly. The basic objectives of this council are to:

- Advise the Government on policies and programmes for older persons.
- Represent the collective opinion of elderly persons to the government.
- Suggest steps to make old age productive and interesting.
- Provide feedback to the government on the implementation of the NPOP as well as on specific programme initiatives for elderly.
- Suggest measures to enhance the quality of intergenerational relationships.
- Provide a nodal point at the national level for redressing the grievances of older persons who are of an individual nature provide lobby for concessions, rebates and discounts for older persons both with the Government as well as with the corporate sector.
- Work as a nodal point at the national level for redressing the grievances of elderly people.
- Undertake any other work or activity in the best interest of elderly people.

The council was re-constituted in 2005 and met at least once every year. At present, there are 50 members in it, comprising representatives of Central and State Governments, NGO's, citizens' groups, retired persons' associations and experts in the fields of law, social welfare and medicine.

Central Sector Scheme of Integrated Programme for Older Persons (IPOP) An integrated Programme for Older Persons (IPOP) is being implemented since 1992 with the objective of improving the quality of life of senior citizens by providing basic amenities like food, shelter, medical care and entertainment opportunities and by encouraging productive and active ageing. Under this scheme financial assistance up to 90% of the project cost is provided to Non-Governmental Organizations for running and maintenance of old age homes, day 226 care centres and mobile medicine units. The scheme has been made flexible so as to meet the diverse needs of the older persons including reinforcement and strengthening of the family, awareness generation on issues pertaining to older persons, popularization of the concept of lifelong preparation for old age, etc. Several innovative projects have also been added which are as follows:

- Maintenance of respite care homes and continuous care homes.
- Sensitizing programmes for children particularly in schools and colleges.
- Regional resource and training centres for caregivers of elderly persons.
- Volunteer Bureau for elderly persons o Formation of associations for elderly.
- Helplines and counselling centres for older persons.
- Awareness Generation Programmes for elderly people and caregivers.
- Running of day care centres for patients of Alzheimer's Disease/Dementia and physiotherapy clinics for elderly people.
- Providing disability and hearing aids for the elderly people.

The scheme has been revised in April 2008. Besides a 227 increase in amount of financial assistance for existing projects, Governments/Panchayati Raj institutions/local bodies have been made eligible for getting financial assistance.

Inter-Ministerial Committee on Older Persons An Inter-Ministerial Committee on Older Persons comprising twenty-two Ministries/Departments and headed by the secretary, Ministry of Social Justice and Empowerment is another coordination mechanism in implementation of the NPOP. Action Plan on ageing issues for implementation by various Ministries/Departments concerned is considered from time to time by the committee.

National Old Age Pension (NOAP) Scheme Under NOAP Scheme, in 1994 Central Assistance was made available. The amount of old age pension varies in the different States as per their share to this scheme. It is implemented in the State and Union Territories through Panchayats and Municipalities. The assistance was available on fulfilment of the following criteria:

- 65 years or more should be the age of the applicant (male or female)
- The applicants have no regular means of subsistence from their own source of income or through financial support from family members or others.

The Ministry is now implementing the Indira Gandhi National Old Age Pension Scheme (IGNOAPS). Under this scheme, Central assistance in form of Pension is given to persons, above 65 years @ Rs. 200/- per month, belonging to a below poverty line family. This pension amount is meant to be supplemented by at least same contribution by the States so that each applicant gets at least Rs. 400/- per month as pension. The number of beneficiaries receiving central assistance, in the form of pension, was 171 lakh as of 31st March 2011.

Further, the Ministry has lowered the age limit from the existing 65 years to 60 years and the pension amount for elderly of 80 years and above has also been increased from Rs. 200/- to Rs. 500/- per month with effect from 1 April 2011.

According to 2008 UNDP study, there are 65% of widows in India are over 60 years old. Of these, only 28% are eligible for pension. However, only 11% annually receive it (Basu, 2010).

National Programme for the health care of Elderly (NPCHE): This programme was launched by Directorate General of Health Services with the vision of: (1) To provide accessible, affordable and high-quality long term, comprehensive and dedicated care services to an ageing population; (2) Creating a new "architecture" for Ageing; (3) To build a framework to create an enabling environment for "a Society for all Ages;" (4) To promote the concept of Active and Healthy Ageing. The programme envisages to operate with the following strategies.

- Community-based PHC approach including domiciliary visits by trained health care workers.
- Dedicated services at PHC/Community Health Centre (CHC) level including provision of machinery, equipment, training, additional human resources, Information, Education and Communication (IEC), etc.

- Dedicated facilities at the district hospital with 10 bedded wards, additional human resources, machinery and equipment, consumables and drugs, training and IEC.
- Strengthening of 8 Regional Medical Institutes to provide dedicated tertiary level medical facilities for the elderly, introducing PG courses in geriatric medicine and in-service training of health personnel at all levels.
- IEC using mass media, folk media and other communication channels to reach out to the target community.
- Continuous monitoring and independent evaluation of the Programme and research in geriatrics and implementation of NPHCE.
- Promotion of public private partnerships in geriatric health care.
- Mainstreaming Ayush – revitalizing local health traditions and convergence with programmes of Ministry of Social Justice and Empowerment in the field of geriatrics.
- Reorienting medical education to support geriatric issues.

In the programme, it is envisaged providing promotional, preventive, curative and rehabilitative services in an integrated manner for the Elderly in various Government health facilities (Fig. 8.4). The package of services would depend on the level of health facility and may vary from facility to facility. The range of services will include health promotion, preventive services, diagnosis and management of geriatric medical problems (out- and in-patient), day care services, rehabilitative services and home based care as needed. Districts will be linked to RGCs for providing tertiary level care. The services under the programme would be integrated below district level and will be an integral part of existing PHC delivery system and vertical at district and above as more specialized health care is needed for the elderly.

International Day of Older Persons The International Day of Older Persons is celebrated every year on 1st October 2009. On 1 October 2009, the Hon'ble Minister of Social Justice and Empowerment flagged off "Walkathon" at Rajpath, India Gate, to promote intergenerational bonding. More than 3000 senior citizens/elderly people from across Delhi, NGOs working in the field of elderly issues and school children from different schools participated in this.

Role of Non-Governmental and voluntary organizations: Presently there are many non-governmental organizations working for the cause of the elderly in India. In India, most non-governmental organizations have concentrated their work among the lower income group and the disadvantaged sections of the society. This is mainly because one third of these people are defined as "capability poor" which means that they do not have access to minimum levels of health care and education for earning a decent living. However, in the first few years of the growth of the NGO's the emphasis was on the abuse of women due to the gender discrimination prevalent in our Indian society. It is only in the last few years when the demographers provided alarming statistics on the growth of the elderly population that a need was felt to work in this area as it was always assumed that the elderly were well taken care of and were safe in the custody of the well integrated joint family system in India. Initial studies show that the elderly are taken care of by the family but the reality and recent ethnographic cases studies also prove that the so called "joint family system" in India is a myth

Health facility	Packages of services
At sub-center level	Health Education related to healthy ageing
	Domiciliary visits for attention and care to home bound/bedridden elderly persons and provide training to the family care providers in looking after the disabled elderly persons
	Arrange for suitable calipers and supportive devices from the PHC to the elderly disabled persons to make them ambulatory
	Linkage with other support groups and day care centers etc., operational in the area
Primary health center	Weekly geriatric clinic run by a trained Medical Officer
	Maintain a record of the elderly using the standard format during their first visit
	Conducting a routine health assessment of the elderly persons based on simple clinical examination relating to eye, blood pressure, blood sugar, etc.
	Provision of medicines and proper advice on chronic ailments
	Public awareness on promotional, preventive and rehabilitative aspects of geriatrics during health and village sanitation day/camps
	Referral for diseases needing further investigation and treatment, to CHC or the District Hospital as per need
CHC	First Referral Unit for the elderly from PHCs and below
	Geriatric clinic for the elderly persons twice a week
	Rehabilitation Unit for physiotherapy and counseling
	Domiciliary visits by the rehabilitation worker for bed ridden elderly and counseling of the family members on their home-based care
	Health promotion and prevention
	Referral of difficult cases to District Hospital/higher health-care facility
District hospital	Geriatric clinic for regular dedicated OPD services to the elderly
	Facilities for laboratory investigations for diagnosis and provision of medicines for geriatric medical and health problems
	10-bedded Geriatric Ward for in-patient care of the elderly
	Existing specialties like General Medicine; Orthopedics, Ophthalmology; ENT services etc., will provide services needed by elderly patients
	Provide services for the elderly patients referred by the CHCs/PHCs, etc.,
	Conducting camps for Geriatric Services in PHCs/CHCs and other sites
	Referral services for severe cases to tertiary level hospitals
RGC	Geriatric clinic (Specialized OPD for the elderly)
	30-bedded Geriatric Ward for in-patient care and dedicated beds for the elderly patients in the various specialties viz. Surgery, Orthopedics, Psychiatry, Urology, Ophthalmology and Neurology etc.
	Laboratory investigation required for elderly with a special sample collection center in the OPD block
	Tertiary health-care to the cases referred from medical colleges, district hospitals and below

PHC=Primary health-care, CHC= Community health center, OPD=Out-patient department, RGC=Regional geriatric centers, ENT=Ear, Nose and Throat

Fig. 8.4 Proposed package of services for elderly at different levels under NPCHE

and the elderly though they live with their sons and their families are neglected and uncared for by them. This scenario led to the emergence and mushrooming of various NGO's working towards the concerns of the elderly.

In recent years several national level and state level voluntary organizations have been set up for promoting the welfare of the elderly, for advocating a general national priority to their problems and needs and for organizing services. The Government describes the services they are providing as residential care, day care, geriatric care, medical and psychiatric care, recreation, financial assistance and counselling. These services are however primarily urban based.

One of the premier voluntary organizations which began work on the cause and care of the older people of our country is Help Age India. It is a secular, non political, non profit, non-governmental organization and is registered under the Societies' Registration Act, 1960, in 1978. Help Age India was formed in 1978 with the active help from Mr. Cecil Jackson Cole, founder member of help the Aged, United Kingdom. In its newsletters and brochures, one can clearly see it has charted out its goals and objectives which are "To create an awareness and understanding of the changing situation and the needs of the elderly in India and to promote the cause of the elderly. To raise the funds for creation of infrastructure through the medium of voluntary social service organizations for providing a range of facilities specially designed to benefit the elderly and thus to improve the quality of their lives." Help Age India is basically a funding organization that looks for partner agencies in the field that are able to implement the various projects and programmes of the organization. The head office of Help Age India is located in New Delhi and it has around twenty-four regional and area offices located all over the country.

Old Age Homes and Day Care Centres: Help Age India has sponsored the construction and maintenance of old age homes in India. These homes cater to the needs of those elderly who are unable to live by themselves and for those who have been abandoned by the family or are neglected and uncapped for by their children. These old age homes provide and cater to the various needs of the elderly so that they can spend the "evenings of their lives" with dignity and respect and not feel a burden to society. There are over 800 old age homes all over India and nearly half of them are being sponsored and funded by Help Age India. Besides old age homes, Help Age India also supports day care centres where the elderly come for a few hours every day or on certain days of the week and spend some time together. These centres combat the loneliness they face and create a sense of "we feeling" among them. In some of the centres being supported by Help Age India in rural areas, they are also places where income generating activities are conducted.

Schemes of Other Ministries

Ministry of Railways

The Ministry of Railways provided the following facilities to senior citizens (elderly).

- Separate ticket counters for the elderly people at various Passenger Reservation System Centres.
- Provision of Lower Berth Quota – provide in AC and Sleeper Classes.
- Provision of 30% discount in all Mails/Express.
- Provision of wheel chairs at stations for the disabled elderly passengers.
- Railway grants 75% concession to Senior Citizens undergoing major heart/cancer operations from starting station to Hospital station for self and one companion.

Ministry of Health and Family Welfare

Central Government Health Scheme provides pensioners of central government offices the facility to obtain medicines for chronic ailments up to three months at a stretch. Ministry of Health and Family Welfare provides the following facilities for the elderly people:

- Provision of separate queues for elderly people in governmental hospitals.
- Set up of two National Institutes on Ageing at Delhi and Chennai.
- Provision of Geriatric clinic in several government hospitals.

Ministry of Finance:

Some of the facilities for senior citizens provided by the Ministry of Finance are:

- Exemption from Income Tax for senior citizens of 60 years and above up to Rs. 2.50 lakh per annum.
- Exemption from Income Tax for senior citizens of 80 years and above up to Rs. 5.00 lakh per annum.
- For an individual who pays medical insurance premium for his/her parents or parents who are elderly or senior citizens, deduction of Rs. 20,000 under Section 80D is allowed.
- An individual is eligible for a deduction of the amount spent or Rs. 60,000, whichever is less for medical treatment of a dependent elderly or senior citizen.

Insurance Regulatory Development Authority (IRDA):

Insurance Regulatory Development Authority (IRDA) vide letter dated 25 May 2009 issued some instructions on health insurance for elderly or senior citizens to CEOs of all General Health Insurance Companies which inter-alia includes:

- Allowing entry into health insurance scheme till 65 years of age
- Provision of transparency in the premium charged.
- Reasons to be recorded for denial of any proposals on all health insurance products catering to the needs of senior citizens.

Ministry of Civil Aviation

Under the Ministry of Civil Aviation, the National Carrier, Air India provides concession in air fare up to 50% for male passengers aged 65 years and above and female passengers aged 63 years and above on production of proof of age and nationality on the date of commencement of journey.

Ministry of Road Transport

The Ministry of Road Transport and Highways has provided reservation of two seats for elderly or senior citizens in front row of the buses of the State Road Transport Undertakings. Some States Governments are providing fare concession to senior citizens in the State Road Transport Undertaking buses for, e.g. in Punjab Elderly women above 60 years enjoy free travel, Free passes are provided to old people who are freedom fighters to travel in fast and express buses in Kerala. Some State Governments also introducing Bus models according to the convenience of the elderly.

Medical Insurance Scheme

The Medical Insurance Scheme known or Mediclaim is available to persons between the age of 5 years and 75 years. Earlier, premium for medical insurance varied from Rs 175 to Rs 5770 per person per annum and the sum insured ranged from Rs 15,000 to Rs 300,000 depending upon the different slabs of sum insured and different age groups. However, with effect from 1 November 1999, these limits of benefits and the premium rates have since been revised. Now, the premium varies from Rs 201 to Rs 16,185 per person per annum and sum insured varies from Rs 15,000 to Rs 500,000 depending upon different slabs of sum insured and different age groups. The policy is now made available to persons between the age of 5 years and 80 years. The cover provides for reimbursement of medical expenses incurred by an individual towards hospitalization/ domiciliary, hospitalization for any illness, injury or disease contracted or sustained during the period of insurance.

However, these social policies do not recognize the social, emotional and health care requirements of older women. Older women in India are often left-out unattended not only in their own homes but also in policy making decisions.

Few Success Stories in the Area of Old Women Welfare

UNFPA and Stree Shakti in their collaboration prepared a document named "Innovative Practices for Care of Elderly Women in India". The aim behind this initiative was to promote the rights of ageing women and showcase effective models that are dedicated to restoring their dignity. Further, it has been said that all the case studies are extraordinary in terms of their approach, outreach and sustainability. These case studies also suggest the potential replicable work in welfare of elderly women.

Sulabh International's work In 2012, Sulabh International initiated the project with the widows of Vrindavan, which has now spread to Varanasi and Deoli, Uttarakhand. Vrindavan has been known to harbour a large number of aged women. These are mostly widows, abandoned by their families, living in poor conditions at ashrams with no health care or sustainable income. They were living in a very pitiful situation that their concerns were taken up by Supreme Court, which requested Sulabh International to plan an intervention in Vrindavan to improve their dreadful condition. Sulabh International made these widows economically independent by providing them with financial assistance. Further, they also made the provision for medical facilities like ambulances and cost of prescription drugs and treatment of ailments. The organization also worked towards their vocational training as well as language classes. A helpline for widows in need of assistance was also launched. The project covered approximately 800 widows across eight ashrays (homes). Because of this project, there is a marked difference in the lifestyle of these women. Now, they live independently, work on various vocational projects and are more aware of their rights. All these are signs of active ageing which Sulabh International has been able to bring about in the lives of these widows.

Ekal Nari Shakti Sangathan (ENSS) is an organization in tradition-bound and highly patriarchal state of Rajasthan for widows and other single women. The establishment of this organization was an attempt to address the social and economic isolation faced by widows in India. Another aim was to challenge the patriarchal system and helps organize women who are abandoned or rejected by their families and societies. Ekal Nari Shakti Sangathan was established in 1999 and currently has 43,006 members from both rural and urban areas of Rajasthan. The organization operates on the philosophy of 'collective power' i.e., if people unite and organize themselves, they can bring about reform in social customs and policies. They handle social problems of women at the community level and issues of entitlement directly with the administration. ENSS aims to help as many single/widowed women as possible to help them claim their rights and lead a dignified life in the community.

The International Longevity Centre-India (ILC-I) is an important voluntary organization in Pune working on issues of Ageing since 2003. ILC has started many projects with the aim of providing a healthy, productive and participatory life to the elderly, especially women. There are currently three projects—Aajibai Sathi Batwa, an innovative community-based project providing partial medical assistance through seeking sponsorship. 'Elders' Volunteers Bureau, a group of senior citizens working on a voluntary basis on various projects that give them financial independence which also helps in addressing loneliness; and Athashri Housing project which are residential complexes built exclusively for the aged. ILC's successful and innovative projects have provided a platform for other NGOs to replicate and enhance them at the national level.

The Calcutta Metropolitan Institute of Gerontology (CMIG), Kolkata was started in 1988 with the objective of promoting research in the field of gerontology and implementing the findings. Kolkata is home to one of the largest number of aged persons, mostly women living in poor conditions. Social security is almost non-existent in the state and very few programmes are initiated by the Government to support these women. Though a research institute, CMIG believes in turning its knowledge and values into actionable goals. It has initiated a wide range of programmes, ranging from day care centres to provision of livelihood and a holistic health care system by running mobile clinics in slum areas. CMIG's unique and successful approach has been recognized by the Ministry of West Bengal for its positive impact on the lives of the elderly in West Bengal.

Nightingales Medical Trust (NMT), Bangalore is one of the first recognized providers of quality "age care" and dementia services to persons suffering from Alzheimer's belonging to all socio-economic groups. In India, dementia is still viewed with ignorance and social stigma. Dementia puts more challenges for older women who are economically dependent on their families. To address this, NMT's innovative telemedicine enabled centre has enhanced the access of elderly persons to high-quality dementia care in a cost effective manner. Apart from that, the specially designed infrastructure and medical facilities at the Centre for Ageing & Alzheimer's provides comprehensive residential care for both short and long-term stays. As a result of its path-breaking work in the field of dementia, NMT has been recognized by Alzheimer's & Related Disorder Society of India (ARDSI) as the promoter of its Bangalore Chapter.

SEWA Bank, Gujarat provides financial support to aged women from lower economic sections of the society. SEWA Bank was conceived as a microfinance organization providing financial aid to women in the non-formal sector but very soon realized that it needed to reach out to elderly women. Hence the Life-Cycle Approach for financial inclusion of women was started, whereby women would be supported throughout their life beginning with household emergencies, children's education, improving their housing or income and preparing for old age. The SEWA Bank is a pioneer in microfinance, serving more than 350,000 women, providing savings, loans and access to insurance and pension products.

Old Age Homes: Focus on Mumbai is a study of four institutions from the city to showcase essential features of old age homes that make them examples of innovative practices. All the institutions studied here have shown good policies of health care, constant presence of caregivers and promotion of a support system among the aged that help them to become more self-sufficient. In addition, some of the institutions have also implemented innovative techniques like intergenerational programmes, involvement of community in care-giving, vocational training and age friendly infrastructure and environment that fosters positive integration of the older generation into these homes. These are important features that old age homes across the country can learn from and adapt to provide better quality of life to their residents.

HelpAge India's Vidarbha Project was implemented to reduce the financial burden on aged women who were victims of the epidemic of farmers' suicides in Maharashtra. In 2005, more than 70% of the farmers' suicides in Maharashtra occurred in the Vidarbha region. HelpAge India, with its primary intervention aimed at providing short-term credit loans to these widowed women, expanded its project to cover nine villages in the area. Beginning with Elder Self-Help Groups (ESHGs) for microfinance, various other interventions were introduced such as income generating training and activities, initiation of government schemes and health care through mobile medical camps. The ESHGs were able to reduce the debt burden on lonely widowed women, resulting in economic independence and sustainable livelihoods. The project was also able to reduce the number of farmer suicides in the area and led to the promotion of women's participation in small business activities, boosting their self-confidence and promoting women's empowerment.

State Initiatives of Kerala: There are few schemes for the aged which are state driven and specific to Kerala. Most states in India are just able to implement programmes run by the Central government on age care, Kerala has gone a step further by taking up the issue of old age, especially older women who are in need of special attention and care. Kerala has been the frontrunner in not only coming out with a State Old Age Policy (2013), it has also amended the Kerala Maintenance and Welfare of Parents and Senior Citizens Act (2007). Schemes for the aged implemented by the state, are innovative, replicable and have had a tremendous impact on the life of the elderly.

Conclusion

These good practices are just a drop in an ocean of despair. They stand as examples for government and NGO's to initiate endeavours that are more sustainable and reach all especially underprivileged women.

It is quite evident from above stated discussion that problems of older women are multifaceted and it requires a consistent effort not only from policy makers but it has to begin right from their home. Existing social policies and programmes should recognize the social, emotional and health care requirements of older women and plan these by keeping gender sensitivity in their mind.

Ultimately India will win if it cares for its women and mothers.

References

About us. Retrieved from https://www.helpageindia.org

Article 41 in the Constitution of India (1949). Retrieved from https://indiankanoon.org/doc/1975922/

Article 41 in the Constitution of India (1949). Retrieved from https://indiankanoon.org/doc/1551554/

Audinarayana, N., Sheela, J., & Kavitha, N. (2002). *Are the elderly women the most deprived among the deprived? A micro level investigation in rural Tamilnadu in aging: Indian perspectives* (L. Tharabhai, Ed., pp. 247–262). Decent Books.

Balagopal, G. (2009). Access to health care among poor elderly women in India: How far do policies respond to women's realities? *Gender & Development, 17*(3), 481–491.

Central Sector Scheme of Integrated Programme for Older Persons (IPOP). Retrieved from http://www.socialjustice.nic.in/SchemeList

Chaturbhuj, S. (1998). *Problems of ageing among the Indian Tribes*. Surup & Sons.
Chokkanathan, S., & Lee, A. E. (2006). Elder mistreatment in urban India: A community based study. *Journal of Elder Abuse & Neglect, 17*(2), 45–61.
Dalal, P. M. (1997). Strokes in the elderly: Prevalence, risk factors and the strategies for prevention. *Indian Journal o f Medical Research, 106*, 332–352.
Dilip, T. R. (2003). *The burden of ill health among older in Kerala: Man in India*, 83.
Elderly population in India and welfare measures for them. Retrieved from https://www.indianeconomy.net/splclassroom/elderly-population-in-india-and-welfare-measures-for-them/
Hiremath, S. S. (2012). Health status of rural elderly women in India: A case study. *International Journal of Criminology and Sociological Theory., 5*(3), 960–963.
India Ageing Report. (2015). https://india.unfpa.org/sites/default/files/pub-pdf/India%20Ageing%20Report%20-%202017%20%28Final%20Version%29.pdf
Perappadan, B. S. (2016, August 16). *Situation worse for old women in India*. Retrieved from https://www.thehindu.com/news/cities/Delhi/%E2%80%98Situation-worse-for-old-women-in-India%E2%80%99/article14572641.ece
Basu, S. (2010, June 30). *India's city of widows*. Retrieved from https://www.theguardian.com/commentisfree/2010/jun/30/india-city-widows-discrimination
Inter-ministerial committee implementing Indian national policies on older persons. Retrieved from http://silverinnings.in/wp-content/uploads/2016/10/list-of-ministries-for-implementation-OF-NPOP.pdf
Joshi, K., Kumar, R., & Avasthi, A. (2003). Morbidity profile and its relationship with disability and psychological distress among elderly people in Northern India. *International Journal of Epidemiology, 32*(6), 978–987.
Kaur, J., Singal, P., Sidhu, L. S. (2004). *Physique and psychosocial stresses in rural and urban Jat Sikh women with special reference to senescence* (Unpublished Phd Thesis). Punjabi University, Patiala.
Lena, A., Ashok, K., Padma, M., Kamath, V., & Kamath, A. (2009). Health and social problems of the elderly: A cross-sectional study in Udupi Taluk, Karnataka. *Indian Journal of Community Medicine: Official Publication of Indian Association of Preventive & Social Medicine, 34*(2), 131.
Innovative practices for care of elderly in India (2016). Retrieved from www.streeshakti.com/pdf-files/A-collection-of-good-practices.pdf
Lusti-Narasimhan, M., & Beard, J. R. (2013). Sexual health in older women. *Bulletin of the World Health Organization, 91*, 701–709.
Maintenance and Welfare of Parents and Senior Citizens Act. (2007). Retrieved from http://www.prsindia.org/billtrack/themaintenance-and-welfare-of-parents-and-senior-citizens-bill-2007-441/
National Old Age Pension (NOAP) scheme. Retrieved from http://www.nsap.nic.in
National policy for older persons year 1999. Retrieved from http://socialjustice.nic.in
National policy on senior citizens 2011. Retrieved from http://socialjustice.nic.in
National Programme for the health care of Elderly (NPCHE). Retrieved from https://mohfw.gov.in/major-programmes/other-national-health-programmes/national-programme-health-care-elderlynphce
Older women in India—A note by Agewell Foundation-India. Retrieved from www.agewellfoundation.org
Parkar, S. R. (2015). Elderly mental health: Needs. *Mens Sana Monographs, 13*(1), 91.
Patwardhan, B., & Gokhale, S. (2003, September 16–18). *Longevity phenomenon in India: Emerging issues and responses*. A theme discussion paper for UNESCAP Expert Group Meeting on Assessing Regional Implementation of Commitments from the World Summit for Social Development, Bangkok, Thailand.
Prakash, I. J. (1999). *Ageing in India*. World Health Organization
Ramachandran, R., & Radhika, R. (2006). Problems of elderly women in India and Japan. *Indian J Gerontology, 20*, 219–234.

Rastogi, S., Gupta, S. R., & Lala, M. K. (2014). A Cross-Sectional Study Done in Geriatric Age Group People Living Under Field Practice Areas of BJMC Ahmedabad to Assess Their Major Health Problems and Its Impact on Their Living. *International Journal of Health Sciences and Research (IJHSR), 4*(7), 56–61.

Roy, K., & Chaudhuri, A. (2008). Influence of socioeconomic status, wealth and financial empowerment on gender differences in health and healthcare utilization in later life: Evidence from India. *Social Science & Medicine, 66*(9), 1951–1962.

Salagre, S. B. (2013). *Health issues in geriatrics.* Retrieved from www.apiindia.org/medicine_update_2013/chap177.pdf

Shah, B., & Prabhakar, A. K. (1997). Chronic morbidity profile among elderly. *Indian Journal of Medical Research, 106*, 265–272.

Shan, S. K., Sahu, T., Sahani, N. C., & Swain, S. P. (2003). Functional status of the older persons Residing in Urban Slums. *Indian Journal of Gerontology*, 17.

Sharma, K. L. (2009). *Dimensions of ageing: Indian studies.* Rawat Publications.

Sharma, K. L. (2003). Health status and care giver of elderly in Rajasthan villages. *Indian Journal of Gerontology., 17*(1 & 2), 401–410.

Singh, D., & Yesudian, P. (2007). After age 60 in India, A Glimpse through Census and NSSO. *The Indian Journal of Social Work., 68*, 545–560.

Soodan, K. S. (1975). *Ageing in India, Calcutta.* Minerva Association Pvt. Ltd.

Sumanth, S. H. (2012). The health status of rural elderly women in India: A case study. *International Journal of Criminology and Sociological Theory, 5*(3), 960–963.

Sushma, V., & Darshan, S. (2004). Health problems of aged widows in Rural Haryana. *Ageing and society*, 14.

The NGO's commitment to the elderly in India. Retrieved from https://www.silverinnings.com/old/docs/Ageing%20Indian/The%20NGO%E2%80%99s%20commitment%20to%20the%20Elderly%20in%20India.pdf

Chapter 9
Emerging Problem of Dementia and Challenges of Care Services

Meera Pattabiraman and R. Narendhar

Abstract Longevity and changing life styles have made "Dementia" a problem rife among the elderly with increased reporting of early onset dementias in India. The number of affected people (5.29 million) is daunting and scarce services to meet the rising demands add to the challenges. The helpline calls have gone up by 100% in the last seven years. The calls mostly seeking support for managing dementia, training of family care givers and increased requirement of professional care facilities confirm that dementia is now a pressing health priority in India. The Dementia India Report 2010 brought out by the Alzheimer's and Related Disorders Society of India highlighted the scarcity of services. While diagnosis is estimated at a very low 10%, treatment and care facilities are negligible. Lack of trained professionals to diagnose treat and mange dementia is a key issue to be addressed holistically. Family care is the most common and the immediate care giver/ family member faces physical, social and economic burdens. The Kerala State Initiative on Dementia (KSID) is a good beginning, with a joint collaboration between the Kerala Social welfare department, Kerala Social Security Mission and ARDSI. KSID is mandated to set up day care centres and fulltime care centres in all districts and equip the health and social workers to get trained in identifying and managing persons with dementia. ARDSI is advocating for a National Plan for comprehensive care through a structured strategy, action plan and allocation of resources to address this emerging need holistically.

Keywords Dementia · Care givers training · Professional care giver services · Diagnosis · Treatment · Family care · Government initiatives · National plan · Holistic action

Background

Dementia in India is largely an unknown health problem among general population, affecting the elderly. Family members having persons living with Dementia,

M. Pattabiraman · R. Narendhar (✉)
Alzheimer's and Related Disorders Society of India (ARDSI), New Delhi, India
e-mail: narendhar@ardsi.org

M. K. Shankardass (ed.), *Gerontological Concerns and Responses in India*,
https://doi.org/10.1007/978-981-16-4764-2_9

invariably end up as forced care givers without a clue to handle and manage them. Incidentally, all affected persons are first-generation cases, so understanding about Dementia and its management is not in their scheme of things or is part of their knowledge base.

Longevity of life, changing life style has made "Dementia" a problem rife among elderly. Dementia is also counted as a life style disorder with increased reporting of early onset Dementias in India. The number of affected people (5.29 million) is formidable and the services available are scarce to meet the rising demands. The impact of Dementia is proportionate to the number of people affected, which in the present situation is much larger than any other disease. Diseases which are much less in number are still given more priority and many national programmes are run by the Government with a view to providing relief to the affected. The impact of Dementia must be understood from the point of the affected person, his/her family and the society, which on getting quantified monetarily, the cost and human efforts shall be larger than any other existing disease in India. Dementia India Report 2010 indicates this aspect by estimating the informal cost by family amounting to 56%, while the societal cost is 29% and the remaining 15% is covered as medical cost. The total societal cost as per this report for 5.29 million dementia affected people shall be around INR 174 billion without any cost escalation of 2010 estimates.

The helpline calls to the National Helpline of ARDSI and its chapters have gone up by 100% in the last seven years. The calls received mostly seek support for treatment from reliable sources, seek training of family care givers, more demands for professional care givers, rise in demand for day care and fulltime care services are key indicators of Dementia cases on the rise. This emerging trend clearly outlines, Dementia is now a pressing health priority within India, which needs to be inclusive of care givers and addressed holistically covering related risk factors.

Challenges and Hurdles to Good Care

Those affected are oblivious, it is the disease which makes them like that, but family care givers undergo a traumatic experience of not being able to understand and often mistake it to obvious mental and behavioural disorders, thus remain recluse reducing their socializing, fearing societal ostracization. This leaves the affected person not getting correctly diagnosed. As the disease severity increases, the care giver finds it difficult to manage and venture for external support and is confronted with very few options for assisted living. The preparedness to accost the impending health burden because of Dementia is thus completely missing at Primary, Secondary and Tertiary care levels.

People with Dementia and their family care givers require continued support at different stages. The symptoms, of all forms of dementia, starts much earlier, however, requisite intervention starts much later and mostly when the condition gets aggravated. This pattern clearly indicates that the primary awareness about the disease is quite low and the health seeking behaviour has never been preventive or protective rather focused on curative and managing the conditions which often reach unmanageable levels. The major barriers can thus be categorized as lack of awareness, which is inclusive of health seeking behaviours and lack of facilities.

Low Awareness and Poor Health Seeking Behaviours

In India, awareness about the disease is deplorably low, stigma and attached discrimination add up to the woes of both patients and their families. Evidently, the key barriers for treatment and care have been found to be:

a. Low awareness about the disease. This leads to the affected person and their family care givers remain ignorant of early symptoms of the disease.
b. Misreading symptoms, considering memory problems as a natural sign of ageing and feel shy to avail medical care due to the fear of getting stigmatized and discriminated.
c. Caring is majorly confined to families of the affected at early stages, with possibility of abuse and neglect and institutional care becomes the essential need at advanced stages as caring becomes unmanageable.
d. In India, generally, people affected with any kind of ailments prefer to go to a private general physician (56%) or resort to across the counter medication available with pharmacies/medicine stores, where symptoms are often misread/misunderstood. The worst part is around 33% of the people do not avail any services and live with the ailment.
e. Affected people generally do not prefer to visit a Government hospital or a multi special poly clinic where experts and requisite facilities are present, essentially owing to the access difficulties and related drudgeries.

Lack of Facilities and Requisite Human Resources

On the other hand, identifying and chalking a patient centric prognosis is lacking due to

a. Poor awareness within the medical fraternity, resulting in only 10% of the affected getting correctly diagnosed.
b. Inadequate para-medical staff and other related human skills and physical resources to assess cognitive impairments, care treatment and lack of such facilities resulting in poor diagnosis.
c. Lack of training at family and professional care levels to deal with people affected by Dementias resulting in mismanagement of affected people.
d. Lack of favourable policies, schemes, social security (such as insurance/elderly privileges) and resource allocations is another area which affects service delivery at all levels.

Efforts Towards Dementia by Variety of Stakeholders

The challenges and barriers require a holistic multi-pronged action from Government, private sector and the general public. The minimalistic possible action from the affected community by forming themselves as a tangible group, in the form of Alzheimer's and Related Disorders Society of India, has been in action for 25 years now, however, in a minor way as depicted in the following section. There are few more agencies that have now come into the arena of Dementia care, but their coverage does not address the real need and requirements of the large affected numbers of patients.

Dementia Services from CSOs

The dementia services in India are limited. Though Alzheimer's and Related Disorders Society of India (ARDSI) established in 1992 and spearheaded dementia advocacy in India, currently the ARDSI could establish 22 chapters across India. These centres are extending Care and Support services, Awareness Generation and is actively engaged in Research and Training. These services extended are model centres and are perpetually resource dependent in nature to keep it sustained.

There are few more organizations also offering dementia care services either independently or in support of ARDSI.

The services exclusively for people with dementia are approximately;

- Day care centres-15;
- Residential care facilities-12;
- Domiciliary care services-6;
- Memory clinics-100;
- Dementia help lines-10.

ARDSI is the only pioneering organization working for this virgin cause in the whole of the country running various services, which tries and address the needs of the affected patients and their family including care givers.

Nevertheless, there are limited non-governmental organizations that are focused on dementia services. There is a significant inadequacy in establishing and running the dementia care giving centres in India when compared to the proportion of dementia cases.

In addition to above, ARDSI also has been engaged in creating evidences on best Dementia care practices by piloting studies to ascertain the efficacy, efficiency, ease of application of a care practice following modern, indigenous and many other patient centric non-pharmacological interventions, including therapies to stimulate and regulate cognition. In addition, few researches were focusing on the prevalence, severity of the disease progression by increasing age, health seeking behaviours, cost burden of care, care giver burn out, Early Dementia diagnosis and loss of productivity, etc.

Dementia India Report brought out in 2010, gave the country a clear estimation of prevalence for 20 years starting from 2006 to 2026 which ranges between 3.09 and 6.35 million persons affected with Dementia.

Dementia India Report 2010 is a compendium of researches till then, which speaks of

- Understanding Dementia
- Number of people with Dementia in India
- The Impact of Dementia
- Services for people with Dementia

STRIDE Project

ARDSI is presently engaged in researches with the London School of Economics, which is a multi-country initiative called "Strengthening Responses towards Dementia in Developing Economies"-STRIDE (2018–2021) in collaboration with NIMHANS. This study shall be looking in detail the aspects of care giver costs and burden with a view to providing inputs to the Government country strategy/action plan.

Dementia India Strategy

ARDSI also conducted a series of regional consultations to emanate responses from multi-stakeholders (comprising doctors, family caregivers, patients, para-medical experts, sociologists, service providers, economists, etc.). The recommendations were consolidated and juxtaposed with the recommendations of Global action plan of WHO and a comprehensive Strategy specific to India was drawn and handed over to the Union Health Minister, calling for action. He has promised to look into it and provide relief by all possible means. ARDSI's efforts do not end here, it shall continue in shaping up the plan with budget and shall seek a role in implementation and monitoring of services to assist people living with Dementia.

Government Initiatives-Kerala State Initiative on Dementia

ARDSI actively took up to public policy advocacy mode and demonstrated its role in extending model services of care and related aspects. These action-based advocacies resulted in local governments adapting to the service models of the society by collaborating with ARDSI as a knowledge partner. Kerala State Initiative on Dementia is the most successful Government run initiative to holistically benefit people living with Dementia, which is now studied for emulation across the country.

Kerala State Initiative on Dementia is a small beginning, where the state Government joined hands with ARDSI and took the issue seriously. KSID is mandated to set up Day care centres and Fulltime care centres in all districts and train the paramedical staff working in old age homes and government hospitals to get trained on managing persons with Dementia. Though it has been established in two districts on a pilot basis and three more districts have been finalized to roll out the services, it is a gradual process and takes its sweet time. ARDSI is advocating a National Plan seeking for comprehensive care through a structured strategy, action plan and allocation of resources to address this emerging need holistically, towards which a suggestive Dementia India Strategy has been prepared and presented to the Government of India seeking a way forward.

Envisaged Solution

The narration above has touched the present status in terms of the number of affected people, difficulties faced in getting correct diagnosis and access to care, cost burden, hitherto efforts by stakeholders including that of ARDSI and a pilot effort by a State Government. However, as a matter of fact, need for services is not in proportion to the projected numbers. The services are scarce and do not match the ever-emerging demands. Given the fact that health care is a state subject, it is quite natural and logical to expect the facilities are created, maintained and extended by the local Governments, while expertise could come from practitioners who have experience in running the services. Health and rehabilitative care have to go hand in hand, which at present is divided into health care and social care domains.

Need for a National Plan

An effective public policy/strategy to holistically address the issue covering all aspects must be in place, along with an action plan and allocation of exclusive resources. Mainstreaming dementia in health care, social justice, social security, transportation, human resources, law, enabling national dementia registry, etc., has to be ensured, enabling integration of dementia into all relevant domains where people living with dementia shall require support, just as in the case of cancer and other life challenging diseases where cure is not possible. People lack access to timely information or advice on how to respond to the disease and related social and emotional challenges. There is a need to mobilize social support to meet the needs of people with dementia in their own homes and within their communities. Sustainable and community-based care initiatives need to be promoted where the patient and their families lead and live in a friendly environment.

Ensuring Dementia Readiness

Dementia readiness has to be ensured at all levels viz., at household levels, awareness among children at schools, primary and private health care levels, at the levels of para-medical staff, at the levels of General Practitioners, as part of medical and nursing care curriculums, at the policy levels and at large at the community/society levels.

Need for Dementia-Friendly Communities

Dementia-friendly community-DFC approach specifically at different stakeholder levels would prove to improve the Dementia readiness aspect envisaged. A continuous effort to educate the public and developing services to improve quality of life of people living with dementia shall prove an informed society and a workforce to handle the requirements of such patients. Professionals trained on the nuances of Dementia care can understand and be skilled in addressing the problems associated with dementia patients. Thus there is a need to create focused dementia care services that can be accommodated within the existing resource settings. The necessary strategies for DFC shall include the following;-

- Developing awareness on dementia among the common public.
- Building capacities of health care professionals about dementia management through training and education.
- Developing diagnostic facilities and ensuring dementia care management with balanced approach including medical and psychosocial care
- Ensuring grouping of community volunteers/workers and dementia-friendly people to provide care and support and keeping it accessible.
- An exclusive strategy for dementia specific to each state and care policy which focusing on diagnostic, care facilities, including less addressed issues like legislation and financial assistance to carers.
- Practicing dementia risk reduction strategies by pursuing complementary programmes focusing NCDs and creating awareness on modifiable risks
- Government health setups should collaborate with stakeholders from non-governmental organizations, voluntary sector and look for public private partnerships.

Memory Clinics

- Establishing memory clinics to ensure early diagnosis at primary health care levels shall prove a breakthrough. A memory clinic would ideally ensure:
- Service provisioning for assessment of memory problems with expert assistance.
- The approach should take up a multidisciplinary mode involving - medical (doctor) nursing care, psychosocial support (from social worker/psychologist, etc.).

- Family getting dedicated attention, which is normally deprived for outpatient.
- Assessment of memory, behaviour, Activity of daily living, etc. in an objective manner.
- A robust MIS with meticulous record keeping, analysis and follow up ensuring a better quality of specialist care.

In addition to the above campaigns, lucid IEC materials, signboard messages, websites, TV talk shows, effective use of modern-day media and social media gears, helplines, etc. shall help to raise the profile of the disease and the process shall optimize the Dementia readiness aspects.

Conclusion

There is very minimal public health care spending in India. Thus creating care facilities is a costly proposition. Dementia care must progress following two pathways of 'Risk reduction' and 'Care Management'. Risk reduction should be ensured by creating awareness to raise the profile of the disease, its condition, suggesting life style changes ensuring change by working on modifiable risk factors, to prevent and check the disease. On the other hand diagnostic facilities have to be created to ensure early diagnosis. This should be complemented with a trained workforce of care givers to meet the need of patient families who can afford paid care.

There are many initiatives and programmes sponsored and implemented by few central Ministries, covering various aspects of dementia. There is, however, need for a national vertical programme for Dementia. The Kerala State Initiative on Dementia and the District level initiatives in Maharashtra focusing Dementia addressing the needs of people living with Dementia comprehensively could be taken as reference. The National programme on health care for elderly, District mental health programme under NHM, National Palliative Programm and NPCDS (NCD), from Ministry of Health needs to be converged along with the National Programme for Older people from the Ministry of Social Justice and Empowerment, to bring about an all-inclusive programme for Dementia care through a specific policy focusing Dementia. Under the National Health Mission, the union Government has taken up promotion of wellness centres at the primary care levels and have inclusion of mental health initiatives, these should be inclusive of Dementia diagnosis and its care at secondary and tertiary levels.

The National Health Mission is devolved to states as State Health Mission, where the districts have to submit a District Implementation Plans-DIPs. These plans, under provision of District Mental Health programme, should invariably include Dementia diagnosis, care and treatment. They should also include care centres, training and care giver support clear indication of a budget. Such specific resource allocation shall ensure care and support to people living with Dementia and their care givers linked to a dedicated MIS specifically to be created for this purpose.

References

ARDSI guidelines for establishing memory clinics, ARDSI DFC notes from www.ardsi.org

Dementia India Report 2010 brought out by Alzheimer's Related Disorders Society of India.

Details of Dementia Services in India are approximate estimates and are in addition to service centers listed in ARDSI website www.ardsi.org. These include services run by Dignity foundation, Nightingales Medical Trust, Silver Innings Foundation etc.

Chapter 10
Social Protection for Ageing Population in India: Concerns and Recommendations

Anurag Priyadarshee and Kavim Bhatnagar

Abstract Social protection is generally described to include response from the state and the civil society towards levels of vulnerability, risk and deprivation that a given society deems unacceptable within its social, political and economic normative structures. We can grasp the political and political economy aspects of social protection more clearly through the framework of social contract between the state and its citizens endeavouring to enhance the wellbeing and augment opportunities accessible to all citizens. Thus, social contract helps place social protection under the scope of State policies in order to promote equality and justice. Due to a rapid increase in life expectancy in India after Independence and corresponding demographic changes, number of people considered to be old has increased significantly. Population data suggest that more than 6.5% of the India consists of 'elderly' people with about 80 million Indians over the age of 65. A vast majority of such elderly population is living a life of stark loneliness and poverty. They depend on the society and the state and leverage their social capital, for their wellbeing and addressing their vulnerability, risk and deprivation. This chapter analyses the social protection measures undertaken for the ageing population in India after Independence. It is observed that the elderly population of India is faced with a situation of highly inadequate social protection. Only a fraction of them is covered by social assistance pension scheme. Even in case of people receiving social assistance pension, the amount is so unreasonably low that they are unable to meet even their most basic needs through that amount. Barring a small minority of people working in organized sector, working age population of the present will be entering an uncertain future in terms of their wellbeing. Due to lack of awareness and poor incomes they are unable to join contributory (social insurance) pension plans. Even when some of them are able to join such plans, the amounts they are able to save towards their pension are so meagre that their retirement benefits are abysmal. It is, therefore, important that policymakers accord the issue due importance and design suitable measures for addressing the situation. It is recommended that the amount of social assistance pension is stepped up to be equivalent to at least

A. Priyadarshee (✉)
Foundation for Holistic Vision, New Delhi, India

K. Bhatnagar
World Food Programme, Dhaka, Bangladesh

M. K. Shankardass (ed.), *Gerontological Concerns and Responses in India*,
https://doi.org/10.1007/978-981-16-4764-2_10

half of the prescribed minimum wages. It is further recommended that the scheme is universalized while excluding the people who are income tax payees or the people who receive pension or any other financial assistance the amount of which is not less than the proposed pension amount under social assistance.

Keywords Ageing population · Social protection · India · Social assistance · Social insurance · Pension schemes · Contributory pension · Poverty

Background: India's Ageing Demography

According to Population Census 2011, about 104 million Indian residents are aged 60 years or above. The Census further reveals that such demography consists of 53 million females and 51 million males. Population growth trends also indicate increasing rate of ageing of the Indian population over the years. While only 5.6% of India's population comprised of people aged 60 and above in 1961, the corresponding figure for 2011 was 8.6%. Old age dependency ratio has also been observed to have been increased from 10.9% in 1961 to 14.2% in 2011. Ageing of the Indian population also exhibits gender and rural-urban divide. Share of aged people among the female population is 9% as against 8.2% of the males being 60 years of age or more. As many as 71% of the elderly population resides in rural areas while only 29% of them reside in urban areas.

United Nations describes a country as 'ageing' if share of its old age population (above 60 years of age) reaches more than 8% of its total population. Thus, India is an 'ageing' country now. Increasing share of elderly people in the Indian population is attributable to reduced fertility rates, improved health care facilities, better nutritional status and consequent improvement in life expectancy.

Indian demographic landscape is at the crossroads of being young and yet ageing rapidly towards joining the majority. While the median age of the entire country is just 25 years, the aged above 60 are rapidly outnumbering the population growth rate and would reach 320 million by the mid of this century. The current scenario that young people are seen everywhere: on the streets, in offices, in shops, on campuses bringing with them a mood that is progressive, optimistic and dynamic is likely to change over the next few decades.

India host approx. 20% of the world's population including 33.33% of the world's poor and one-eighth of the world's elderly. Most belong to informal sector and work till they die without no or little old age security. In their old age, they are compelled to depend on their children who usually have their own challenges in life. However, aged old the joint family structure that dominated in India is on the verge of dismemberment. However, with migration and better opportunities elsewhere, the new social norm has eroded the family-based system to support old age care for the poor. India being the second most populated country in the world is projected to overtake China in about half a decade to become the world's most populous country. By 2050, life expectancy at birth is projected to reach 74 years. Fertility rates in India have already declined to 2.6 children per woman, less than one-half the early 1950s rate of 5.9 children per woman (Haub & Gribble, 2011).

Old Age Vulnerability

A majority of India's informal sector working poor, especially low-income women workers in urban and rural India, are highly vulnerable to old age poverty since they are not only excluded from any formal pension provisions but also unable to access any regulated insurance and retirement savings product at an affordable transaction cost. Empirical evidence suggests that while there is limited existence for coverage of 'risk of life' (life insurance), the mitigation of 'risk of longevity' (pension) is mostly unheard of. With 17 years of life expectancy at 60, workers will need to accumulate enough savings during their working life to support themselves for nearly 15–20 years when they are too old to work (Bhatnagar, 2014). However, their fragile labour market attachments and modest intermittent incomes, coupled with the absence of a low cost and easily accessible long-term savings mechanism and above all the concept of pension, so conspicuously missing, puts retirement planning out of reach of most of these workers. This presents a bleak outlook for the next generation of India's elderly and clearly suggests that old age poverty will continue to be an intractable public policy challenge. For a majority of these low-income workers and equally for the States and Central Government, therefore, a vital issue is the management of the longevity risk with the cessation of earnings in old age.

Increased Dependence

Demography of India is changing rapidly resulting in falling fertility rates, improving life expectancy, ultimately leading to higher elderly population. With young people becoming more aspirational and families becoming more nuclear, the support system of the elderly is slowly disintegrating. In addition, low savings and absence of pension support are adding to the woes of this part of the population who is too old to work. A good 45% of elderly males and 75% of elderly females are completely dependent. According to the India Human Development Survey (IHDS) of the National Council of Applied Economic Research (NCAER). Elderly females have it worse as they tend to have lower incomes due to discrimination at work, employment interruptions due to pregnancy and child care, lower accessibility to formal sources of finance and so on.

Demographic Catastrophe in Offing

With 320 million senior citizens by 2050, India might be heading for a socio-economic demographic catastrophe if the younger population fails to create pension savings today. Striking demographic changes have occurred during the previous and current century with the increase in the number and proportion of elderly in the Indian population. With the improvement in health care industry and life expectancy, however, the elderly are also experiencing more of the cumulative effects of multiple chronic diseases and disabilities leading to increased expenses in old age. The growing needs of the aged population require the availability of more caretakers and money at their disposal and commitment to geriatric care. Yet, numerous reports have documented a widespread insensitive or negative attitude held by the younger cohort toward ageing and the care of the elderly. Such biases may, in part, be due to the general societal attitude toward the aged and they may further reflect the traditional non-orientation of beliefs, customs and values, which emphasizes the care and management of older generation by the younger cohort. Financial constraints in old age and a similar crunch of resources among their children add fuel to the fire.

India's ageing population is expected to grow at more than double the rate of the general population. According to Census 2011, India has 10.8 million senior citizens (above 60 years of age). This number is expected to increase substantially in the coming years with a rise in the life expectancy to 65 years from 42 years in1960. In fact, it is predicted that between the years 2000 and 2050, the population of India will grow by 55%. However, the population above 60 years and 80 years will grow by 326% and 700% respectively.

By the mid of the current century, India shall have 19.3% of its population in the age groups that have crossed 60 years of age and 13.7% (5.71% in 2020) who have crossed 65 years of age. In other words, over the next 3 decades, the population of 65 + years old would almost touch 2.4 times what it is today (Fig. 10.1).

Social Protection: A Theoretical Overview

Social protection is generally described to include 'public actions taken in response to levels of vulnerability, risk and deprivation which are deemed socially unacceptable within a given polity or society' (Norton et al., 2001: 7). The basic idea of such protection is 'to use social means to prevent deprivation and vulnerability to deprivation' (Dreze & Sen, 1991: 5). Social Protection thus has a 'strong poverty focus' (Barrientos & Lloyd-Sherlock, 2002: 1). According to Avato et al., (2009: 456), social protection 'includes interventions and initiatives that support individuals, households and communities in their efforts to prevent, mitigate and overcome risks and vulnerabilities and that enhance the social status and rights of the marginalized'.

Social protection measures are crucial to alleviate such shocks and vulnerabilities at the individual, household and community levels. Dreze and Sen (1991: 3–4)

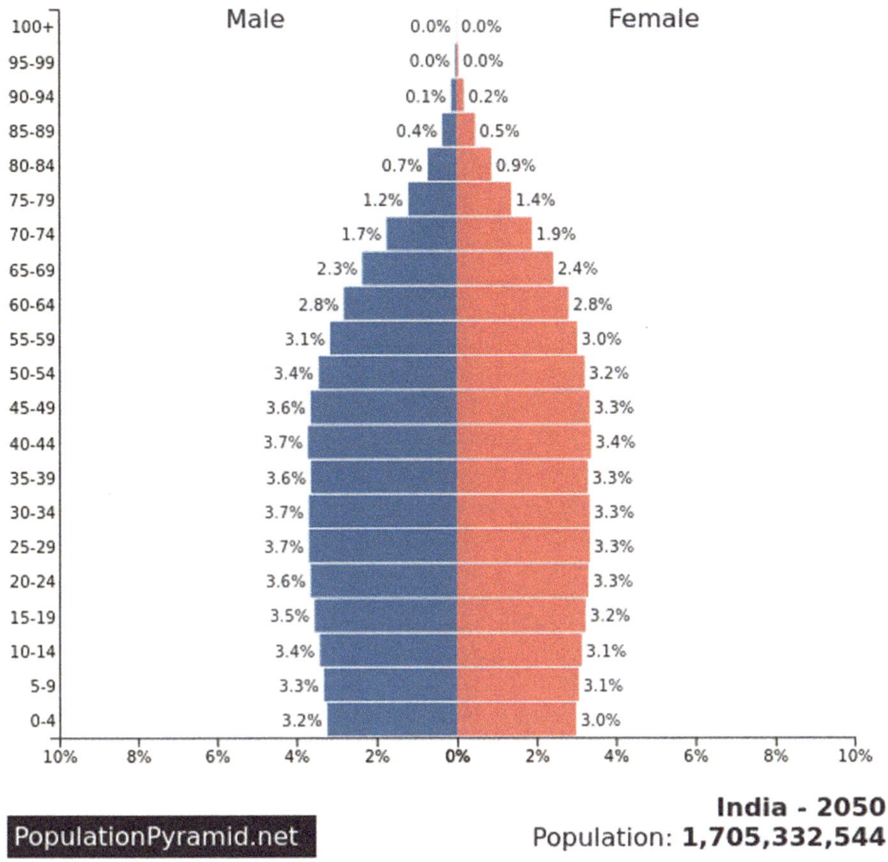

Fig. 10.1 Projected distribution of Indian population in the year 2015

argue that there may be a protection aspect to these measures and a promotional aspect. The former endeavours to protect the living standards, assuming tremendous importance during social and economic threats such as famines. The latter aspect aims to improve the general standard of living by proactively addressing deprivation and vulnerabilities. The objectives of both aspects may be very different from each other but their implementational framework and planning may not be completely independent of each other. Moreover, their successes tend to be cyclical, feeding into the other. For instance, achievements attributed to the promotional aspects may warranty easing down of implementation of protection aspects (e.g. higher incomes may make individual insurance pinch less). Sabates-Wheeler and Devereux (2008: 69) extend such classification to categorize the social protection measures in four ways, viz. provision, preventive, promotive and transformative measures. According to them, the provision measures aim to lessen and mitigate deprivation, while the preventive measures attempt to prevent the incidence of deprivation and include various poverty alleviation measures. Promotive measures help improve incomes and capabilities 'through a range of livelihood-enhancing programmes targeted at both households and individuals'. The transformative measures target exclusion and social injustices.

Different agencies have been promoting various aspects of social protection under different terminologies according to their ideological standpoints and their development strategies (Paitoonpong et al., 2008). In 1952, ILO proposed a comprehensive definition of social security with its Social Security (Minimum Standards) Convention, 1952 (No. 102), which included nine core contingencies, such as old age and death, widowhood, sickness, employment injury, invalidity, maternity, unemployment, provision of medical care and meeting increased financial needs for families with children, to be addressed through social security. This definition encompassed two strands of social protection, social insurance that is largely contributory and social assistance that is non-contributory (Arun & Arun, 2001). The word "social" specifically connotes that the market alone cannot be relied on to address such contingencies (Unni & Rani, 2003). Perceived adverse effects on the incomes, livelihoods and general life conditions of workers due to structural adjustment programmes undertaken in low-income countries in the 1980s and 1990s gave rise to social safety nets. The World Bank promoted a concept of social funds as means to finance the social safety net programmes. Social protection is an umbrella term that includes all these concepts and has a sharper focus on poverty reduction (Lund & Srinivas, 2000).

Munro (2008: 27) mentions that social protection policies have been traditionally justified using following three discourses. The risks and market failures discourse justifies social protection by attributing informational issues in addition to credit, human capital and labour market failures as reasons for failures in insurance markets. The rights-based discourse calls on the state's responsibility to provide legally-implementable social and economic rights to its citizens. On the other hand, needs-based discourse pushes for social protection measures to reduce poverty and deprivation by focussing on the practical and moral arguments of poverty alleviation. Constraints faced by people living in poverty can be explained in a lot of different ways, thus giving rise to different social protection measures used to address those constraints (Barrientos and Hulme 2008a). Therefore, the overall objective of social protection can be to lessen market failures, fulfil basic needs of the citizens, or employ rights-based approach to address deprivation. The chosen approach depends on policymakers and the strategies they deploy to ensure social protection. For instance, the modern welfare State came into being due to the market failure-induced demand to increase the economic and social role of the State.

Graham (2002) opines that we can make better sense of the political and political economy aspect of social protection when we study them in the light of a social contract between the State and citizens. This social contract delineates the State's responsibility to enhance overall wellbeing of citizens and provide them with access to opportunities equally (Barrientos and Hulme 2008b). Social contract as a concept is convincingly used to argue in favour of mandating the State to promote equality and prevent injustice (Jayasuriya 2002) through measures such as social protection.

Even though India's formal sector was fortified with labour regulations on account of workers' struggles, implementation of other social protection measures in the unorganized sector were entrenched in the cognizance that economic success by itself cannot ensure inclusion (Priyadarshee, 2011).

The social protection schemes can be grouped under: social insurance, social assistance and labour market regulations. Social insurance includes initiatives that offer protection against eventualities such as sickness, maternity, unemployment or old age. Social assistance schemes provide relief to people living in poverty, while labour market regulations ensure workers receive fair wages and basic rights among other things (Barrientos and Hulme 2008a: 3). Social protection measures developed as an overarching set of programmes to address multidimensional aspects of poverty in around late 1980s and early 1990s. At the same time, these measures were also touted to be insufficient in addressing all concerns and were criticized as 'residualist and paternalistic' (Sabates-Wheeler & Devereux, 2008: 64).

Social protection for the elderly population needs to consist of elements of both social assistance and social insurance. It will be in the form of elderly care in terms of their housing, health care and other aspects of their general wellbeing. In addition, it will be in the form of pensions that ensure regular incomes to meet their daily needs when they are no longer in a position to be in the paid employment. Such pensions could be provided by the State (social assistance pensions) or be based on a combination of their savings and contribution of their employers or the State (social insurance pensions-retirement pensions). This article deals with both types of old age pensions.

Evolution of Social Protection for the Elderly Population in India

According to the Article 41 of the Constitution of India, "the State shall, within the limits of its economic capacity and development, make effective provision for securing the right to work, to education and to public assistance in cases of unemployment, old age, sickness and disablement and in other cases of undeserved want." Social Security and social insurance figures in item 23, while old age pensions figure in item 24 of the Concurrent List within the Seventh Schedule of the Constitution of India.

Government of India launched an 'Integrated Programme for Older Persons (IPOP)' in the year 1992, which was revised and further improvised in the years 2008 and 2015 by including provisions such as establishment of old age homes. In the year 1999, a National Policy on Older Persons (NPOP) was announced and an Act namely, 'The Maintenance and Welfare of Parents and Senior Citizens Act' was enacted in 2007. The Act made it obligatory and justiciable to provide maintenance of the senior citizens by their children and relatives. The Act has Penal provisions in case of abandonment of senior citizens and allows them to revoke transfer of properties in case of negligence by their relatives. The Act further provided for establishment of old age homes and adequate medical facilities for senior citizens. In the year 2012, Government of India established National Council for Senior Citizens (NCSrC).

The Central Ministry of Social Justice and Empowerment is the nodal ministry for the welfare of the aged population in the country. The Ageing Division in the Social Defence Bureau of the Ministry has been entrusted with the task of policymaking and programme implementation for the senior citizens in collaboration with state governments and the concerned non-governmental agencies.

Ministry of Health and Family Welfare is implementing a programme named National Programme for Health Care of the Elderly (NPHCE) since 2010, which provides separate, specialized and comprehensive health care to the senior citizens at various levels of State health care delivery system including outreach services. Central Government contributes 75% of the implementation cost of the programme while remaining 25% is borne by the concerned state governments.

Income tax incentives have been provided to elderly people. They are also allowed to earn higher rates of interest on their savings under senior citizen savings schemes.

Senior citizens are allowed fare concessions on various modes of public transport.

As far as social assistance pensions are concerned, various state governments launched social pension schemes for vulnerable groups including the elderly people much before the issue attracted the central government's attention. In the year 1995, the central government introduced National Social Assistance Programme (NSAP) as a Centrally Sponsored Scheme, which was converted into Additional Central Assistance (ACA) Scheme in the year 2002. National Old Age Pension Scheme (NOAPS) was one of the social assistance schemes constituting NSAP. NOAPS was renamed as Indira Gandhi National Old Age Pension Scheme in the year 2007.

Success of non-governmental and state governments' efforts towards contributory pensions motivated the government of India to launch a New Pension Scheme Lite (NPS Lite) across the country in the year 2010. In 2015, the NPS Lite was replaced by Atal Pension Yojana (APY). The government also extended its National Pension System (NPS), which was until the targeting only the government employees, to all the citizens of India between the age of 18 and 60, in the year 2009.

Despite these efforts, only a handful of Indians (7.4%) form beneficiaries of any kind of pension programme. Studies also show that the people in India are themselves not inclined to prepare for their retirement, making the country a 'very young and immature pension industry'. Not surprisingly, India spends a mere 1.45% of its Gross Domestic Product (GDP) on social protection programmes and policies. This proportion of expenditure on social protection is among the lowest in Asia (including Thailand, China, Nepal and Sri Lanka which have a much higher portion earmarked for such schemes).

The following sections of the article describe the impact of the old age pension programmes and analyse various issues associated with social insurance and social assistance pension programmes in India in detail.

Old Age Pensions and Reduction of Poverty

Various studies suggest that pension schemes significantly reduce incidence of poverty among the aged population. Giang (2013) estimates that in Vietnam older population may have encountered a higher rate of poverty by 50% if they were not allowed any retirement or social pensions. As an example, poverty rate for the people in the age bracket of 60 to 69 might have grown to 23% from 10.2% if they were not allowed retirement benefits. It might have further increased to 26.6 if they were further denied social assistance pension. His research also reveals that such poverty-reducing impact of pensions is significantly more pronounced in case of rural population than in case of urban elders.

While analysing data of National Sample Survey (NSS) 61st round (2004–2005) and 64th round (2007–2008) Kaushal (2014) also found that IGNOAP programme reduced poverty among the recipient households in India. She further found that a part of pension amount was also spent on health care and education of children thus concluding that the pensions may have resulted in "intergenerational payoffs" in addition to improvements in elderly wellbeing.

Such poverty-reducing impact of pensions has also been observed to be improving with passage of time. Giang (2013) notes that in 2004 old age poverty would have grown from 19.5–22.4% without retirement benefits. In 2008, however, it would have increased to 24.1% from 13.3%. Causal factors for such temporal trends in old age poverty reduction due to pensions may relate to the observed increase in old age dependency ratio with time.

Contributory Retirement (Social Insurance) Pensions

Evolution of Contributory Pensions

The evolution of contributory savings by the poor, specifically targeted for old age owes the early initiate of SEWA Bank in India way back in April 2006. It was initially termed as micro pension which was a fair, safe, secure and sustainable method for retirement during old age, customized to serve the needs of working poor, especially women with limited savings and flexibility in contributions. It was safe from the prying hands of middlemen or intervening agencies, in addition to being economical.

While the movement sparked with women savings on their own, without the support from the State of Federal Government, it was interesting to observe that a few state governments and later the central government started taking keen interest in designing and implementing such contributory schemes with their support and ownership. This, however, was a slow and gradual process of evolving a consensus on contributory pension system in India.

SEWA Bank Initiative (2006)

SEWA Bank in Ahmedabad encouraged young women with low salaries such as rag pickers, domestic workers, vegetable vendors, etc. to put aside small amounts of money to secure their old age pension funds (Bhatnagar, 2012). The savings were managed by the oldest mutual find, UTI under their Retirement Benefit Pension Fund (RBPF) at the backend. The unorganized sector women started saving as low as a dollar a month, exclusively for their old age. SEWA Bank was supported by technical assistance from Invest India group that had been working on designing the pensions for the poor.

Rajasthan Vishwakarma Scheme (2008)

The year 2008 marked a turning point in social security in India with the launch of its First Co-Contributory Pension Scheme targeting low-income informal sector occupational groups in the state of Rajasthan. Vishwakarma Unorganized Sector Pension Motivational Scheme was initiated by the Rajasthan State Government. It aimed to match the contributions of the worker for up to Rs 1000 per year per worker. This amount was delivered straight to the individual retirement accounts (IRAs) of the workers with no perceived leakages, marking the beginning of targeted delivery of social security benefits (Bhatnagar, 2012).

Andhra's Abhyahastam (2009)

The state of Rajasthan had successfully displayed that 'Poor are Pensionable' and the model with certain modifications was further developed by the state of Andhra Pradesh and other states in India. Abhyahastam, a micro pension scheme was launched by the Andhra Pradesh Government in February 2009 that was intended to cover more women belonging to more than 100,000 SHGs being set up and monitored by the Society for Elimination of Poverty (SERP) of the Department of Rural Development, Government of AP. These women members of the SHGs were supposed to contribute Re. 1.00 per day or Rs 360 per annum towards their pension fund and were assured of a minimum income of Rs 500 per month. The women having a higher corpus would receive higher pensions, depending on their corpus value.

NPS Lite and Swawlamban (2010)

Year 2010 was another landmark in the history of contributory pensions in India. Learning from the experiences of Contributory Pension of SEWA Bank and Co-Contributory Pension programme of Rajasthan and Andhra Pradesh, the Government of India introduced the New Pension Scheme Lite (NPS Lite) across the country. "NPS Lite" was constructed to incur low administrative and transactional costs in order to make small investments viable. The implementation modalities of the NPS Lite worked on a "group" model, though the contributions and accounts were individual. It also planned to piggy-back on the outreach achieved and capacity generated by Government-run programmes, MFIs, NGOs, NBFCs to address the savings requirements of low-income workers. Each eligible group or "Aggregator" in the model was tasked with enrolling customers at the ground level, collect, re-conciliate and transfer individual contributions as well as delivery of services and information dissemination (Bhatnagar, 2012). Eventually, most of the Government projects of the states as well as banks including the RRBs were provided with the status of aggregator-ship under the NPS Lite.

The "Swavalamban Scheme" of the Indian Government provided monetary benefit of Rs 1000 per year for first 5 years to all eligible NPS Lite account holders. The NPS Lite and Swavalamban schemes targeted economically weaker sections of society and marginal investors. All Indian citizens between 18 and 60 years were eligible to enrol. The investment amount per year was left at the discretion of the subscriber. Unorganized workers could simply open an account through their Aggregator and get an NPS Lite account. The scheme was securely regulated by Pension Fund Regulatory and Development Authority (PFRDA), monitored periodically by NPS Trust and contained transparent investment norms. It was efficient and provided an economical cost structure with no requirement of a minimum cutoff amount either per annum or per contribution (Bhatnagar, 2012).

Atal Pension Yojana (2015)

Atal Pension Yojana (APY) replaced the previously implemented NPS Lite Swavalamban Yojana[1] in May 2015, as the national level, contributory elderly pension scheme for informal workers. It targets beneficiaries within the age group of 18–40 years. APY is also administered by the PFRDA and implemented through all nationwide banks.

Benefits under (APY) are applicable to all bank account holders. The Central Government would also co-contribute 50% of the total contribution or Rs 1000 per annum, whichever is lower, for each subscriber joining APY before 31st December 2015, for a 5-year period (Financial Year 2015–2016 to 2019–2020). The subscribers

[1] The Swavalamban Scheme subscribers over the age of 40 are allowed to opt out of the scheme by withdrawing the entire savings in a lump sum.

should not be members of any statutory social security scheme and should not be income tax payers (Government of India, n.d.).

Under the APY, the monthly pension would be available to the subscriber and after them to their spouse and after their death, the pension corpus would be returned to the subscriber's nominee. Under the APY, the subscribers would receive the fixed minimum pension of Rs 1000 per month to Rs 5000 per month, at the age of 60 years, depending on their contributions, which itself would be based on the age of joining the APY. Therefore, in this way, Government guaranteed the benefit of minimum pension. However, if higher investment returns are received on the contributions to APY, higher pensions would be paid to the subscribers (Government of India, n.d.).

This scheme has been linked to 'Pradhan Mantri Jan Dhan Yojana (PMJDY)' scheme and the contributions made into the PMJDY bank accounts are being deducted automatically. A majority of these bank accounts contained no funds initially. Government is working towards reducing the number of such zero-balance accounts. The national Aadhaar ID number is the primary 'know your customer' document to identify beneficiaries, spouses and nominees, helping prevent entitlement-related disputes in the long term. A copy of ration card or bank passbook acts as an address-proof document.

Subscribers are eligible to request for their 'guaranteed minimum monthly pension' or a higher amount if the returns are more than the guaranteed returns as embedded in APY, after turning 60 years of age. Spouse is the default nominee who gets the same amount of monthly pension upon the original beneficiary's demise. Upon the death of the spouse, the appointed nominee will be eligible for return of pension wealth accumulated till the age of 60 of the subscriber.

A subscriber joining the scheme of Rs 1000 monthly pension at the age of 18 years would be required to contribute Rs 42 per month. However, if he joins at age 40, he has to contribute Rs 291 per month. Similarly, a subscriber joining the scheme of Rs 5000 monthly pension at the age of 18 years would be required to contribute Rs 210 per month. However, if he joins at age 40, he has to contribute Rs 1454 per month. Therefore, it is always better to join early in the Scheme. The contribution levels, the age of entry and the pension amounts are available in a Table 10.1.

National Pension System

National Pension System (NPS) is a voluntary, defined contribution (DC) retirement savings scheme designed to enable the subscribers to make optimum decisions regarding their future through systematic savings during their working life. It is administered and regulated by the Pension Fund Regulatory and Development Authority (PFRDA), created by an Act of the Parliament of India. It was initiated with the decision of the Government of India to stop defined benefit (DB) pensions for all its employees who joined on or after 1 January 2004. While the scheme was initially designed for government employees only, it was opened up for all citizens

Table 10.1 Guaranteed pension amount receivable under APY

Monthly, quartely and half-yearly contributions under APY for different minimum guaranteed amount of pension at different age entry and return of the corpus amount to the nominee

		Minimum guaranteed pension of Rs. 1000/month			**Minimum guaranteed pension of Rs. 2000/month**			**Minimum guaranteed pension of Rs. 3000/month**		
Return of corpus amount to the nominee		**Rs. 1.70 Lakh**			**Rs. 3.40 lakh**			**Rs. 5.10 Lakh**		
Age at entry	Vesting period	Monthly instalment	Quaterty instalment	Half yearly instalment	Monthly instalment	Quaterty instalment	Half yearly instalment	Monthly instalment	Quaterly instalment	Half yearly instalment
18	42	42	12S	248	84	250	496	126	376	744
19	41	46	137	271	92	274	543	138	411	814
20	40	50	149	295	100	298	590	150	447	885
21	39	S4	161	319	108	322	637	162	483	956
22	38	59	176	348	117	349	690	177	527	104S
23	37	64	191	3/8	127	378	749	192	572	1133
24	36	70	209	413	139	414	820	208	620	1228
25	35	76	226	449	151	450	891	226	674	1334
26	34	82	244	484	164	489	968	246	733	1452
27	33	90	268	531	1/8	530	1050	268	799	1582
28	32	97	289	572	194	578	1145	292	870	1723
29	31	106	316	626	212	632	1251	318	948	1877
30	30	116	346	685	231	688	1363	347	1034	2048
31	29	126	376	744	252	751	1487	379	1129	2237
32	28	138	411	814	276	823	1629	414	1234	2443

(continued)

Table 10.1 (continued)

Monthly, quartely and half-yearly contributions under APY for different minimum guaranteed amount of pension at different age entry and return of the corpus amount to the nominee

33	27	151	450	891	302	900	1782	453	1350	2673
34	26	165	492	974	330	983	1948	495	1475	2921
35	2S	181	539	1068	362	1079	2136	543	1618	3205
36	24	198	590	1169	396	1180	2337	594	1770	3506
37	23	218	650	1287	436	1299	2573	654	1949	3860
38	22	240	715	1416	480	1430	2833	720	2146	4249
39	21	264	787	1558	S28	1574	3116	792	2360	4674
40	20	291	867	1717	582	1734	3435	873	2602	5152
		Minimum guaranteed pension of Rs. 4000/month			**Minimum guaranteed pension of Rs. 5000/month**					
Return of corpus amount to the nominee		**Rs. 6.80 Lakh**			**Rs. 8.50 Lakh**					
Age at entry	Vesting period	Monthly instalment	Quaterty instalment	Half yearly instalment	Monthly instalment	Quaterly Instalment	Half yearly Instalment			
18	42	168	501	991	210	626	1239			
19	41	183	54S	1080	228	679	1346			
20	40	198	590	1169	248	739	1464			
21	39	215	641	1269	269	802	1588			
22	38	234	697	1381	292	870	1723			

(continued)

Table 10.1 (continued)

Monthly, quartely and half-yearly contributions under APY for different minimum guaranteed amount of pension at different age entry and return of the corpus amount to the nominee										
23	37	254	757	1499	318	948	1877			
24	36	277	826	163S	346	1031	2042			
25	35	301	897	1776	376	1121	2219			
26	34	327	975	1930	409	1219	2414			
27	3332	356	1061	2101	446	1329	2632			
28	32	388	1156	2290	485	144S	2862			
29	31	423	1261	2496	529	1577	3122			
30	30	462	1377	2727	577	1720	3405			
31	29	504	1502	2974	630	1878	3718			
32	28	551	1642	3252	689	2053	4066			
33	27	602	1794	3553	752	2241	4438			
34	26	659	1964	3889	824	2456	4863			
35	25	722	2152	4261	902	2688	5323			
36	24	792	2360	4674	990	2950	5843			
37	23	870	2S93	5134	1087	3239	6415			
38	22	957	2852	5648	1196	3564	7058			
39	221	1054	3141	6220	1318	3928	7778			
40	20	1164	3469	6869	1454	4333	8581			

of India between the age of 18 and 60 in 2009. NPS is administered and regulated by the PFRDA.

NPS seeks to encourage citizens to build a saving habit to ease the financial burden of retirement by making available opportunity to access a sustainable and adequate retirement income for every Indian. NPS collects all the savings made by individuals into a pension fund. This fund is then invested by professional fund managers, regulated by PFRDA, into diversified portfolios of the government bills and bonds, corporate shares, etc. This fund will eventually garner returns and grow over the years.

The choice of investments and fund manager remains with the individuals and NPS offers a variety of such options, under regulatory restrictions, whereas the returns completely depend on the market forces. Once a customer opens her account with NPS, she is given a unique Permanent Retirement Account Number (PRAN). The scheme is structured as follows:

a **Tier-I account** is non-withdrawable permanent retirement account. Accumulations are deposited and invested as per subscriber's discretion and PFRDA regulations.

b **Tier-II account** is a voluntary withdrawable account. This is only setup in case of an active Tier-I account in the subscriber's name. Subscribers can withdraw as per their needs.

NPS also provides seamless portability across jobs and across locations, unlike all current pension plans, including that of the EPFO. It would provide hassle-free arrangements for the individual subscribers. Finally, NPS is regulated by PFRDA, with transparent investment norms, regular monitoring and performance review of fund managers by NPS Trust.

Issues of Daily Wage Labourers in Informal Sector

Contributory pensions aim to prevent old age poverty for those who are in the working age group of say, 18–50. Daily wage workers are seldom in a position to save for their old age since their immediate consumption takes a higher priority over the need to save. This cohort earns in the day and spends by night and they, therefore, have no means to save for tomorrow. This becomes critical as even though they do not "retire" like their counterparts in the formal sector, however, they would still need to plan for contingencies in the future, particularly relating to ill-health, which leads to dwindling incomes during old age.

Retirement Savings—Never on the Horizon

Providing opportunities to the working poor to build up savings for retirement through thrift and self-help should be an important public policy goal. Yet, 'barely 5% of this group is presently saving for retirement and less than one in five have some form of insurance' (MoF, 2007). Even for this cohort, which is 'actively saving for their old age, the savings accumulations are as modest as an average savings corpus of those above 45 years at Rs 25,000 or less' (IIMS Dataworks et al., 2008). Hence, in the best case scenario, even for those presently saving for their old age, is that they will manage enough preretirement savings to support themselves for no more than two years when they decide to stop working or are unable to work.

For the general population, assets particularly gold, land and property serve as guaranteed security for old age retirement. However, this is not an option for people in poverty. They generally have low estimate of their capacity to utilize savings to secure their retirement and also have little experience on how to utilize said savings for the same.

Poor Annuity Markets

'With underdeveloped annuity markets and poor financial literacy, people in India face considerable challenges in planning their retirement security. Many elderly citizens are stuck with lives of never-ending work, a fate that may befall millions in the coming decades. One can see a miserable preview for those who do not have the pensions that previous generations enjoyed' (Qazi, 2019). While the capital markets have been providing consistent returns over the past decade, the short term fluctuations and major downtrend such as the one in 2008 cannot be ruled out.

Urgent Need to Reform

India's older population will increase dramatically over the next three decades. The share of India's population ages 60 and older is projected to climb from 8% in 2010 to 19% in 2050, according to the United Nations Population Division (UN, 2011). This profound shift in the share of older Indians comes with great challenges that require immediate attention. These challenges are likely to be taking place in the context of already changing family relationships, dismemberment of joint family structure in both urban and rural India, urban migration leaving the old and poor behind, poor agricultural outcomes, limited job opportunities and severely limited old age income support, either self or from the Government, urgently calls with it a variety of social, economic, demographic and health care policy reforms changes challenges.

The Evidence from the Indian Retirement, Incomes and Savings Survey, 2005 and the Ministry of Finance and the Invest India Incomes and Savings Survey, 2007 suggest that a significant proportion of India's working poor are willing and capable of saving for their old age. But to achieve an above poverty pension, they needed supplementary savings from the government along with a secure environment where their modest savings are channelled to customized long-term savings products and earn high real returns at a low transaction cost. Most of these issues have been resolved since the launch of the National Pension Scheme (NPS) for the working poor.

Latent Need for Pension

Interestingly, while there could be a huge latent 'need' for pension among the informal sector workers with low salaries, there is little to no such 'demand' as the concept of 'pension for poor' is non-existent in India. Pension at best is considered a prerogative of few civil servants and employees covered and eligible under the 'Employees' Pension Scheme' of the EPFO. Thus, pension literacy plays a predominant role in transforming a 'latent need' into a 'demand' (Bhatnagar, 2012).

Two strategies for converting need into demand are identified. One, a longer term programme, involves raising the level of 'want', or perceived need, through attitude change. The other has a more immediate impact and involves increasing the rate at which perceived needs are converted into demands by reducing organisational barriers. It is argued that, potentially, a quarter of the adult population is susceptible to demand expansion under the second strategy. Although racial and social class differentials in perceived need would be unaffected by such a programme, inequality in demand would be reduced. A number of quite specific initiatives are suggested. First, the retentiveness of the pension system as need for social and economic security in old age can be increased, especially among marginal groups, through the establishment of a more egalitarian partner relationship, by the exercise of human relationship skills, through behavioural strategies for increasing compliance and through improved access. Secondly, improved geographical access can be achieved through tapping the 'captive' populations present in two major institutional areas, the SHGs and farmers clubs or Cooperatives. This requires mobility in deployment of resources and flexibility in negotiating the organisation and financing of care. It is only once the 'need' for pension in old age is established that one finds that people start owning the scheme. By owning the scheme one finds that people start contributing on a regular basis and not just on an initial one. Finally, more rational visit schedules, organisational arrangements and payment systems need to be developed in the average contribution practice.

Breaking the Dormancy—A Paradigm Shift in Thinking

Need Assessment is perhaps the foremost goal and precursor of creating awareness on old age income in/security. It is a shift towards a more customer-focused approach, where design is not the shiny layer around a crappy product, but a new way of thinking

In the traditional approach to market research, one would ask statistically average people to respond to a survey that asks them what they want. But Henry Ford already noticed that consumers are not able to express themselves properly when he remarked ***"If I'd asked my customers what they wanted, they'd have said a faster horse"***. That's why these techniques rarely come up with any important insights and are only useful for pointing towards incremental innovation. They will never come up with those ground-breaking, paradigm-shifting, game-changing breakthroughs that make us think '*why didn't anyone think of that before?*'

Indira Gandhi National Old Age (Social Assistance) Pension Scheme

The Scheme

Central Government is currently providing a pension amount of Rs 200 per person per month to people above 60 years of age and Rs 500 per person per month above 80 years of age under Indira Gandhi National Old Age Pension Scheme (IGNOAPS). The pension is, however, admissible to the people located below poverty line (BPL) only. The scheme provides for the concerned state governments to supplement this amount through their own resources. They are free to increase the number of beneficiaries or quantum of assistance provided they meet the excess expenditure from their own resources. Different state governments are, therefore, augmenting the scheme differently in terms of amounts of pensions as well as its coverage.

Although its umbrella programme, NSAP was launched as a Centrally Sponsored Scheme, it was transferred to State Plan in the year 2002–2003. Accordingly, the funds are released as Additional Central Assistance (ACA) by the Ministry of Finance to Finance Departments of the state governments. In case of union territories, the funds are released by the Ministry of Home Affairs. State Finance Departments in turn release funds to the implementing Departments. Funds are allocated by the Planning Commission and monitoring of implementation is with the Ministry of Rural Development.

Currently, only about 30 million people are covered under IGNOAPS out of about 104 million old people in the country.

Inadequate Coverage

India's population of 103.8 million elderly people (aged 60 or above) as per the Census 2011 figures is the second largest of such population for any country in the world. Reports of the National Commission for Enterprises in the Unorganized Sector (NCEUS) suggest that as much as 93% of India's total workforce is engaged in informal employment and is deeply steeped in poverty (NCEUS, 2007). These workers receive low wages and very little, if any, other benefits. No pension or any other retirement benefits are available to them. The Unorganized Sector Workers' Social Security Act, enacted in 2009, is only enabling legislation. The Act does not enforce any concrete social protection measures. Thus, there has been no improvement in the situation even after promulgation of the Act.

Due to these reasons, they keep on working as long as their health permits them to work. According to the Census 2011 data, 66.4% of the men in rural India and 46.1% of men in urban India continued to work even after attaining 65 years of age (MOSPI, 2016). Elderly people who cannot work continue to be engaged in unpaid domestic work while receiving support from the joint family system. Such joint family support is also shrinking rapidly due to migration of working age people and other changes in social and family structures. This leaves them without any social support.

In contrast to this situation, the coverage of population under IGNOAPS was 21.3 million in 2011–2012 as against the total population of 103.8 million old people (Jha & Acharya, 2013). This clearly implies that a large majority of elderly people in need of financial support are out of the ambit of IGNOAPS.

Due to this, a Task Force constituted by the Ministry of Rural Development, Government of India (the coordinating Ministry for NSAP) recommended that the coverage of the entire NSAP should be expanded by 1 April 2017 to cover all beneficiaries then proposed to be covered under the National Food Security Act (MoRD, 2013). This would have covered about 75% of the rural households and 50% of the urban households. The Task Force further recommended that such coverage should be expanded to be universal within a well-defined timeframe.

Implementation of the Scheme: Identification of Beneficiaries

As mentioned earlier the old age pension in India is restricted to be given to the people below poverty line (BPL). Thus, the correct identification of beneficiaries depends on the correctness of the list of BPL households. Numerous studies on the subject (e.g. Priyadarshee & Hossain, 2010) point out significant inclusion as well as exclusion errors in the BPL lists. Thus identification of old age pension beneficiaries also suffers from inclusion and exclusion errors.

Acknowledging the inaccuracies of the BPL lists and their limitations as an eligibility condition for NAOPS benefits several states have designed their own criteria for granting old age pensions. Thus, eligibility criteria for obtaining old age pensions have come to be different in different states. This creates confusion among the beneficiaries and also poses implementation and monitoring challenges for the programme.

This problem may be overcome effectively if the old age pension is made applicable universally excluding the people already in receipt of adequate retirement pensions or those paying income tax.

Implementation of the Scheme: Deficient Deliveries

Implementation of the scheme also suffers from several delivery efficiencies. Although it differs from state to state the administrative capacity for implementation and monitoring is not adequate in most of the states. A massive programme was launched by the government of India in collaboration with the state governments to open bank accounts of the beneficiaries and credit the pension benefits directly in the accounts of the beneficiaries through an identification process based on their Aadhar numbers. However, several technical glitches are reported form the field and it becomes very difficult for the beneficiaries to withdraw their money without making several rounds to the banks or the banking correspondents.

In addition, there are several instances of pension amount not being credited into the beneficiary accounts due to incomplete/wrong information entered by the person who filled application form (e.g. Agrawal, 2016). Such errors may relate to misspelling names, entering incorrect personal details such as their addresses or even making a mistake in writing account numbers (which now contain several digits in case of all the banks due to computerization of their operations). In such cases, undisbursed money goes to some suspense account in the bank. Even if the error is corrected the pensioners do not get their arrears as the process within the banks to transfer amounts from the suspense accounts to the individual accounts is quite tedious and the pensioners do not have wherewithal to influence banks to carry out this process. Government, in any case, cannot pay the same amount twice. To compound the matter, the personnel of government implementing agencies do not have knowledge about how to solve such issues and are unable to help or guide the beneficiaries.

The MoRD Task Force (MoRD, 2013) had recommended that the government of India should formulate standard procedure for recovery of undisbursed pension amounts from the banks. This recommendation does not seem to have been implemented and the problem still persists in the field.

Inadequacy of Pension Amount

All discussions on the subject invariably conclude that the pension amounts under IGNOAPS are highly inadequate in meeting the requirements of the beneficiaries.

Inadequacy of pension amounts is reflected in the fact that many among the pensioners continue to work as long as they are physically capable of doing. Kaushal (2013) finds that "the employment effects of the pension programme to be modest and much less than what has been observed in studies of most high- and middle-income countries". According to Kaushal (2013)'s calculations the pension amount needed to be at least Rs 1000 per month in 2007–2008 in order to make any dent in old age employment. Such an amount would have been more than three times the national average of the pension, state and central components taken together, in 2007–2008.

The MoRD Task Force (MoRD, 2013) recommended increasing the pension amount payable to 60–79 years age group from Rs 200 to 300 with effect from financial year 2013–2014. It further recommended that the pensions should be indexed to inflation on annual basis from 1 April 2014 using the criteria adopted for fixing dearness allowance for the central government employees. It recommended that the pension amounts should be stepped up to Rs 500 for 60–79 age group and Rs 1000 for the people above 80 years of age if the amounts after being indexed for inflation are lower than these amounts. The Task Force requested the government of India to issue advisory to state governments to augment such pension amounts with at least equal contribution from their side.

The government of India has, however, expressed its inability to raise the pension amount in response to a petition moved before the Supreme Court while mentioning that it cannot draw money from other sources (PTI, 2018). The petition had requested the Court to direct the Government of India to increase the old age pension amount to Rs 3000 per month per person.

Proposed Pension Amount Based on Poverty Line Per Capita Expenditure

According to the Rangarajan committee report, the minimum per capita average expenditure for being above the poverty line was Rs 1407 in urban areas and Rs 972 in rural areas in the year 2011–2012. By providing a weightage of 70% to the rural areas and 30% to the urban areas, on the basis of population distribution, the national average comes out to be Rs 1102.5 (Rs 1103 after rounding off). If this amount is indexed for inflation it will be Rs 1706 in today's terms.

Proposed Pension Amount Based on Minimum Wages

Minimum wages in the country are decided differently for different occupations and for different types of localities. The agriculture sector commands a minimum of the minimum wages, which are further lowest in the 'C' class localities. As per the latest orders on the subject, the minimum wage for an agriculture worker in 'C'

Table 10.2 Financial implications of expanded coverage under IGNOAPS with increased pensions

Amount of monthly pension (Rs)	Population to be covered (million)	Total pension amount to be disbursed (million)	Annual cost as % of GDP
2000	106.3 (90%)	212,600	0.14
	94.5 (80%)	189,000	0.12
1500	106.3 (90%)	159,450	0.10
	94.5 (80%)	141,750	0.09
1000	106.3 (90%)	106,300	0.07
	94.5 (80%)	94,500	0.06

class locality is Rs 321 per day (Chief Labour Commissioner-Central, 2018), which corresponds to Rs 8025 per month if the labourer works for 25 days in a month. Even if it is assumed that such workers will be getting work for 20 days only in a month, their monthly income while drawing minimum wages would be Rs 6420. If the old age pension is allowed to be half of the minimum wages for only 20 days of work in a month it will amount to be Rs 3210. In such a situation it is recommended that the pension amounts under IGNOAPS should be raised to at least Rs 1000 for the people in the age bracket 60–79 and to Rs 2000 for the people aged more than 80 years of age with a provision of at least equal contribution from the state governments.

Financial Implications of an Increased Pension Amount with Wider Coverage

We recommend that the social assistance pension should be given to all the people above 60 years of age excluding the people who are income tax payees or the people who receive pension or any other financial assistance the amount of which is not less than the proposed pension amount under social assistance.

In order to estimate the financial implications of the above proposal two scenarios have been considered. Scenario one: where 90% of the total elderly population is covered by the social assistance pension. Scenario 2: where 80% of the total elderly population is covered by the pension. Table 10.2 calculates the financial implications for both the scenarios for uniform pension amounts of Rs 2000, 1500 and 1000 across the entire elderly population.

As the accurate data regarding elderly people is not available after 2011, official projection of elderly population (available at https://data.gov.in/catalog/percentage-elderly-persons-total-population[2]) has been relied on for the following calculations.

[2] It has projections for the years 2016, 2021 and 2026.

Accordingly, old age population figure for the year 2016 was 118.10 million. India's GDP in the year 2016–2017 at the current prices was Rs 152,510,280 million.[3]

Thus, in the most generous case scenario, the government of India will need to spend about 0.14% of the total GDP on IGNOAPS. It currently spends about 0.04% of the GDP while poor countries like Botswana and Nepal spend much more for the purpose. France spends 11.5% of its GDP towards cash benefits to its elderly citizens. Germany spends 8.5%, Italy spends 12.3%, while Sweden and Finland spend 7.4% and 8.2% respectively. Even a country such as Brazil spends about 4.5% of its GDP towards old age pensions (Jha & Acharya, 2013).

Government of India has already made it clear that it does not have resources to fund any increase in the IGNOAPS. But, is it so difficult? Jha and Acharya (2013) calculate that between the years 2005–2006 to 2012–2013 the money forgone in terms of exemption and incentives in corporate income tax, personal income tax, excise duty and customs duty amounted to between 5 and 7% per annum of the GDP of the country. There are robust arguments against such exemptions and their claimed social and economic benefits, discussion on which is beyond the scope of this article. However, if corporates and others can be allowed incentives at such a high rate the elderly people of the country may be spared about 0.15% of the GDP amount.

India's current tax to GDP ratio was 11.6% in the fiscal year 2017–2018 (CMIE, 2018), which is quite low going by international standards. Due to this, the government of India has been admitting time and again that there is scope of improving this ratio (for e.g. Srivats, 2018). International experience also suggests that direct tax component within the entire tax collection, which was 49.65% in 2016–2017, is quite low and there is a reasonable possibility to increase it. The additional requirements for IGNOAPS may therefore be financed by such improved tax incomes.

Concluding Remarks

Rapidly ageing population of India is faced with a situation of highly inadequate social protection. Barring a small minority of people working in organized sector, working age population of the present will be entering an uncertain future in terms of their wellbeing. Due to lack of awareness and poor incomes, they are unable to join contributory pension plans. Even when some of them are able to join the amounts they are able to save towards their pension are so meagre that their retirement benefits are abysmal. On the other hand, only a fraction of them will be covered by social assistance pension scheme. Even in case of people receiving social assistance pension, the amount is so unreasonably low that they will not be able to meet their very basic needs through that amount.

It is, therefore, important that policymakers accord the issue due importance and design suitable measures for addressing the situation. Although social security is on

[3] available at: https://community.data.gov.in/all-india-gross-domestic-product-at-current-prices-from-2011-12-to-2016-17/. Accessed on 9 December 2018.

the concurrent list, the central government needs to take primary responsibility for providing adequate social protection for the elderly in India, as in the Indian federal structure the central government has much larger financial resources than the state governments. The central government's apathy towards social security in general and welfare of the elderly in particular is reflected in the fact that while NSAP was launched as a centrally sponsored scheme it was later moved to be Additional Central Assistance (ACA) from the Finance Ministry to the Finance Departments of the state governments. Recently, the government categorically denied to consider any upward revision of IGNOAPS pensions. Such attitude of the central government towards the people who contributed to build this nation through their working lives is even more deplorable in view of the fact that India spends much less on old age pensions and social security measures than other poorer countries.

References

Agrawal, V. (2016). The elderly in India are made to live on Rs. 500 a month. But there's a bigger problem. *YKA-Youth ki Awaaz*. Retrieved from https://www.youthkiawaaz.com/2016/01/old-age-pension-schemes-india/

Arokiasamy, P., Bloom, D., Lee, J., Feeney, K., & Ozolins, M. (Forthcoming). Longitudinal aging study in India: Vision, design, implementation, and some early results. In James P. Smith & M. Majmundar (Eds.), *Aging in Asia: Findings from new and emerging data initiatives*. The National Academies Press.

Arun, S., & Arun, T. (2001). Gender issues in social security policy in Kerala,India. *International Social Security Review, 54*(4), 93–110.

Avato, J., Koettl, J., & Sabates-Wheeler, R. (2009). Social security regimes, global estimates, and good practices: The status of social protection for international migrants. *World Development, 38*(4), 455–466.

Barrientos, A., & Hulme, D. (2008). Embedding social protection in the developing world. In A. Barrientos & D. Hulme (Eds.), *Social protection for the poor and the poorest: Concepts, policies and politics* (pp. 315–330). Palgrave Macmillan.

Barrientos, A., & Hulme, D. (2008). Social protection for the poor and the poorest: An introduction. In A. Barrientos & D. Hulme (Eds.), *Social protection for the poor and the poorest: Concepts, policies and politics* (pp. 1–18). Palgrave Macmillan.

Barrientos, A., & Lloyd-Sherlock, P. (2002). *Non-contributory pensions and social protection* (Discussion paper 12). Issues in social protection. ILO.

Bhatnagar, K. V. (2014). Return and retirement funds for Indian migrant working women in ECR countries. In *Global Diasporas and Development* (pp. 355–368). Springer.

Bhatnagar, K. V. (2012, July). Bangladesh old age income social in/security: On razor's edge. *American Chamber, 5*(3), 24–32.

Chief Labour Commissioner-Central. (2018). File No. 1/38 (1)/2018-LS-II, dated 28 September 2018. Retrieved from https://clc.gov.in/clc/node/586

CMIE. (2018). Gross tax revenue to GDP ratio on a rise since 2015–16. *Centre for Monitoring of Indian Economy*. Retrieved from https://www.cmie.com/kommon/bin/sr.php?kall=warticle&dt=2018-02-05%2012:14:08&msec=846

Dreze, J., & Sen, A. (1991). Public action for social security: Foundations and strategy. In E. Ahmed, J. Dreze, J. Hills, & A. Sen (Eds.), *Social Security in developing countries* (pp. 3–40). Oxford University Press.

Giang, T. L. (2013). Social protection for older people in Vietnam: Role, challenges and reform options. *Malaysian Journal of Economic Studies, 50*(2), 207–219.

Government of India. (2006). *Report on social security for unorganized workers.* National Commission for Enterprises in the Unorganized Sector.

Government of India. (n.d.). *Atal Pension Yojana: A Guaranteed pension scheme of Govt. of India.* Retrieved from https://www.india.gov.in/spotlight/atal-pension-yojana

Haub, C., & Gribble, J. (2011). The world at 7 billion. *Population Bulletin, 66*(2).

IIMS Dataworks, NABARD, SADHAN, ISMW & IIMPS. (2008). *Towards a financially inclusive financial system: financial services demand and utilisation by India's low income workforce.*

Jha, P., & Acharya, N. (2013). Social security for elderly in India: A note on old age pension. *Helpage India Research & Development Journal, 19*(2), 3–15.

Kaushal, N. (2014). Economics of public pension: Analysing India's old-age pension scheme. *Ideas for India.* Retrieved from https://www.ideasforindia.in/topics/urbanisation/economics-of-public-pension-analysing-indias-old-age-pension-scheme.html

Kaushal, N. (2013). *How public pensions affect elderly labour supply and well-being: Evidence from India* (Working Paper 19088. NBER Working paper series, National Bureau of Economic Research), Cambridge, MA.

Lund, F., & Srinivas, S. (2000). *Learning from experience: A gendered approach to social protection for workers in the informal economy. STEP and WIEGO.* ILO.

MoF (2007). *Invest India income and savings survey.* Ministry of Finance, Government of India.

MoRD. (2013, March). *Proposal for comprehensive national social assistance programme,* Report of the Task Force. Ministry of Rural Development, Government of India.

MoSPI. (2016). *Elderly in India 2016.* Central Statistics Office, Social Statistics Division, Ministry of Statistics and Programme Implementation, Government of India.

Munro, L. T. (2008). Risks, needs and rights: Compatible or contradictory bases for social protection. In A. Barrientos & D. Hulme (Eds.), *Social protection for the poor and the poorest: Concepts, policies and politics* (pp. 27–46). Palgrave Macmillan.

NCEUS. (2007). *Report of National Commission for enterprises in the unorganised sector.* Retrieved from www.nceus.gov.in

Norton, A., Conway, T., & Foster, M. (2001). *Social protection concepts and approaches: Implications for policy and practice in international development. Centre for Aid and Public Expenditure* (ODI Working Paper, No 143). Overseas Development Institute.

Paitoonpong, S., Abe, S., & Puopongsakorn, N. (2008). The meaning of "social safety nets. *Journal of Asian Economics, 19*, 467–473.

Priyadarshee, A. (2011). Evolution of social protection: A political economy perspective. *The Indian Economy Review, 8* (Quarterly issue 16 May–15 August 2011), 118–127.

Priyadarshee, A., & Hossain, F. (2010). Decentralisation, service delivery, and people's perspectives: Empirical observations on selected social protection programmes in India. *International Journal of Public Administration, 33*(12), 752–756.

PTI. (2018, November 30). Can't draw funds from other places for old age pension: Centre to Supreme Court. *The Economic Times.* Retrieved from https://economictimes.indiatimes.com/news/politics-and-nation/cant-draw-funds-from-other-places-for-old-age-pension-centre-to-supreme-court/articleshow/66886911.cms

Qazi, M. (2019). Micro-pensions can boost security for India's elderly poor. *The Asian Age.* Retrieved from https://www.asianage.com/india/all-india/210119/micro-pensions-can-boost-security-for-indias-elderly-poor.html

Sabates-Wheeler, R., & Devereux, S. (2008). Transformative social protection: The currency of social justice. In A. Barrientos & D. Hulme (Eds.), *Social protection for the poor and the poorest: Concepts, policies and politics* (pp. 64–84). Palgrave Macmillan.

Srivats, K. (2018, June 18). Need to improve tax GDP ratio by 1.5 percentage points: Jaitly, 2018. *The Hindu.* Retrieved from https://www.thehindubusinessline.com/economy/need-to-increase-tax-gdp-ratio-by-15-percentage-points-jaitley/article24191374.ece

Unni, J., & Rani, U. (2003). *Regional overview of social protection of informal workers in Asia: Insecurities, instruments and institutional arrangements* (Discussion Paper Series, No. 14), Gender & Development. Economic and Social Commission for Asia and the Pacific. Retrieved from http://www.unescap.org/esid/gad/Publication/DiscussionPapers/14/Paper14.pdf

Chapter 11
Elderly as Family Caregivers: Burden and Challenges in India

Ankita Kumari and T. V. Sekher

Abstract Older people are caregivers rather than care–recipients in many respects, where they provide emotional, personal and financial support to younger generations. The primary focus of this study is to examine the nature and extent of older adults (50+ years) involvement in caregiving activities and the impact of caregiving on caregivers. The study used data from the WHO sponsored "Study on Global AGEing and Adult Health (SAGE)" in India. It was evident that caregiving responsibilities at home had adverse consequences on elderly. Age, gender, traditions, economic status and the complexity of the situation determine the caregiving roles in most Indian households. It is important to ensure that caregivers can fulfil their roles without compromising their own health, leisure and well-being.

Keywords Elderly · Caregiving · Impact of caregiving · Study on Global AGEing and Adult Health (SAGE) · India

Introduction

Ageing: Global and Indian Scenario

One of the most distinctive demographic phenomena experienced by the world today is population ageing, wherein a large share of population constitutes the older persons (aged 60 years and above). The world population is ageing at a very rapid pace and this is very clearly evident in developed countries. People are considered old when they observe certain changes in their activities as they are more prone to diseases, ill health and sickness and their body becomes weak and less energetic.

The United Nations defines a country as "Ageing" or "Greying Nation" where the proportion of people over 60 years of age has reached at least 7% of the total population. The United Nations has projected that by 2050, approximately 2 billion global population will be elderly and out of that 80% of them will be residing in the developing nations. According to India's National Policy on Older Persons (Govt. of

A. Kumari · T. V. Sekher (✉)
International Institute for Population Sciences (IIPS), Mumbai, India

M. K. Shankardass (ed.), *Gerontological Concerns and Responses in India*,
https://doi.org/10.1007/978-981-16-4764-2_11

India, 1999), senior citizens are defined as those who are of age 60 years and above. So, a major challenge of this century for India and for all developing countries will be the ageing of their population and its inevitable consequences.

There has been a constant growth in the elderly's population across the globe, but the pace of growth has recently accelerated (United Nations, 2011). All the developed countries have already reached an advanced stage of ageing and the developing countries are following its way to a similar scenario alarmingly. Globally, elderly population is growing faster than all younger age groups. By 2017, there was an estimated 962 million people aged 60 years and above across the world, comprising 13% of the total global population and the UN report stated that the population was growing at a rate of about 3% per year. It has been projected that there will be one elderly accounting for every six persons globally. By the middle of the twenty-first century, one in every five people will be aged 60 years or over (United Nations, 2017).

India, now home to 1.3 billion people, is projected to overtake China in less than a decade to become the world's most populous country (PRB, 2012). There has been an increase in the population of India from 683 million in 1981 to 1.21 billion in 2011, with approximately 9% of the total population accounting for aged 60 years and above (Census of India, 2011). Bloom (2012) calls the share of India's population aged 50 years and older relatively small (16%) and anticipated that in future, India might experience rapid growth in their share of its older population. The growth rate of elderly population is three times higher than the overall population, clearly implying that ageing of the population will be a major challenge for India in the coming decades. With the number progressively increasing, gradually India is moving towards becoming an aged country, as the current youth population is expected to last only few more decades to come. The elderly population of India has increased from 12.1 million in 1901 to approximately 104 million in 2011. According to official population projections, it has been anticipated that the elderly population will increase to approximately 140 million by 2021 and more than 315 million by 2050 (Govt. of India, 2011). The amount of supportive socio-economic and emotional infrastructure needed to take care of this fast-growing segment of population is huge and governments are least prepared to face this challenge.

India's Cultural Context and Aspects of Caregiving

India is a country where culture and traditions have been valued considerably where people use to live with their families, relatives and elder ones under the same roof with integrity and harmony. The role of a caregiver in India was naturally accepted in the society where people believed in joint family system and respected older generation, family values and its virtues. In general, the elderly is dependent on the younger family members for physical assistance and psychological support. For caregiving, they are not just dependent on a single person, as all the family members take turns in providing care (Radhakrisna, 2013). But this scenario has undergone significant changes-many old parents are staying alone fending for themselves and living with insecurity and old age problems without anyone to look after them.

Due to various changes in demographic structure of Indian population over time, there have been changes observed in social, cultural and family structure too.

- The joint family system prevalent earlier in India has changed into more nuclear families. Young people are migrating due to various reasons and this has affected the family structure in recent decades, even in rural areas.
- As the life expectancy of the Indians has been increasing, the population of very old has also increased over time. Thus, the children, who are potential caregivers, are also old and contribute to caregiving tasks besides the fact that they also need support and care from their children.
- In India, the age at marriage has increased and the fertility level has decreased considerably in last decades. The women are becoming more educated and their participation in labour market has brought a huge change in family situations too.

The young adults in order to build their careers are delaying their marriage. Once married, they prefer to delay the pregnancy as much as possible to concentrate on their work. Since young adults prefer to work nowadays even after their marriage and pregnancy, they are left with no choice but to rely on their parents to take care of their children. Thus, in many households, the elderly is contributing more as a caregiver than as a care recipient.

As Bookman and Kimbrel (2011) observed that demographic changes that occur in a country like delayed marriage and childbearing for young adults, decreased family size and changes in family composition and structure are complicating the challenges for care provision and caregiving tasks. Increased longevity among elders extends the years of caregiving by their adult children and may require their grandchildren to become caregivers as well. But nowadays, the dual-earner couples or the single-parent household has replaced the previously dominant family type of a sole wage-earner father with a wife/mother who stayed at home to raise children. Now, most of the households have working mothers/wifes. This changes the overall outlook of caregiving dimension. So, the young married couple, who were responsible for taking care of their children and the elderly are not present in the household anymore to carry out their responsibilities of caregiving. Thus, the number of grandparents looking after their grandchildren is increasing.

Based on this scenario, this paper is an attempt to reflect upon the caregiving role of elderly. Elderly are viewed as burden because of their decrease in participation in labour force and household activities and most importantly, their deteriorating health demands the attention of family members to take care of them. But, we often forget the fact that these elderly have been providing care and continues to do so in many different ways to their younger ones.

Caregiving is an act of care given by an individual who helps and assists others with activities of daily living or medical tasks without being paid. Caregiving is defined as providing unpaid assistance for the physical and emotional needs of another person, ranging from partial assistance to 24-h care, depending on the condition of the care recipient (Clark & Weber, 1997).

The time spent in providing care can be divided into—shorter or longer duration depending on the conditions of the care recipient. Longer sessions of caregiving roles can impact the social life of the caregiver who is constantly involved in taking care of the person facing co-morbidities or disabilities. Short term care does not have much significant effect on the caregivers as it is manageable and does not require the caregiver to give up on all other important roles and priorities in life. The caregiving roles can be taken up by anyone in the family or people around—child, parents, grandparents, close relatives, or even friends. Caregiving can differ in terms of the type of care (physically, emotionally, or financially) being provided, depending on who requires the care- child, adult, or elderly. Caregivers can provide a wide range of services, depending on the degree of disability, economic situation and living environment of the older person. Caregiving activities include assisting an individual in managing their day to day life activities such as eating, bathing, dressing, laundry, movement, or managing medications, etc. The caregiver can also take up the responsibilities to manage financial and legal matters pertaining to care-recipient's needs.

Although a caregiver can be anyone, a spouse, child, friend, or neighbour, usually it is a woman and in a conventional Indian family context, caregiver is mostly a married women providing care to each member of her family. According to a study done by Clark and Weber (1997), there are approximately 2 million women as a part of sandwich generation, simultaneously taking care of their children as well as their parents. In India, the caregiver's role is usually taken up by the spouses and majority of these caregivers are women who possess the ability to manage time for their caregiving responsibilities, have patience and tolerance to take up the nursing roles and have a tendency to help out her loved ones. The individuals who take up the responsibilities to provide care to the people suffering with multiple morbidities and disabilities are considered great assets to their family and society (Schultz & Beach, 1999). Although neighbours and friends may help, about 80% of help in the home (physical, emotional, social and economic) is provided by family caregivers. The magnitude and kind of family caregiving depend on various factors, i.e. economic resources, household composition, relationship status, one's own time and energy, health status and other essential needs of the other family members. Family caregiving can be demanding and can range from minimal assistance (e.g. checking in intermittently) to complex fulltime care. A study pointed out that, family caregiving can be time consuming and can take up to a minimum of 4 h a day to take care of everything (Clark & Weber, 1997).

Caregiving can be distinguished broadly into two categories—formal and informal. Usually, formal caregiving is a paid service provided by health professionals, institutions, or sometimes welfare organizations who assist individual in taking care of them in case they are incapable to look after themselves. Informal caregiving can be defined as unpaid services provided by family members, relatives and close friends who usually take care of all their needs.

Furthermore, Caregivers can be categorized as—primary caregivers and secondary caregivers. The individuals who take up the main responsibility of caregiving and are directly involved in providing care to the care-recipients are known as Primary Caregivers. Secondary caregivers can be termed for those individuals who indirectly provide care by assisting the primary caregivers in managing their caregiving responsibilities. The secondary caregivers are less involved in providing personal care (ADL) such as bathing, dressing, toileting, etc. but can assist in the instrumental activities of daily living (IADL) such as managing medications, transportation, paying bills, etc. These secondary caregivers can be another family member, a distant relative, a close friend, or a neighbour of the care-recipients. Caregiving has two aspects in our society. When we think about care, an immediate thought that passes through our mind is that care needs to be given to older people but it's not always like that. Sometimes it's the younger ones who are getting the love, attention and care from the elderly. But the care and support provided by them are often overlooked.

Informal caregiving is very common in Indian society. In most of the households, three generations are living together and they give care to the needy members such as children, old or the disabled. According to a study of Indian families, Gupta (2009) found that although financial assistance is aided by family members in a multigenerational family system, might not necessarily support the main primary caregivers in providing personal care such as eating, bathing and toileting. This study also pointed out that level of burden pertaining to caregiving is directly related to number of caregiving tasks provided by the caregiver and thus, the burden increases with the increase in these tasks. The higher the age of the caregiver, the greater the burden in providing care for the elderly. Consistent with other studies, women caregivers experience greater burden as compared to men caregivers in India and this might hold true for old age caregivers too. The Indian female caregivers in all age groups feel that they are expected to provide care for their parents, in-laws, spouse, children, grandchildren, etc. and is not much of their choice but rather more of a duty to abide by the caregiving responsibilities, which is considered much of a normative custom in India.

There are several aspects where very little research has been done in the Indian context, on the issue related to caregiving to and by the elderly.

So, the objectives of the present study are as follows:

- To examine the extent and nature of caregiving activities among older adults and elderly in India.
- To understand the assistance received by the elderly in carrying out the task of caregiving.
- To study the impact of caregiving responsibilities on caregivers.

Materials and Methods

The research is based on the data available from Study on Global AGEing and Adult Health (SAGE), Wave-1 survey in India, which was carried out in 2007. SAGE was implemented in six countries—China, Ghana, India, Mexico, South Africa and

Russian Federation—during 2007–2010. SAGE is a longitudinal, cross sectional, household, face-to-face survey, which the World Health Organization (WHO) initiated. SAGE-India was implemented in six states—Assam, Karnataka, Maharashtra, Rajasthan, Uttar Pradesh and West Bengal. The target population in the SAGE survey is those aged 18 years and above with an emphasis on population aged 50+ years. A multistage stratified clustered sample design was used uniformly in all the countries. SAGE Wave 1, India, included a total of 11,230 samples distributed as: 4670 samples for persons in the age group 18–49 years (Men—1045 and Women—3625) and 6560 samples for persons aged 50+ years (Men—3304 men and Women—3256) (IIPS & WHO, 2013).

Dependent variables: The dependent variables considered for the present analysis is the type of care (five types- Financial, Social, Health, Physical, Personal), Personal care (six types-Bathing, Eating, Dressing, Toileting, Moving, Incontinence), Duration of care, Average Time spent, relationship and the impact of the caregiving.

Independent variables: The various independent variables used in the study are as follows:

- Age Group: Considering the older adults with age starting from 50 years and above, i.e. 50–59, 60–69 and 70+. The 50–59 age group is considered as the reference category.
- Sex: The variable is categorized as males and females and males are considered as the reference category.
- Place of Residence: Rural and Urban. Urban is considered as the reference category.
- Marital Status: This variable is categorized into three different categories—Never Married, Currently Married and Divorced/Separated/Widowed. Never married is considered as the reference category in the analysis.
- Educational Status: The variable is categorized into four categories as—No Formal Education, Primary School Education, Secondary School Education and High School Education & above. No formal education is considered as the reference category.
- Wealth Tercile: The wealth tercile was categorized into three as—Lowest, Middle and Highest. Lowest wealth tercile is considered as the reference category.

For the purpose of analysis, we are considering all the persons in the age group of 50 years and above in this study. The word 'elderly' and 'older adults' have been used interchangeably in this study meaning all adults aged 50 years and above.

Both bi-variate and multi-variate analyses were carried out. Overall, the percentage distribution for the respondents aged 50 years and above in context to various dependent variables has been calculated using bi-variate analysis to show the prevalence of the elderly people providing care. All the covariates have been tested for association with the dependent variable using bi-variate technique and only those variables which are found to be significant, have been used further in the analysis by using logistic regression.

Binary Logistic Regression is used to estimate the differentials among the various types of care provided to the adults by the older adults in accordance with various

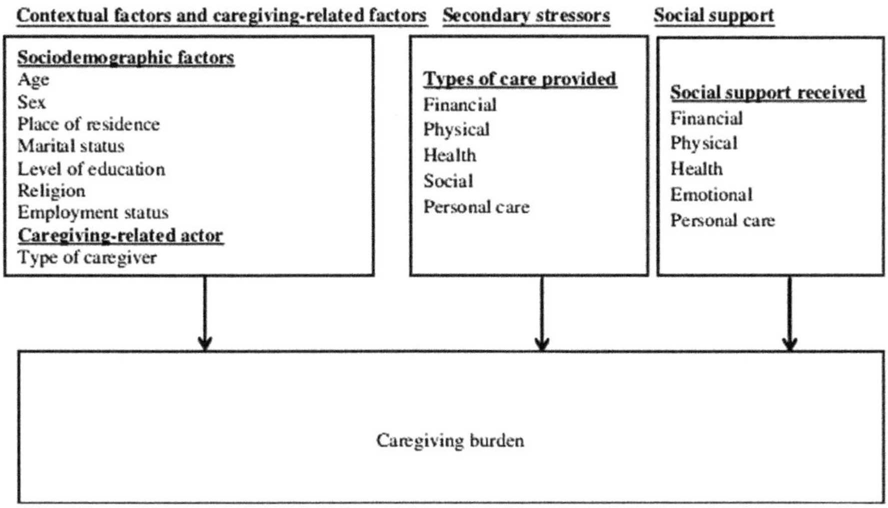

Fig. 11.1 Conceptual framework (Conde-Sala et al., 2010; Sanuade & Boatemaa, 2015)

background characteristics. Similarly, Ordered Logistic Regression is used to analyze the impact of the caregiving responsibility on caregivers by their background characteristics.

Conceptual Framework on Burden of Caregiving

The conceptual framework, adopted in this study, emphasizes the interdependence and independence of all factors related to stress of family caregivers (Conde-Sala et al., 2010; Sanuade & Boatemaa, 2015). This includes contextual stressors, primary stressors, secondary stressors and social support (Fig. 11.1).

Results and Discussions

Here, we have looked into various aspects of caregiving, by exploring the different types of care, i.e. financial care, social/emotional care, health care, physical care, personal care and the duration of time spent in providing the care. We have also explored the extent and nature of various caregiving activities and the roles played by elderly.

The results (Table 11.1) shows five different types of care, i.e. financial, social, health, physical and personal provided by the elderly (aged 50 years and above) by background characteristics of the older adults- age, sex, place of residence, marital status, education and the wealth status. It can be seen that with increasing age, a

Table 11.1 Percentage distribution of older adults according to type of care provided by background characteristics, India

Background characteristics	Type of care provided					Total number
	Financial	Social	Health	Physical	Personal	
Age group						
50–59 years	5.1	4.7	6.5	4.8	4.3	2939
60–69 years	4.2	4.1	5.3	3.9	4.3	2235
70+ years	2.8	2.0	2.2	1.8	2.3	1386
Sex						
Male	6.0	3.7	4.9	3.7	2.5	3304
Female	2.7	4.3	5.6	4.1	5.4	3256
Place of residence						
Urban	3.7	2.1	4.5	2.5	4.5	1676
Rural	4.7	4.7	5.6	4.5	3.7	4884
Marital status						
Never married	4.4	2.6	4.7	5.4	4.7	64
Currently married	5.1	4.5	6.0	4.4	4.2	4862
[a]Div./[b]Sep./[c]Wid.	2.0	2.2	2.8	2.1	2.9	1634
Education level						
No education	3.4	3.6	4.7	3.2	4.0	3365
Primary	5.0	3.8	5.3	4.4	4.4	1675
Secondary	5.1	5.4	7.1	5.2	4.3	654
High school and above	6.4	5.4	7.0	6.4	3.8	866
Wealth tercile						
Lowest	4.6	4.5	5.0	4.0	3.6	2624
Middle	5.1	2.6	6.4	3.4	5.5	1313
Highest	3.7	4.0	5.0	4.0	3.5	2623

[a]Divorced
[b]Separated
[c]Widowed

decreasing trend of providing all types of care is prevalent among the elderly in India. As people get older (reaching 70 years and above), there is a drastic fall in the percentage of elderly providing care. The major reasons could be that since their capabilities, health and financial status deteriorates, their ability to provide care also gets affected. In India, generally, it is expected that financial and physical care will be extended more by the male caregiver in comparison to female caregivers and it is evident, that the amount of financial care provided more by males (6%) than females (3%) as compared to any other type of care whereas, females have provided more of the other type of care especially the personal care (5%).

Similarly, it is expected that caregiver's marital status is likely to influence their extent of care provided to others. So, it was observed from Table 11.1, that currently married elderly have provided more of the financial (5%), social/emotional (5%) and health care (6%) whereas, never married are providing more of the physical and the personal care to the other family or non-family members. Divorced/Separated and widowed are less likely to provide any type of care as they themselves might be dependent on others in all aspects. Further, elderly with more educational background provided more care to others and for almost all the types of care except for the personal care, which decreased slightly for the more educated ones. Educational status has an influence on caregiving tasks as more educated elderly are capable to provide care to others due to better understanding and capability to handle the situation that emerges while providing care to other people, be it their children, grand children, or other relatives and friends.

Table 11.2 provides state-level variations in different types of care provided by older adults to others. Overall, 4% of older adults reported assisting financially and taking care of social needs (4%), 5% supported in health-based matters and approximately 4% of them reported extending support each for physical assistance and personal care. Looking at the state level, it was quite clear that, older adults residing in Maharashtra, Rajasthan and Uttar Pradesh were more likely to extend support in terms of caregiving, while West Bengal reported least amount of support being provided in all the aspects of care given by the older adults.

The state of Rajasthan and Uttar Pradesh has higher percentage of elderly providing care and that could be possible as these states have a more rural share of population where families are close knitted and more influenced by traditional customs of family values.

Now, the dependent variable is the type of care (financial, social, health, physical, personal) which is dichotomous in nature and is categorical, we applied Binary Logistic Regression in order to check the relationship of the dependent variable with six different independent variables to capture the effects of the confounding factors on the dependent variables. Binary logistic regression is used to determine the effects of various types of care according to background characteristics (Table 11.3). Elderly in the age group 60–69 years, 70 years and above are less inclined

Table 11.2 Percentage distribution of older adults according to types of care provided by States and India

Type of care	States						INDIA (pooled)
	Assam	Karnataka	Maharashtra	Rajasthan	Uttar Pradesh	West Bengal	
Financial	2.0	4.0	5.5	5.7	5.8	0.5	4.4
Social	2.5	3.9	2.7	7.0	5.9	0.4	4.0
Health	3.6	5.7	6.4	5.4	6.4	1.8	5.3
Physical	5.2	4.1	2.4	4.8	5.3	2.1	3.9
Personal	2.5	4.0	5.2	5.5	3.5	2.5	3.9

Table 11.3 Binary logistic regression on types of care provided by the older adults by background characteristics

Explanatory variable	Financial		Social		Health		Physical		Personal	
	Odds ratio	*p*-value	Odds ratio	*p*-value	Odds ratio	*p*-value	Odds ratio	*p*-value	Odds ratio	*p*-value
Age group										
50–59 years®										
60–69 years	0.82	0.29	1.01	0.95	0.85	0.33	0.81	0.23	1.03	0.88
70+ years	0.46***	0.00	0.75	0.22	0.60**	0.03	0.59**	0.03	0.78	0.33
Sex										
Male®										
Female	0.19***	0.00	1.12	0.50	1.31*	0.10	1.18	0.36	2.63***	0.00
Place of residence										
Urban®										
Rural	0.82	0.36	1.45*	0.06	0.93	0.71	1.43*	0.08	0.68*	0.07
Marital status										
Never married®										
Currently married	1.26	0.13	2.53	0.41	0.77	0.75	0.28	0.16	0.41	0.31
[a]Div./[b]Sep./[c]Wid.	0.29	0.17	2.09	0.52	0.61	0.57	0.22*	0.10	0.35	0.24
Education level										
No education®										
Primary	0.93	0.72	0.57***	0.01	0.85	0.40	1.04	0.86	1.35	0.43
Secondary	1.07	0.82	0.96	0.90	1.03	0.91	0.99	0.98	0.73	0.31
High school and above	0.99	0.96	0.79	0.40	1.82	0.46	1.09	0.78	0.54*	0.07
Wealth tercile										

(continued)

Table 11.3 (continued)

Explanatory variable	Financial		Social		Health		Physical		Personal	
	Odds ratio	*p*-value	Odds ratio	*p*-value	Odds ratio	*p*-value	Odds ratio	*p*-value	Odds ratio	*p*-value
Lowest®										
Middle	0.76	0.24	0.81	0.33	1.02	0.94	0.77	0.25	1.42	0.71
Highest	0.79	0.25	1.13	0.52	1.02	0.91	1.00	1.00	0.74	0.13
Constant	6.22	0.05	0.20	0.16	1.02	0.98	1.51	0.66	1.18	0.86

***1% significant, **5% significant, *10% significant

[a]Divorced

[b]Separated

[c]Widowed

towards supporting financially and all the other types of care except for the social support. Female elderlies are less likely to provide financial care compared to the male elderly, whereas in all other types of care females are more likely to provide care especially personal care. Rural elderly are less likely to provide financial, health and personal care respectively while more likely to provide social and physical care as compared to the urban elderly. On average, educated people are less likely to provide care in comparison to the uneducated elderly. Lastly, it can be inferred that elderly belonging to middle-income group is more likely and those belonging to highest income group is less likely to provide personal care.

The personal care provided by any individual to others which are hands-on care with activities of daily living (ADL) are bathing, eating, dressing, toileting, moving and incontinence. Table 11.4 shows personal care provided by the elderly (50 years and above) by background characteristics. It can be seen that with the increase in ages, especially male elderly, follows a declining trend in providing personal care. Female elderly provided maximum personal care as compared to male elderly. Females are the main providers of personal types of care—bathing (3.9%), eating (3.5%), dressing (3.8%), toileting (4%), moving (2.4%) and incontinence (1.6%) than the males. Irrespective of age, women in India are expected to take care of and provide care to all members of the household. A noticeable finding is that the unmarried older adults provided more personal care, be it bathing (4.7%), eating (4.7%), dressing (4.7%), toileting (4.7%), or moving (2.6%) as compared to married elderly. Educational status of the elderly does not affect much in care providing tasks.

Table 11.5 provides the state-level variations in the personal care provided by older adults to others in the household. Overall, 2.6% of older adults provided bathing care, 2.5% helped in eating, 2% in dressing, 2.3% with toileting and 2% helped moving around. At state level, older adults residing in Uttar Pradesh, Rajasthan and Karnataka reported that they were more likely to support by helping in various types of personal care whereas, West Bengal reported lowest percentage of older adults providing different types of personal care to others.

The study also tried to capture the duration of care given by the elderly (aged 50 years and above). The time spent by the elderly caregivers in providing help to others with their activities of daily living (ADL) like bathing, toileting, dressing, etc. or instrumental activity of daily living (IADL) like helping in managing financial problems, taking them to doctors, etc. depends upon the kind of assistance they are receiving. Care can be given for short as well as long duration depending upon the situation.

The analysis shows that with increasing age, the percentage of people providing care for long duration of time decreases. Gender differentials can be acknowledged here, as we see that for longer duration of time (for more than one month), higher percentage of females are providing care in comparison to their male counterparts. In fact, rural elderly are seen to contributing more time in caregiving as compared to urban elderly. Elderly tend to elongate their duration for providing care irrespective of whether they are illiterate or highly educated (Table 11.6).

Table 11.7 shows the average time spent per day by the elderly in providing care. Higher percentage of the oldest (70+) seems to spend less number of hours

Table 11.4 Percentage distribution of older adults according to the type of personal care provided by background characteristics, India

Background characteristics	Type of personal care provided						Total number
	Bathing	Eating	Dressing	Toileting	Moving	Incontinence	
Age group							
50–59 years	3.0	3.0	2.8	3.2	2.4	1.4	2939
60–69 years	2.7	2.8	2.4	3.3	1.9	1.5	2235
70+ years	0.8	1.7	1.5	0.5	0.7	0.4	1386
Sex							
Male	1.1	1.8	1.0	1.4	1.4	0.9	3304
Female	3.9	3.5	3.8	4.0	2.4	1.6	3256
Place of residence							
Urban	2.2	3.8	3.2	3.4	1.7	1.6	1676
Rural	2.6	2.2	2.1	2.4	2.0	1.1	4884
Marital status							
Never married	4.7	4.7	4.7	4.7	2.6	0.8	64
Currently married	2.5	2.8	2.5	2.8	2.0	1.3	4862
[a]Div./[b]Sep./[c]Wid.	2.3	2.2	1.7	2.3	1.4	1.0	1634
Education level							
No education	2.8	2.4	2.1	2.3	1.4	0.8	3365
Primary	2.7	3.1	2.5	2.4	2.5	1.2	1675
Secondary	2.7	2.8	1.9	2.1	3.1	1.4	654
High school and above	2.1	2.9	1.5	2.8	2.1	1.5	866
Wealth tercile							
Lowest	2.5	1.7	1.9	2.5	2.0	1.1	2624
Middle	2.7	4.8	3.6	3.3	2.0	2.2	1313
Highest	2.4	2.7	2.3	2.6	1.7	0.9	2623

[a]Divorced
[b]Separated
[c]Widowed

for caregiving (less than 3 h in a day) while the others contribute for longest period of time, exceeding more than 12 h sometimes. As expected, males spend lesser hours in comparison to females. With an increase in the amount of hours spent in caregiving, percentage of female caregivers with respect to male caregivers increases too. Overall, older adults in rural areas are spending more time than urban residents providing the care. Higher percentage of currently married older adults overall has spent maximum hours daily to provide care. Less educated and middle-income group elderly has contributed the most in time-spent daily for providing care to the adults.

Table 11.5 Percentage distribution of older adults according to types of personal care by States and India

Type of personal care	States						INDIA (pooled)
	Assam	Karnataka	Maharashtra	Rajasthan	Uttar Pradesh	West Bengal	
Bathing	2.1	3.3	1.3	3.8	2.9	1.8	2.6
Eating	2.2	2.6	2.6	4.1	2.4	0.8	2.5
Dressing	2.1	2.2	1.9	2.0	2.4	1.2	2.0
Toileting	1.5	2.6	1.5	3.3	2.6	1.6	2.3
Moving	1.5	1.6	2.1	3.4	2.1	0.9	2.0
Incontinence	0.1	1.1	1.3	1.3	0.9	0.9	1.0

In the course of providing care, many a time, people have to face lots of difficulties and have to sacrifice their own personal needs. So, we are going to discuss the major impact of caregiving on the older adult caregivers and find out that in the process of providing the care, whether they are receiving any assistance or support and if at all they are receiving such assistance then, who are those people assisting them in doing so? Therefore, we look into the different types of assistance received by the elderly for providing care. These may vary from financial help to physical or personal help.

Table 11.8 shows the various types of assistance received by the older adults in providing care by their background characteristics. The most common type of support or assistance received by elderly caregivers is financial help and with an increase in age, an increasing trend of receiving support or assistance can be seen. The oldest adults (70+) have received maximum help in almost all types of assistance. Female elderly have received maximum assistance from others compared to the male caregivers in all aspects. Illiterate elderly have received the maximum assistance compared to educated elderly. Highest proportion among middle-income groups has received the most support and assistance for caregiving.

Now, the question arises that who is providing the assistance to these older adults in caregiving. Table 11.9 will show who exactly helps these older adults in their caregiving tasks. With increasing age, female elderly has received the maximum assistance from other family members who live outside the household; rural elderly have received most of the assistance from the family members outside and from the neighbours. With an increase in education level, there was a declining trend in the percentage of elderly receiving assistance from family members outside the households, neighbours and the community. Older adults belonging to middle-income groups received more help from everybody.

The various impact of caregiving on the caregivers is also very important to understand. For capturing the impact of caregiving, we have considered few aspects like whether the caregivers were able to have enough food to eat, or were having enough sleep or not or they were left with enough energy after the caregiving task or not. We also consider whether they were paying attention towards their own health care and were able to visit their friends and relatives, just the way they were

Table 11.6 Percentage distribution of older adults according to time spent for caregiving by background characteristics, India

Background characteristics	Duration of time spent for caregiving				Total number
	1 month	1–3 months	3–6 months	More than 6 months	
Age group					
50–59 years	5.6	1.9	1.1	5.1	2939
60–69 years	4.5	2.1	1.1	5.1	2235
70+ years	4.0	1.2	0.9	3.7	1386
Sex					
Male	5.3	1.8	0.9	4.6	3304
Female	4.5	1.9	1.3	5.0	3256
Place of residence					
Urban	4.5	1.4	1.0	3.9	1676
Rural	5.0	2.0	1.1	5.1	4884
Marital status					
Never married	3.1	3.1	3.1	0.0	64
Currently married	5.4	1.9	1.1	5.4	4862
[a]Div./[b]Sep./[c]Wid.	3.5	1.7	0.8	3.1	1634
Education level					
No education	5.5	1.8	1.2	4.7	3365
Primary	6.9	2.2	0.7	6.0	1675
Secondary	5.5	0.9	0.9	3.1	654
High school and above	3.6	1.5	0.7	3.4	866
Wealth tercile					
Lowest	4.5	1.5	1.2	5.1	2624
Middle	5.6	1.7	1.1	3.7	1313
Highest	4.9	2.2	0.9	5.0	2623

[a]Divorced
[b]Separated
[c]Widowed

able to do so before they were not burdened with caregiving tasks. A composite score was generated using all the variables mentioned with the help of principal component analysis and this composite score is further categorized into three different categories—mild, moderate and severe difficulties.

Table 11.10 shows the impact of caregiving on the caregivers by age group, sex, place of residence and marital status. More of the oldest-old (70+) respondents have reported as experiencing severe difficulty in providing care compared to the

Table 11.7 Percentage distribution of older adults according to average time spent (per day) for caregiving by background characteristics, India

Background characteristics	Average time spent per day for caregiving				Total number
	Less than 3 h	3 h to less than 6 h	6–12 h	More than 12 h	
Age group					
50–59 years	8.5	3.8	1.2	0.2	2939
60–69 years	8.7	3.4	0.9	0.1	2235
70+ years	9.2	1.5	0.3	0.2	1386
Sex					
Male	9.7	2.8	0.5	0.2	3304
Female	7.7	3.5	1.4	0.2	3256
Place of residence					
Urban	7.6	2.9	0.8	0.0	1676
Rural	9.2	3.3	1.0	0.3	4884
Marital status					
Never married	0.8	3.2	3.6	0.0	64
Currently married	9.2	3.5	0.9	0.2	4862
[a]Div./[b]Sep./[c]Wid.	7.2	2.0	0.8	0.0	1634
Education level					
No education	9.1	3.0	1.0	0.1	3365
Primary	10.0	4.2	1.0	0.2	1675
Secondary	8.0	2.1	0.5	0.2	654
High school and above	5.8	2.9	0.5	0.3	866
Wealth tercile					
Lowest	8.4	3.0	1.0	0.2	2624
Middle	10.2	3.5	1.0	0.1	1313
Highest	8.4	3.2	0.7	0.3	2623

[a]Divorced
[b]Separated
[c]Widowed

older adults of 50–59 years who constitute the higher proportion facing mild difficulty. Rural elderly have faced more difficulties in caregiving. Less educated elderly reported severe difficulties while providing care.

Ordered Logistic Regression is used to analyze the impact of caregiving on the caregivers by their background characteristics. It is quite clear that the elderly in the age group 60–69 years and 70 and above years are more likely to experience the impact of caregiving on them. This indicates that the impact of caregiving increases with an increase in age. Females are more likely to face the difficulties of caregiving in comparison to their male counterparts. Both middle and the highest income groups

Table 11.8 Percentage distribution of older adults according to the types of assistance received for caregiving by background characteristics, India

Background characteristics	Type of assistance received				
	Financial	Social	Health	Physical	Personal
Age group					
50–59 years	1.3	0.3	0.5	0.2	0.3
60–69 years	1.7	0.6	0.4	0.3	0.4
70+ years	1.8	0.4	1.0	1.3	0.2
Sex					
Male	1.4	0.3	0.3	0.3	0.2
Female	1.6	0.6	0.8	0.7	0.4
Place of residence					
Urban	1.5	0.1	0.7	0.6	0.0
Rural	1.6	0.5	0.5	0.5	0.4
Marital status					
Never married	0.0	0.0	0.0	0.0	0.0
Currently married	1.6	0.4	0.3	0.2	0.3
[a]Div./[b]Sep./[c]Wid.	1.4	0.5	1.5	1.4	0.5
Education level					
No education	1.8	0.4	0.7	0.7	0.3
Primary	1.7	0.3	0.4	0.2	0.4
Secondary	1.1	0.4	0.4	0.3	0.3
High school and above	0.5	0.4	0.5	0.5	0.4
Wealth tercile					
Lowest	1.3	0.4	0.8	0.7	0.3
Middle	2.4	0.5	0.4	0.3	0.3
Highest	1.3	0.4	0.4	0.3	0.4

[a]Divorced
[b]Separated
[c]Widowed

are less likely to have adverse impacts as compared to those belonging to the lowest income group (Table 11.11).

It is evident that women are more prone to caregiving burdens as compared to men. In Indian families, the women have to follow the traditional norms and culture associated with caregiving where they are obliged to look after every member of the household. It has become a stereotypical attitude of people from all sections of the society that women are the ones who have to take up all the responsibilities of the household and look after their parents, grandparents, in-laws and children. It's not

Table 11.9 Percentage distribution of older adults according to those who received assistance by their background characteristics, India

Background characteristics	Caregivers received assistance from:			Total number
	Family members (Outside HH)	Neighbours/community	Others	
Age group				
50–59 years	1.3	0.9	0.2	2939
60–69 years	1.8	0.7	0.2	2235
70+ years	1.3	1.5	0.8	1386
Sex				
Male	1.3	0.9	0.4	3304
Female	1.6	1.2	0.3	3256
Place of residence				
Urban	1.0	0.9	0.7	1676
Rural	1.6	1.0	0.2	4884
Marital status				
Never married	0.0	0.0	0.0	64
Currently married	1.5	0.9	0.4	4862
[a]Div./[b]Sep./[c]Wid.	1.4	1.3	0.2	1634
Education level				
No education	1.5	1.1	0.1	3365
Primary	1.1	0.5	1.0	1675
Secondary	1.4	0.5	0.3	654
High school and above	0.6	0.1	0.0	866
Wealth tercile				
Lowest	1.4	0.9	0.2	2624
Middle	1.8	1.1	0.9	1313
Highest	1.3	0.7	0.2	2623

[a]Divorced
[b]Separated
[c]Widowed

that the men do not provide care or support, but their liability for it is not the same as compared to the women. Very few men seem to provide physical or personal care but contribute more in providing financial care.

Table 11.10 Percentage distribution of older adults according to the impact of caregiving by background characteristics, India

Background characteristics	Impact of caregiving			Total number
	Mild difficulty	Moderate difficulty	Severe difficulty	
Age group				
50–59 years	8.7	5.4	1.1	2939
60–69 years	8.3	5.2	0.7	2235
70+ years	6.8	3.4	2.0	1386
Sex				
Male	8.9	4.6	1.0	3304
Female	7.4	5.4	1.4	3256
Place of residence				
Urban	6.7	5.0	1.0	1676
Rural	8.8	5.0	1.3	4884
Marital status				
Never married	2.6	2.3	2.6	64
Currently married	8.9	5.2	1.1	4862
[a]Div./[b]Sep./[c]Wid.	6.0	4.1	1.3	1634
Education level				
No education	8.4	5.2	1.0	3365
Primary	7.4	6.4	2.1	1675
Secondary	9.1	4.1	0.6	654
High school and above	8.0	2.2	0.6	866
Wealth tercile				
Lowest	7.5	5.0	1.2	2624
Middle	9.0	5.8	2.0	1313
Highest	8.5	4.4	0.7	2623

[a]Divorced
[b]Separated
[c]Widowed

Conclusion

Family remains the central organizing unit for economic, emotional and care support for individuals in India. In India, families are considered to be the most significant genesis of care for dependents regardless of age and gender. Even though elderly is considered a burden in our society because of their physical incompetence but they can also prove to be an asset by providing financial, emotional and personal support to their loved ones in times when the family system is breaking apart and there

Table 11.11 Ordered logistic regression on the impact of caregiving on caregivers (aged 50+) by background characteristics, India

Explanatory variable	Impact of caregiving	
	Odds ratio	*p*-value
Age group		
50–59®		
60–69	1.01	0.28
70+	1.05*	0.08
Sex		
Male®		
Female	1.58***	0.00
Place of residence		
Urban®		
Rural	1.04*	0.09
Marital status		
Never married®		
Currently married	0.27*	0.09
[a]Div./[b]Sep./[c]Wid.	0.31	0.14
Education level		
No education®		
Primary	1.11	0.51
Secondary	0.79	0.30
High school and above	0.64*	0.06
Wealth tercile		
Lowest®		
Middle	0.72*	0.07
Highest	0.72**	0.04

***1% significant, **5% significant, *10% significant
[a]Divorced
[b]Separated
[c]Widowed

are significant socio-economic changes happening around, which includes increased incidence of marital dissolution, women's workforce participation and single parenthood (Kamiya & Timonen, 2011). In countries with poor provision of public childcare services which in general is meant to provide help and support to the dual earning parents or even a single parent, grandparental care to young grandchildren turns out to be a boon for the families.

Sometimes, it becomes pertinent to apprehend from an individual's perspective, "to what magnitude is a family support needed by/from them in times of need?" in order to understand whether the caregiving is available or absent for that individual or whether they have the capability to provide care to other individuals. The dynamics of caregiving and care receiving are inter-related irrespective of age group or gender depending on our present needs and availabilities on various grounds. Sometimes, it may be voluntary while sometimes the situation may demand it. So, it was beneficial to look into this aspect of caregiving on behalf of older adults as to how and in what situations these older adults themselves are vulnerable to care and support but have to look after others as well. Caregivers may be old and have health problems of their own to deal with in addition to the demands of caregiving (Ekwall et al., 2007). So, it was imperative to acknowledge how these elderly deal with the responsibilities of caregiving even though they also belong to the care receiving age groups.

After going through a detailed analysis and post adjusting for the probable confounding effects of selected caregiver characteristics, this study found that there are significant gender differentials among the caregivers in care provision challenges. Gender is a consequential predictor of experiencing major difficulties in caregiving challenges. When we look at an Indian family scenario, with enormous traditions and cultural values, it plays a major role in defining the caregiving situation. Basically, male members are considered as the bread earners while females look after the household chores, including looking after the older parents. We also found that elderly women caregivers experienced greater burden and difficulties in comparison with elderly men in India. This may be also due to the demanding roles for women both inside and outside of their homes.

From the analysis, it was evident that male elderly usually provided financial support which decreased with the increasing age. Higher percentage of females have contributed to other types of care especially, personal care. This indicates that women have to look after the household and also play the role of primary caregiver in most of the households. They are the ones who experienced greater challenges and difficulties under familial obligations in caregiving. Elderly women caregivers were more likely to be in need of assistance economically. Rural elderly are more into the task of providing care rather than their urban counterparts. Family members provided the maximum support in terms of financial assistance to the caregivers. The adverse impact of caregiving includes not having enough food, sleep, energy, proper health care and having no time for visiting friends and other relatives as reported by the respondents. However, a very small percentage of elderly had admitted that they were severely affected, while most of them reported as mildly affected by their caregiving responsibilities.

Family caregiving (unpaid caregiving) has long been thought of as a 'women responsibility', which ultimately results not only in gendered but also financial and health inequities (Giesbrecht et al., 2012). An important aspect of this study was to illustrate that older men and women are not only the receivers of care and support but also the caregivers for their families. One critical aspect of an ageing society is that with an increase in life expectancy and healthier functioning into older ages, older men and women are able to contribute towards the well-being of their families and communities. "Older people are not only at the receiving end of the support but also contribute to the dynamic and interdependent aspects of social institutions" (Cong & Silverstein, 2008; Silverstein et al., 2002). "The bi-directional force is often less recognized as societies begin to have larger older populations with a resultant undue emphasis on the burden of older people in rapidly evolving societies such as in India"

(Berkman et al., 2012). Given the increasing burden of caregiving on older adults, policies and programme initiatives are required to ensure that caregivers can fulfil their responsibility without compromising their own health, leisure and well-being.

References

Berkman, L. F., Sekher, T. V., Capistrant, B., & Zheng, Y. (2012). Social networks, family, and care giving among older adults in India. In J. P. Smith & M. Majmundar (Eds.), *Aging in Asia: Findings from new and emerging data initiatives*. National Academies Press.

Bloom, D. E. (2012). Population dynamics of india and implications for economic growth. *Harvard Program on the Global Demography of Aging, Working Paper* 65. Accessed at www.hsph.harvard.edu/pgda/working.htm

Bookman, A., & Kimbrel, D. (2011). Families and elder care in the twenty-first century. *The Future of Children, 21*(2), 117–140.

Census of India. (2011). *Provisional Population Totals*. Office of the Registrar General, Ministry of Home Affairs.

Clark, J. A., & Weber, K. A. (1997). *Challenges and choices: Elderly caregiving*. University of Missouri.

Conde-Sala, J. L., Garre-Olmo, J., Turró-Garriga, O., Vilalta-Franch, J., & López-Pousa, S. (2010). Differential features of burden between spouse and adult-child caregivers of patients with Alzheimer's disease: An exploratory comparative design. *International Journal of Nursing Studies, 47*(10), 1262–1273.

Cong, Z., & Silverstein, M. (2008). Intergenerational time-for-money exchanges in rural China: Does reciprocity reduce depressive symptoms of older grandparents? *Research in Human Development, 5*(1), 6–25.

Ekwall, A. K., Sivberg, B., & Hallberg, I. R. (2007). Older caregivers' coping strategies and sense of coherence in relation to quality of life. *Journal of Advanced Nursing, 57*(6), 584–596.

Giesbrecht, M., Crooks, V. A., Williams, A., & Hankivsky, O. (2012). Critically examining diversity in end-of-life family caregiving: Implications for equitable caregiver support and Canada's compassionate care benefit. *International Journal for Equity in Health, 11*(1), 65.

Government of India. (1999). *National policy on older persons*. Ministry of Social Justice and Empowerment.

Government of India. (2011). *Situation analysis of the elderly in India*. Central Statistics Office Ministry of Statistics and Programme Implementation.

Gupta, R. (2009). Systems perspective: Understanding care giving of the elderly in India. *Health Care for Women International, 30*(12), 1040–1054.

IIPS and WHO. (2013). *Study on Global Ageing and Adult Health (SAGE), Wave1, India*. International Institute for Population Sciences, Mumbai and World Health Organization.

Kamiya, Y. & Timonen, V. (2011). Older people as members of their families and communities. In A. Barrett, G. Savva, V. Timonen, & R. A. Kenny (Eds.), *Fifty plus in Ireland 2011*. The Irish Longitudinal Study on Ageing.

Population Reference Bureau. (2012). Today's research on aging, No. 25. http://esa.un.org/unpd/wpp/index.html

Radhakrisna, S. (2013). *Help for the caregiver*. Retrieved from: http://www.thehindu.com/sci-tech/health/help-for-thecaregiver/article5116330.ece. The Hindu.

Sanuade, O. A., & Boatemaa, S. (2015). Caregiver profiles and determinants of caregiving burden in Ghana. *Public Health, 129*(7), 941–947.

Schultz, R., & Beach, S. R. (1999). Caregiving as a risk factor for mortality: The caregiver health effects study. *The Journal of American Medical Association (JAMA), 282*(23).

Silverstein, M., Conroy, S. J., Wang, H., Giarrusso, R., & Bengtson, V. L. (2002). Reciprocity in parent–child relations over the adult life course. *The Journals of Gerontology Series B: Psychological Sciences and Social Sciences, 57*(1), S3–S13.

United Nations. (2011). *World Population Prospects*, 2010 Revision. Population Division. United Nations.

United Nations. (2017). *World Population Ageing 2017—Highlights.* Department of Economic and Social Affairs, Population Division. United Nations.

Chapter 12
The Role of 'Weak Social Bonds' in Perpetuating Fear of Crime: An Investigation of the Aged in Lucknow

Anindya J. Mishra and Avanish Bhai Patel

Abstract Fear of crime is a matter of serious concern among the elderly. Yet it remains one of the least researched areas in Indian gerontology. This chapter looks at the phenomenon of fear of crime in the aged through primary data collected by mixed methods approach from 220 respondents in the district of Lucknow in Uttar Pradesh. The major contributing factors of fear of crime in the aged are prior victimisation, incivility and vulnerability. The findings of the study have also been analysed through the lenses of 'social bond theory' which focuses on how the breakdown of traditional social structures and weakening social bonds have exacerbated the phenomenon of fear of crime in the aged. To address this issue of fear of crime among the elderly, social initiatives, for instance, age friendly communities, neighbourhood watch programmes, helpline services in every district and Elderly Policy Councils have been recommended.

Keywords Fear of crime · Victimisation · Incivility · Vulnerability · Social bond theory · Elderly

Introduction

There is a tremendous growth of elderly population in India. A significant proportion of India's population is living at the age of sixty and beyond. The elderly are facing a lot of troubles in their day to day lives. The crime rate against the elderly has shot up considerably in recent times. There are more reported cases of elder abuse nowadays.

Criminal activities and abusive behaviour that the aged are subjected to can be in the shape of grievous hurt, mistreatment, homicide and robbery. They are also subject to ill-treatment, psychological torment, bodily harm mental and insult and humiliation from the family members and community (Khan & Handa, 2011; Rufus

A. J. Mishra (✉)
Indian Institute of Technology, Roorkee, India
e-mail: anindya.mishra@hs.iitr.ac.in

A. B. Patel
Alliance School of Law, Alliance University, Bengaluru, India

M. K. Shankardass (ed.), *Gerontological Concerns and Responses in India*,
https://doi.org/10.1007/978-981-16-4764-2_12

& Shekhar, 2011). Owing to this, the fear of crime has become a disconcerting issue among the elderly. The crime statistics in India reveal that there were 21,410 incidents of reported crime in 2016, as against 20,532 in 2015, thus leading to a 4.3% variation in crime against elderly. From the list of crimes perpetrated against the elderly as reflected in the official statistics viz. cheating, murder and robbery, the state of Uttar Pradesh leads in reported incidents of murder (National Crime Records Bureau, 2016). The current study attempts to investigate the major determinants of the 'fear of crime' in the aged and it also tries to explore the linkage between 'social bonding and fear of crime' with the support of primary data collected from fieldwork in Lucknow, a northern Indian city.

The usage 'aged' applies to stage of life well past middle age. The term 'aged' does not have an exact definition as its meaning changes from one society to the other. The people can be regarded as aged because of evident alterations in their social actions and duties after a certain age. People above the age of 60 are treated as aged in India. National Policy on Older Persons (1999) considers those people who have crossed the boundary of sixty as elderly (Government of India, 2011). Similarly, the Maintenance and Welfare of Parents and Senior Citizens Act, 2007 describes "an elderly or a senior citizen as a person who has attained the age of sixty years or above" (Government of India, 2007). Moreover, according to the Central Board of Direct Taxes, citizens are treated as old once they cross the age of 65. The United Nations Organisation recognizes people over 60 years as aged (Group for Economic and Social Studies 2009, 20). People have often attributed the label of 'the aged' or 'the old' from 55, 60 or 65 years onwards (Donder et al., 2012). The present study has considered those as elderly who are 60 years and above.

Fear of crime has become very common among the elderly, particularly those living in urban areas. Before beginning a discussion on fear of crime, we should understand the notion of fear of crime. Ferraro and LaGrange (1987) have provided a standard description of fear of crime. They have defined, "fear of crime is an emotional response of dread or anxiety that a person associates with crime". Similarly, Garafalo (1981) has explained in detail that "fear of crime is an emotional reaction characterized by a sense of danger and anxiety produced by the threat of physical harm, elicited by perceived cues in the environment that relate to some aspect of crime for the person." The term fear embraces and engulfs a bewildering array of feelings, perspectives and risk estimations. Fear of crime may be felt in public emotions, thought, personal risk and criminal victimisation.

A Brief Review of Select Literature

The aged treat fear of crime as a grave matter that affects them personally. The sharp rise in fear of crime is linked to changing social environment and perceived feeling of insecurity. Fear of crime affects behaviour patterns, life satisfaction and happiness of the people (Miethe & Lee, 1984).

The determinants of fear of crime are such variables which decide the level of fear of crime in people. The crime statistics in a locality, earlier victimisation, incivility, vulnerability and defensibility determine the level of fear of crime in people. The crime statistics in a locality is known as a contributing cause of fear of crime. The level of anxiety about crime is decided by the crime statistics in a locality and it is observed that urban areas are more affected due to crime rate and the urban people have additional fear of crime than rural people (Miethe & Lee, 1984, 400). Further, it has been claimed in many studies that previous ill-treatment is a reason for deep-seated fear of crime. Social scientists have established a strong relationship between fear of crime and prior experience of crime. The sufferers of crime have a stronger feeling of fear of crime (Donder et al., 2005). The incivility in the locality is another significant factor of fear of crime. Incivility refers to "those unusual conditions and events which are active in neighbourhood and breaches social order and control of the neighbourhood" (Vandeviver, 2011). Incivilities are of two types. One is social incivility and the other one is physical incivility. Social incivility denotes unsettling actions such as people hanging around aimlessly, problematic people living nearby, stray canines, disruptive youngsters, mobs, vagrants and public drinking. Physical incivility includes messy neighbourhoods, for instance, deserted automobiles, damaged goods, empty buildings and crumbling houses (Franklin et al., 2008). Moreover, vulnerability may also be known as a determinant of fear of crime. Vulnerability in the sphere of fear of crime implies that flaws exist in the immediate surroundings which are considered intimidating by the dwellers. Such flaws in the immediate surroundings allow the anti-social elements to carry out unlawful actions in those areas. Apart from this, prior cases of wrong-doings in the area, presence of poorer people and usual suspects residing in the locality also determine vulnerability. They also determine fear of crime in people (On-fung et al., 2009). Moreover, neighbourhood help groups, participation in community happenings and movement of people influence degree of fear of crime. Donder et al. (2005) have emphasized the role of neighbourhood factors as playing a significant part in the origin of fear of crime in the aged. They have explained that those elderly, who reside in a group and report more neighbourhood participation, consider themselves secure than those aged persons who are not staying in a group or in a community. Solitude and absence of involvement in community life are strongly linked to fear of crime.

The Group for Economic and Social Studies (2009) has investigated the relationship between the old and the criminals in India's four big cities and described various kinds of crime against the older persons. These crimes may be defined as crime against the body (homicide, attempted homicide, bodily harm and abductions), crimes against the property (larceny, theft and stealing) and financial crimes (forgery, deceit, felonious treachery). Those old people who are rich tend to be more susceptible to manipulation, demands and bodily intimidation for property and monetary benefits from near and dear ones and from their family members, relatives and harmful outsiders.

Patel (2010), using content analysis, has conducted research on crime against the older persons in a central Indian city. Her work discovered that neighbours, relatives and family members, particularly, sons and daughters-in-law commit crime against the elderly. The domestic help are found to be engaged in offences in certain instances. She described the following factors instrumental in crime against the aged: property and land disputes, solitary stay, police indifference to felony against the aged and village disputes. Moreover, another research on crime against the aged revealed that 44.71% crime against the aged was killing of old people (Mishra & Patel, 2013). The research further indicated that near and dear ones and people living in the vicinity were found to have committed crimes against the aged in 42.35% instances. The above literature suggests an increase in offences against the aged that has definitely disturbed the lifestyle and feeling of safety and security among the older population. Hence fear of crime among the aged is acknowledged as a matter of grave concern by Indian policy makers and academia in current era.

Kalavar et al. (2013) have done research on 150 elderly persons in four big cities of South India. This study was conducted on those older persons who were staying in paid old age homes. The research indicated that lifestyles in urban areas have undergone transformation and new value systems have emerged. The alterations in these value systems are the source of discord and tension between older parents and adult children. Such intergenerational discord is responsible for rise in elder abuse. The study has also found that the aged are not cared for at home and are abused by their sons and daughters-in-law. Because of it, they like to reside in paid old age homes. Furthermore, the survey has reported that the elderly feel very happy and secure in old age homes and besides it, they involve in same group activities which bring positive feelings regarding safety.

Durkheim, backed by empirical research, validated a strong linkage between modernisation and crime and this relationship has been taken forward by the modernisation theory (Nallaet al., 2011). Modernisation theory suggests that urbanisation and industrialisation are instrumental in escalation in crime figures, financial disparity, movement of people from villages, lack of jobs, breakdown in social bonding, crime and fear of crime which are the unintended social outcomes of economic progress and its attendant processes such as modernisation, industrialisation and urbanisation (Nalla et al., 2011). An in-depth study on the fear of crime has been conducted by Nalla et al. (2011). Their paper has found that financial prosperity has brought rapid urbanisation. Rapid urbanisation has increased problems such as unrestrained rise in populace, movement from villages to towns, impoverishment and slums. Consequently, crime rate has also increased due to these problems. Therefore, prior victimisation and regional and local causes are connected with foretelling of fear of crime. Moreover, the decaying of the mechanism of cultural value systems increases fear of crime in the society. The findings show that victimisation such as sexual assault of victims, robbery and fraud increase degree of fear of crime. They have further found that degree of fear of crime is higher in urban areas (fear of robbery and assault) than in rural areas.

The criminal scholars stress the fact that this issue of rise in crime against the aged has less to do with legal loopholes and more to do with changing normative order. Therefore, the topic has important sociological relevance. They opine that these cases of crime and abuse are the consequence of growing segregation of the aged in recent times (Das, 2009).

Major studies on fear of crime have been done through the framework of psychology. But it can also be analysed in an in-depth manner from a sociological perspective. The major factors of fear of crime such as social bond, vulnerability, incivility and prior victimisation are studied through the sociological angle.

Aim of the Research

This paper endeavours to investigate fear of crime in the aged dwelling in both towns as well villages of Lucknow district. The study has two important purposes:

1. To understand some of the major determinants of fear of crime against the aged which include earlier offences (those who have been victimized earlier), vulnerability (it refers to the status of social network and physical condition of an individual) and incivility (talks about the social values and physical surrounding of the society).
2. To examine the linkage between social bonding and fear of crime among the elderly. Social bond is the relationship of the elderly with their family members and the society at large. This objective discusses the aspects of social bonds such as attachment, involvement, faith and commitment. The purpose of this objective is to investigate how weak social bonds contribute to fear of crime and elder abuse.

Theoretical Framing

A sociological understanding of the current study emphasizes that fear of crime in the aged is the result of social changes as well as changes in traditional social structure. Our traditional social structure is declining fast day by day due to migration, urbanisation, modernisation and technological development. These factors are seen to impact the occurrence of elder abuse and crime against the elderly. The findings of the current survey can be comprehended in the context of the social bond theory.

The social bond theory has been derived and propounded by Travis Hirschi in the year of 1969. Although social bond theory has been used with relation to juvenile delinquency in this study the social bond theory has been applied in relation to crime against the elderly and fear among them because old age is one of the most critical times in the life of a human being. During this critical time, a person requires robust and constructive community relation to represent society in the best way possible. Social bond theory is an important way of approaching social relations and also disorganising trends in community. It also emphasizes how social interactions and troubles in personal and community life can be explicated within societal framework. Hirschi has defined social bond as "the connection between individual and the society." Social bond has four dimensions—attachment, commitment, involvement and faith. The construction of social bond is an intricate procedure which starts from the family as it is the primary normative base of customary practices in the community. This formation of social bond sets up the familiar association of a person with family members, relatives, friends and neighbours. Hirschi argues that "weak social bond is synonymous with greater susceptibility to mental disorders in an individual's life. Some disorders connected to a lack of social bond are depression, anxiety, anti-social behaviour and suicidal tendencies."

Further, social bond theory affirms that when social bond is broken or declines, the crime rate rises fast and also neighbourhood becomes insecure. The social bond theory has dominant perspectives about criminal behaviour and its consequences. This theory has been examined and analysed multiple times in criminal scholarship of Sociology (Durkin et al., 1999, 451). Moreover, a study has been conducted in Kwahu which is related to social bonds and elderly, which found the lack of interest and respect of the young generation towards the elderly people (Geest, 2004, 2007). Further, diminishing social interaction is considered as the evident signal of failure to grow old happily which increases bodily and cognitive deficiencies and cause every day difficulties and mental agony. Absence of regular touch with family members, near and dear ones and mates is perceived as individual setback (Geest, 2011).

Some of the major elements of social bond are attachment, involvement, faith and commitment. Attachment is the first and the most prominent element of social bond theory. It touches upon the ties of a person and other members of community and family. Attachment maintains the degree of relation in which an individual has emotional ties to other people in society. According to social bond theory those who have strong attachment, do not have fear about crime. Such people think that they will share every problem with others, which give them emotional support and bring the feeling of safety. Attachment to family members has more importance because the quality of attachment within a family provides greater security to the family.

The second dimension of social bond theory is involvement. Involvement refers to the participation of individuals in social or family activities. Involvement in social or family activities decides the level of social networks. When the individuals communicate their thoughts through social activities with others, they know about their social importance and have a "we feeling" which raises feeling of safety. Involvement in social activities also removes isolation and loneliness. According to social bond theory when people do not involve themselves in social activities, their social networks begin to weaken. Weakening of social networks augments fear and abusive behaviour in the community due to absence of social networks.

The third component of social bond is faith. Faith is a state or habit of mind in which trust is placed in some people. Faith is the conformity of traditional morals and ethics. Here conventional value system refers to family members, relatives, friends and members who regulate our social ties as per the norms of society. According to social bond theory when our faith weakens from the conventional value system, social problems such as fear, isolation, loneliness and depression begin to rise. Moreover, weakening of conventional value system decreases the importance of social relation as well as family relation (Durkin et al., 1999, 452).

Commitment is the fourth and last dimension of social bond. Commitment implies the sense of a grounding force. It means when individuals commit themselves to a

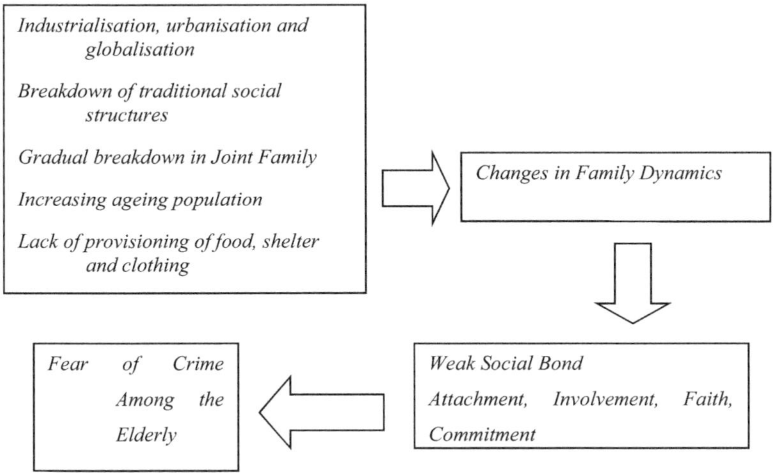

Fig. 12.1 Theoretical framing

social group (social service, religious activity, yoga, informal group, etc.), they are introduced to the reality of society and they get social force to face social problems. Commitment to a social group is a sense of social responsibility as well as duty (Fig. 12.1).

A Note on the Field of Study

The current study was conducted during the time period of 5 months in 2012–13 in Lucknow district, which is part of Uttar Pradesh. Maximum number of migration has taken place in Lucknow district of Uttar Pradesh. Such movement of people due to employment prospects has led to unforeseen rise in inhabitants in the region, proliferation of slum areas and presence of diversity of people in the Lucknow city. The above-mentioned factors are, directly or indirectly, instrumental in diminishing the social bond among the members of the close-knit community as well as the reasons for intergenerational conflict. The authors contend that there is upsurge in crime against older persons and fear of crime among them due to such issues. National Crime Records Bureau (2013) database indicated that the city of Lucknow was at the receiving end of maximum crime compared to other bigger cities in India. In Lucknow, there were a large number of reports of crime against the aged in newspapers in the preceding years to the field study. The crime pertains to these cases are related to homicide, bodily harm, stealing, larceny and ill-treatment of older persons. Keeping in consideration the sharp rise in various types of offences against the aged in the city, the authors attempted to investigate the diminishing social bond among family members and the causes triggering fear of crime in the aged.

Method

The current research has employed mixed method approach that calls attention to "the use of more (qualitative and quantitative) than one approach to the investigation of a research question in order to enhance confidence in the ensuing findings" (Davies, 2013). We have tried to use the basic tenets of "convergent parallel mixed methods design" to study the issues of maltreatment of older persons and attend to the cavity in research in this field. The method includes autonomous gathering of different datasets and their scrutiny through separate theoretical perspectives. The process involves: (i) qualitative information stemming from focused interviews (ii) quantitative data resulting from interview schedule. After that, making use of narrative and descriptive analysis, the results are examined. The reasoning "applied to the selection of this methodology and particular typology, in addition to the strengths identified above, is in offering researchers complementary data on the same topic in order to generate greater understanding" (Davies, 2013) (Fig. 12.2).

A Brief Profile of the Respondents

For the purpose of the study, 220 elderly respondents were chosen through convenience sampling. It is one of the methods of non-probability sampling where the researcher approaches those people who are easily accessible. The researcher studies people who readily agree to be respondents (Ahuja, 2009). For example, the study on fear of crime among the aged was conducted in the rural and urban areas of Lucknow. The elderly who were interviewed were located in recreational areas, places of worship, bazaars and rural plantations. Only those elderly were interviewed who gave their consent and agreed to longer period of sittings.

Face-to-face interviews were conducted with 220 respondents for the study. These respondents were staying in both towns and villages of the district of Lucknow. The demographic profile of the respondents who were interviewed reveals that 45.9% (101) belong to the age category of 70–79 years. While 36.3% (80) elderly respondents belong to the age group of 60–69 years, only 17.8% (39) of the elderly belong to the age group above 80 years. In terms of the gender distribution, there were higher numbers of female respondents, i.e. 62.3% (137) of the entire set of respondents in contrast to 83 male respondents who constituted 37.7% of the total sample. Equal numbers of elderly respondents (110) were interviewed from both towns and villages.

In terms of the occupation of the respondents, the study found that the elderly were engaged as farmers (19.1%), government/medical officers (15.5%), teachers (14.5%), clerks (10.0%), businessmen (7.3%) and street vendors (5.9%). Nearly 27.7% of the elderly interviewed were unemployed and were financially dependent on their children. Further, the study also found that 25.9% elderly earned 1000–5000 rupees per month, 7.7% earned 6000–10,000 rupees, 14.5% earned 11,000–15,000

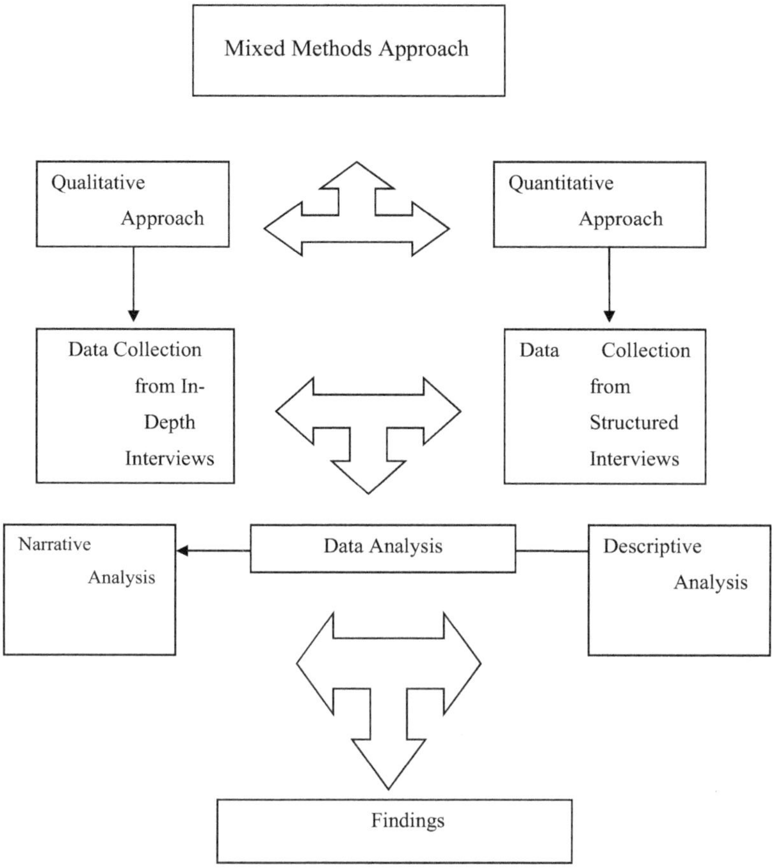

Fig. 12.2 Mixed methods approach

rupees, 15.9% earned 16,000–20,000 rupees and 8.2% earned 21,000 rupees. 27.7% elderly did not have any income resources.

Regarding the marital status of the older people studied, the married aged formed 59.1% of the entire group. More married elderly (65.5%) were from villages as contrasted to towns (52.7%), widows/widowers formed the next group of the elderly (39.1%). According to the data collected, there were more widows (50.6%) than widowers (32.1%).

The study found that 92.7% elderly had children, while only 53.2% of them were staying with their children. The rural-urban difference suggests that 60.9% rural elderly were staying with children as compared to merely 45.5% urban elderly. Further, the study indicates that slightly higher percentages of elderly males (57.7%) were staying with their children as compared to elderly females (45.8%). Those elderly who were not staying with their children were either living with their spouses (57.2%) or in old age homes (26.2%) or were living alone (16.6%). The study found that there were various reasons for the elderly not staying with their adult children. These reasons were migration of children, conflict between the elderly and their children or death of a spouse.

As regards ownership of property, 61.8% of the elderly (136) had property such as land (39.7%), shop (13.9%), house (26.5%) and other property related things such as cattle (19.9%). Moreover, 80.0% (176) of the elderly had savings in different sources such as bank account (45.5%), life insurance (22.7%), post office accounts (16.5%) and *kisanpatra*, a small plan for the farmers by Government (15.3%).

Tools of Data Collection

In this study, technique of interview schedule was used for the data collection. The interview schedules were distributed to the elderly respondents in rural-urban Lucknow. Interview schedule is known as the most important tool of primary data collection because in the field researchers collect the data themselves through interview schedule and show real circumstances of sample and researchers. This enables them to prepare questions according to the nature and the objective of the study. The interview schedule has been prepared to measure variables such as age, gender, education, income, marital status, social bonds, prior victimisation, vulnerability, incivility and elder abuse. The interview schedule also included components such as fear level within the residence and outside it and a general understanding of local perception about crime both at local and national level. Observation as a technique of data collection was also used as far as possible. Observation is also a specific tool for primary data collection and a direct method of study. The researchers observe participants' ongoing behaviour in a natural situation. The purpose of this type of research is to gather more reliable insights.

Analysis of the Data

The semi-structured interview schedule had both close-ended and open-ended questions. There were close-ended questions such as "do you have attachment with your family members?", "do you feel safe during walking alone at night in your neighbourhood?", "has crime been committed against the body?", "do you feel that you are physically vulnerable?" The responses contained options from "strongly agree" to "strongly disagree." A number was assigned to each response without any weightage. In case of open-ended questions, the main themes were noted down and were subsequently analysed.

Besides it, focus group discussion and narrative analysis have also been employed as additional tools to allow the analysis and interpretation of data collected by means of the interview schedule. Moreover, the data has been analysed with aid from the related work. The existing research on the theme was utilized to understand and analyse the results of the current study.

Major Findings of the Study

Elder abuse, as has been discussed earlier is the neglectful and offensive conduct that comprises physical, emotional, verbal and financial exploitation of the aged and such behaviour deprives the elderly of their respect and dignity.

The findings of the study shed light on two major dimensions of the fear of crime in the aged. First of all, it deals with the causes influencing fear of crime in the aged. These include social, environmental and psychological dimensions of the fear of crime in the aged. Elderly. Social and environmental factors cover prior victimisation, vulnerability, incivility, crime rate and crime news while psychological factors include stress, phobia and happiness to examine fear of crime in the aged.

Secondly, the study investigates the relationship between the aged and their family members, relatives and neighbours within the framework of social bonding. This part of the chapter examines social bonding of the aged using the concepts of attachment, involvement, belief and commitment. Their constant touch with children, relatives, friends and neighbours have also been assessed. The perception of the aged regarding the attention and esteem they receive from their near and dear ones and the youth of the areas they reside in is also discussed here. Besides, all the major findings have been analysed so as to make a comparative analysis of the aged from villages and towns as well as male and female respondents.

The study found that 51.4% elderly admitted to being abused by the family out of which majority (65.1%) were women. Demand for meeting basic needs was the major reason for abuse by the family. 26.4% elderly in the sample of 220 admitted to being abused in the neighbourhood. A greater percentage of rural elderly (38.2%) were abused by the family as compared to other groups. The interviews revealed that living alone and isolation by children who migrate to nearby towns and cities for better job prospects exacerbates the scope of crime against the rural aged. The study also indicates that the aged were ill-treated vocally (31.8%), emotionally (36.4%), economically (22.7%) and bodily (29.5%). Some of the causes for the victimisation of the elderly were property (30.0%), absence of personal care (30.5%), dearth of essential requirements (30.5%) and absence of medical attention (20.0%). Further, it was found that the daughters-in-law were the primary perpetrator of abuse (25.9%), followed by sons (20.9%), neighbours (20.5%), brothers/nephews (20.0%), domestic help (4.1%) and grandchildren (1.8%).

Factors Determining Fear of Crime Among the Elderly

Prior Victimisation: Prior victimisation implies that those who have been ill-treated before or suffer due to earlier offences committed against them. It can take the form of crime against the body (with 62.2% of the elderly respondents reporting to being targets of grievous hurt, 20.7% of them being subject to attempts to murder and 16.9% related to sexual harassment), crime against property (36.4% of 220 respondents were victimized for property) and mental abuse (53.2% reported to being subjects of verbal and emotional abuse, neglect and maltreatment). These are the most prominent forms of crimes through which prior victimisation takes place directly. Also 43.6% respondents were fearful due to indirect victimisation. In such cases fear of crime was induced through interaction and narrative accounts of people who have been directly victimized. There are researches corroborating the link between the fear of crime and prior victimisation (Kanan & Pruitt, 2002; Dammert & Malone, 2003). Simply put, people who have been ill-treated beforehand, have intense of fear of crime.

Vulnerability: Vulnerability can be defined as diminished capacity of an individual to anticipate and recover from the impact of physical or social problems. There are two types of vulnerability, namely, physical and social vulnerability.

Physical vulnerability refers to individuals' physical disability because of which they are not able to protect themselves from victimisation. In the study, 89.1% elderly said that they were physically vulnerable. The gender differences indicate that 96.4% elderly females felt more physically vulnerable in comparison with elderly males (84.7%). Further, village-town comparison indicates that 94.5% aged from the villages felt that they were physically weaker in comparison with urban elderly (89.1%).

Social vulnerability refers to weak social ties. Due to weak social ties, individuals feel isolated and alienated in the family and the society. In the study, 57.7% elderly reported feeling socially vulnerable. Further, gender differences show that 66.3% elderly females felt socially vulnerable as compared to 52.6% elderly males. Moreover, village-town comparison suggests that aged from towns (62.7%) perceived themselves as more socially vulnerable as compared to the rural elderly (52.7%). Khan (2004), has discussed in this regard, how the presence of 'family self' among the rural poor accounts for their greater interaction with family members and neighbours. In urban society the 'individual self' predominates, wherein lesser interaction with family members and neighbours, isolation due to greater heterogeneity of population contribute to weak social ties.

Incivility

Incivility denotes the defects in immediate social surroundings and in immediate neighbourhood which breaches the community values signalling a decline of social order and control in the neighbourhood. Incivility indicators have a direct and positive relationship with crime and fear of crime (Wilson & Kelling, 1989; Parker & Ray, 1990; Sampson et al., 1997). There are two types of incivility, namely, physical and social incivility. In the study, 50.5% elderly felt that physical incivility was a grave matter in their neighbourhood. There were no noteworthy gender variances regarding physical incivility in the neighbourhood. In terms of rural-urban difference, 54.5% rural elderly and 46.4% urban elderly reported experiences of physical incivility. The respondents reported that instances of physical incivility including littering (35.1%), rundown houses (41.4%) and graffiti (23.4%) existed in their neighbourhood.

Social incivility refers to anti-social elements which are active in the neighbourhood and affects norms and values of the society. Regarding social incivility, 60.0% elderly respondents felt that social incivility was a grave matter in their neighbourhood. When the village-town variances were factored in, it was found that 66.4% rural aged considered that social incivility was a grave matter in their locality in comparison with 53.6% urban aged. No gender difference was detected in the responses of the elderly. Moreover, the elderly respondents reported many forms of social incivility which were existing in their neighbourhood. They included loitering youth (43.9%), tramps (24.3%) and drug abusers/alcoholics (31.7%).

Social Bond and Fear of Crime Among the Aged

Attachment: Attachment refers to the social linkage between the individuals and other people of the family and the society who reside around them. The study found that 70% elderly respondents felt that attachment to the family members was weakening as compared to 28.2% respondents who felt that attachment was strong to the family members and 1.8% respondents did not answer the questions on attachment. There were 61.8% respondents who argued that nowadays attachment to the relatives was declining as compared to 34.1% elderly who did not agree that attachment to relatives was declining and 4.1% elderly were neutral on the issue of attachment to the family members and relatives. Majority of the elderly respondents, i.e. 80.5%, asserted that attachment to the neighbours was decreasing fast whereas 16.4% elderly did not feel so and 3.2% elderly did not react to this question.

An elderly respondent narrated his experience of attachment with family members: "I stay with my wife at home. We have strained relationships with our sons and their families who live nearby. They rebuke us saying that we have become old and lost our sanity. We keep blabbering all the time doing nothing."

Involvement: On the issue of involvement, which is another dimension of social bond, it was found that 46.8% elderly respondents were involved in family matters for important discussions and decision-making as compared to 30.5% respondents answered in negative that they were involved in any family decision making. There were 22.8% respondents who chose not to answer this question. On neighbourhood activities, 29.1% of elderly replied that they were being called to participate in neighbourhood activities and they also enjoyed decision making power in social activities as compared to 56.4% elderly who did not think they were involved in any way in such social activities. Around 14.5% of the elderly did not have any comment on the issue of involvement.

Another elderly respondent recounted his experience of involvement in family and social decision making: "I am retired from bank. My sons follow my decisions at home. My daughter who is married and stays in another city seeks my help when she is in trouble. I am involved in social activities in the neighbourhood and people share their problems with me. This makes me feel that I am bonded with the society around me."

Faith: Faith is a state of mind of human behaviour which decides the dimensions of the relationship towards the family members, relatives, friends and neighbours. The study has found that 63.2% elderly respondents felt that they did not have faith in family members as compared to 35.0% respondents who said they had faith in family members and 1.8% respondents did not answer the question. Further, when the gender comparison is made regarding faith, 57.7% elderly males felt that they have less faith in the family members as compared to 72.3% elderly females who think that their faith in the family members is declining. Moreover, there is almost no difference in the opinion patterns of elderly interviewed from villages and towns as 63.6% urban elderly replied that their faith was declining in the family while 62.7% rural elderly felt the same.

Responding to the question of faith, an elderly respondent recounted thus:

I stay with my wife at home. We do not have children. We depend on our younger brothers and their sons for help. My younger brother illegally occupied my land and house and bothers me and my wife. My personal experience tells me that we cannot believe relatives anymore.

Commitment: Commitment is an important component of the social bond because it integrates the individuals directly in the social institutions like family and society. These institutions include social service, religious activities, political activities and *chaupal* (it is a kind of get-together of villagers at village centre). But due to the lack of commitment in the social institutions, many problems such as isolation and alienation are faced by the individuals. In the study, 62.3% elderly respondents answered that they were part of social activities such as social service, religious activities, political activities, yoga and informal groups as compared to 36.8% respondents who were not committed to social activities and 0.9% respondents were neutral about this. Further, it was found that 35.5% urban elderly were not committed to social institutions while 64.5% urban elderly were committed to social institutions. Similarly, 38.2% rural elderly did not have any commitment to social activities but 60.0% rural elderly said that they were committed in social activities and 1.8% rural elderly were neutral on this issue. Moreover, there was not much to choose from male and female elderly as 34.3% elderly males were not committed in social institutions while 41.0% elderly females did not have interest in committing themselves to any social activities. Further, it was found that of the elderly who were committed to different social institutions, 38.6% elderly were committed to religious activities and 35.0% elderly were committed to *chaupal*. Besides it, many elderly were committed to social service (8.7%), political activities such as campaigning and meetings (8.1%) and yoga (9.4%).

The Way Forward

The study clearly unravels a change in family dynamics which are no longer based on love, care and affection. There is an advent of material and practical approaches to relationships which can fracture social bonding and impact the mental health of the elderly. It appears that most families may care for their aged members, for their own individualistic pursuits, such as acquisition of property rather than out of love and care. The respondents in the study show signs of alienation and isolation. They also recount narratives of psychological and physical torture, for example, humiliation and deprivation of their basic needs of food, clothing, shelter and medical help. The "individual self" taking precedence over "social self" has further led to the weakening of social bonding (Khan, 2004). Such weakening of social bonding makes the elderly apprehensive about their security. This also heightens their perception of fear of crime. The increasing crime rate in the locality, abuse in family and neighbourhood, direct and indirect experiences of victimisation, instances of incivility, physical and social vulnerability assume pivotal role in determining fear of crime in the aged residing in villages and towns of Lucknow.

Patel and Mishra (2018) suggest that certain strategies should be adopted in residential areas and at personal level which can help in increasing social bonding:

i. Social initiatives like developing gated apartments suitable for the aged and keeping vigil by police in vulnerable localities can help to build safer communities
ii. A helpline service for the elderly in every district
iii. Elderly policy councils in every province of India for formulation of strategies to encourage bonding between generations.

This study brings to the notice of the policy makers and the academia to the serious issue of fear of crime in the aged that has disturbed their feeling of safety and security because of weak social bond, elder abuse, prior victimisation, vulnerability and incivility. The research into viewpoints of adult children regarding intergenerational relationships will be a worthwhile exercise. There should be future studies on the causes of dispute within family. This will throw further light on elder abuse and fear of crime in the aged.

To conclude people who have been at the receiving end of prior offense, experience intense fear of crime. Their perception of crime and fear of crime among them is in stark contrast to the aged who have not experienced crime. The dimension of comparison of victimized and non- victimized aged can be explored in upcoming research. This may yield the factors and nature of fear of crime in the aged which may guide the policy makers and law enforcement agencies to tackle various kinds of elder abuse.

Further inquiry can begin in academia to understand the process through which law and order authorities initiate lessening fear of crime in the aged. There should be more research regarding the instruments of law that can be adopted to safeguard the well-being of the aged.

References

Ahuja, R. (2009). *Research methods*. Rawat Publications.

Dammert, L., & Malone, M. E. T. (2003). Fear of crime or fear of life? Public Insecurities in Chile. *Bulletion of Latin American Research, 22*(1), 79–101.

Das, P. K. (2009). Crime against the elderly: A critical analysis. *Help Age India-Research & Development Journal, 15*(2), 21–33.

Donder, L. D., De Witte, N., Dury, S., Buffel, T., & Verte, D. (2012). Individual risk factors of feeling of unsafety in later life. *European Journal of Ageing*.

Durkin, K. F., Wolfe, T. W., & Clark, G. (1999). Social bond theory and binge drinking among college students: A multilevel analysis. *College Student Journal, 33*, 450–461.

Ferraro, K. F., & LaGrange, R. L. (1987). The measurement of fear of crime. *Sociological Inquiry, 57*, 70–101.

Franklin, T. W., Franklin, C. A., & Fearn, N. E. (2008). A multilevel of the vulnerability, disorder and social integration models of fear of crime. *Journal of Social Justice Research, 21*, 204–227.

Garafalo, J. (1981). The fear of crime: Cues and consequences. *The Journal of Criminal Law and Criminology, 72*(2), 839–857.

Geest, S. V. D. (2004). They don't come to listen: The experiences of loneliness among older people in Kwahu, Ghana. *Journal of Cross-Cultural Gerontology, 19*, 77–96.

Geest, S. V. D. (2007). Complaining and not complaining: Social strategies of older people in Kwahu Ghana. *IFA Global Ageing, 4*(3), 55–65.

Geest, S. V. D. (2011). Loneliness and distress in old age: A note from Ghana. In M. Tankink & M. Vysma (Eds.), *Travels in search of (re)connection*. AMB Publishers.

Government of India. (2007). *Maintenance and welfare of parents and senior citizen Act*. Ministry of Social Justice and Empowerment.

Government of India. (2011). *Situation of elderly in India*. Central Statistics Office: Ministry of Statistics and Programme Implementation.

Group for Economic & Social Studies. (2009). *Rising crime against elderly people and responsibility of police in metros*. New Delhi.

Hirschi, T. (1969). *Causes of delinquency*. University of California Press.

Kannan, W. J., & Pruitt, M. V. (2002). Modelling fear of crime and perceived victimisation risk: The (in)significance of neighbourhood integration. *Sociological Inquiry, 72*(4), 527–548.

Kalavar, J. M., Jamuna, D., & Ejaz, F. K. (2013). Elder abuse in India: Extrapolating from the experiences of seniors in India's Pay and Stay Homes. *Journal of Elder Abuse and Neglect, 25*, 3–18.

Khan, A. M. (2004). Decay in family dynamics of interaction, relation and communication as determinant of growing vulnerability among elders. *Indian Journal of Gerontology, 18*(2), 173–186.

Khan, A. M., & Handa, S. (2011). Exploring older persons' perception about old age and different forms of elder abuse. *Help Age India-Research and Development Journal, 17*(2), 7–19.

Miethe, T. D., & Lee, G. R. (1984). Fear of crime among older people: A reassessment of the predictive power of crime-related factors. *The Sociological Quarterly, 25*(3), 397–415.

Mishra, A. J., & Patel, A. B. (2013). Crimes against the elderly in India: A content analysis on factors causing fear of crime. *International Journal of Criminal Justice Science, 8*(1), 13–23.

Nalla, M. K., Joseph, J. D., & Smith, R. H. (2011). Prior victimization, region and neighborhood effects on fear of crime in Mumbai, India. *Asian Journal of Criminology, 6*, 141–159.

National Crime Records Bureau. (2011). *Crime in India report*. Ministry of Home Affairs.

National Crime Records Bureau. (2016). *Crime in India 2016: Statistics*. Ministry of Home Affairs. Retrieved from http://ncrb.gov.in/StatPublications/CII/CII2016/pdfs/Crime%20Statistics%20-%202016.pdf

On-fung, C., Cheng, K. H. C., & Phillips, D. R. (2009). *Paper presented at the annual meeting of the British Society of Gerontology*.

Parker, K. D., & Ray, M. C. (1990). Fear of crime: An assessment of related factors. *Sociological Spectrum, 10*, 2940.

Patel, M. (2010). Crimes against the elderly. *Indian Journal of Gerontology, 24*(3), 395–402.

Patel, A. B., & Mishra, A. J. (2018). Shift in family dynamics as a determinant of weak social bonding. *The Indian Journal of Social Work, 79*(1), 83–98.

Rufus, D., & Shekhar, B. (2011). A study on victims of elder abuse: A case study of residents of old age homes in Tirunelveli district. *Help Age India-Research and Development Journal, 17*(3), 29–39.

Sampson, R., Raudenbush, S., & Earls, F. (1997). Neighbourhoods and violent crime: A multilevel study of collective efficacy. *Science, 277*, 918–924.

Vandeviver, C. (2011). *Fear of crime in the EU-15 and Hungary.* Retrieved from https://biblio.ugent.be/publication

Wilson, J. Q., & Kelling, G. L. (1989). Making neighbourhoods safe. *Atlantic Monthly*, 46–52.

Chapter 13
Voluntary Organisations Working for Older Persons in India: A Case Study of HelpAge India

Anupama Datta

Abstract '*Vridhashram*' is a term most people in India are familiar with, most of these are found in what is called the *'tirthsthan'* or towns associated with attaining nirvana after death. Some were also established in other towns and cities mainly for single or destitute women. These charitable organisations were a response to the notion of how to lead the last phase of life along with destitution, penury and want in case of sickness. By and large, older persons were respected members of the family who were ensured life and death with dignity. In this era, longevity was low, family size was big and general ethos were respect and care of older persons. However, time changed and so did the other factors; the first non-family actor to intervene in the matter was the government who formulated and implemented policies and schemes for old age security. In the 1980s voluntary sector organisations as we know them today rushed in to respond to the needs of the growing elderly population. The nature, composition and work of these organisations have changed over the years with change in demographic, socio-economic and political situations. The history of HelpAge India, set up in 1978, is co-emergent with these developments. It is not only a pioneer in the field; but, also by far, the only pan India organisation that provides direct and indirect support to older persons. With each decade the organisation faced different challenges and its response followed the trajectory of these needs and demands of the elderly in the country.

Keywords Charitable organisations · Voluntary sector · Government · Support to older person · Challenges and responses

Introduction

In the ancient times in India, life was divided into four phases in the Varnashrama: Brahmacharya, Grihastha, Vanaprastha and Sanyasa. It was based on an assumption that each individual would have life of about 100 years. In modern terms it was

---

A. Datta (✉)
Head, Policy Research and Advocacy, HelpAge India, New Delhi, India
e-mail: anupama@helpageindia.org

M. K. Shankardass (ed.), *Gerontological Concerns and Responses in India*,
https://doi.org/10.1007/978-981-16-4764-2_13

period of preparation and training as a student, then life as a householder and after all the social responsibilities of the individual were completed satisfactorily, s/he would disengage from this world and start preparation for the purification of the soul by way of meditation or activities for benefit of others. However, this was only the ideal and real life was different. But the basic spirit of the system, disengagement continued to guide the behaviour of the people at large. Many people, in old age, withdrew from active life and went as pilgrims to Varanasi and Haridwar to live a reclusive life and die peacefully. The widows were sent to pilgrimage centres like Mathura and Vrindavan and Kashi at any age and were supposed to live a reclusive life in service of God. These destitute and older persons were serviced in the cities by charitable institutions that were mainly religious in nature and run by either affluent masses with liberal donations or religious trusts.

Till early twentieth century when life expectancy was low and family was taking care of the needs of the older persons, the need for such organisations was low and manageable. However, with increasing longevity and decreasing family sizes and shift from joint to nuclear families, large scale migration, both intra and inter country, things began to change. Institutional care that was only the need for destitute older persons and was planned and run for them became the need for a much larger segment of the population.

The Indian Constitution mentions social security in Article 41 stating: The state shall, within the limits of its economic capacity and development, make effective provision for securing the right to work, to education and to public assistance in cases of unemployment, old age, sickness and disablement and in other cases of undeserved want.

The social pension system was started by some state governments in 1950s along with old age care homes. But these were more by way of exception than rule. Up until the 1980s, Govt. of India maintained that older persons were looked after by the family in India and there was no need for government intervention. In the Vienna Assembly, the then PM of India Mrs Indira Gandhi said,

> *If we look at the demographic figures for the 1960s to 1980 we see that shift is gradually taking place but not visible enough for the government to do policy intervention.*

Comparative Data 1961–1991

Age groups	1961	1971	1981	1991
All ages	438,936,918	548,159,652	665,287,849	838,567,936
60–64	11,239,775	14,374,032	18,167,562	22,748,976
65–69	4,851,934	7,001,249	9,514,421	12,858,499
70–74	4,415,078	5,878,564	8,196,143	10,554,081
75–79	1,720,383	2,245,708	3,162,497	4,145,573

(continued)

(continued)

Age groups	1961	1971	1981	1991
80+	2,484,939	3,200,178	4,126,764	6,374,511
Total	24,712,109	32,699,731	43,167,387	56,681,640

Source Census of India 2001

It was only in 1999 that Govt. of India adopted the National Policy on Older Persons. It was a step in the right direction in pursuance of the UN General Assembly Resolution 47/5 to observe 1999 as International Year of Older Persons.

In the last decades of the twentieth century and two decades of the 21st, things have changed dramatically and we see some activity on the part of governments both central and the state to deal with this challenge. In 1995, the Government of India announced National Social Assistance Scheme under which there was a provision to give non-contributory pensions to destitute older persons. The eligibility criteria included poverty along with destitution. The Government of India also adopted the Integrated Programme for Older Persons. It was a grant in aid scheme that included provision for giving 75% grant to voluntary organisations to set up and run residential facilities for older persons. The scheme is still part of central government's efforts to fund services for older persons, but it has undergone many changes.

It is important to state the relevant provisions (para 72–77) of NPOP here that pertains to services for older persons and the role of voluntary organisations in providing those services.

> The State alone cannot provide all the services needed by older persons. Private sector agencies cater to a rather small paying segment of the population. The National Policy recognizes the NGO sector as a very important institutional mechanism to provide user friendly affordable services to complement the endeavours of the State in this direction.
>
> Voluntary effort will be promoted and supported in a big way and efforts made to remedy the current uneven spread both within a state and between states. There will be continuous dialogue and communication with NGOs on ageing issues and on services to be provided. Networking, exchange of information and interactions among NGOs will be facilitated. Opportunities will be provided for orientation and training of manpower. Transparency, accountability, simplification of procedures and timely release of grants to voluntary organisations will ensure better services. The grant-in-aid policy will provide incentives to encourage organisation to raise their own resources and not become dependent only on government funding for providing services on a sustainable basis.
>
> Trusts, charities, religious and other endowments will be encouraged to expand their areas of concern to provide services to the elderly by involving them on ageing issues.
>
> Older persons will be encouraged to organize themselves to provide services to fellow senior citizens thereby making use of their professional knowledge, expertise and contacts. Initiatives taken by them in advocacy, mobilization of public opinion, raising of resources and community work will be supported.
>
> Support will be provided for setting up volunteer programmes which will mobilize the participation of older persons and others in community affairs, interact with the elders and help them with their problems. Volunteers will be provided opportunities for training and orientation on handling problems of the elderly and kept abreast of developments in the field to promote active ageing. Volunteers will be encouraged to assist the home bound elderly, particularly frail and elderly women and help them to overcome loneliness.

> Trade unions, employers' organisations and professional bodies will be approached to organize sensitivity programmes for their members on ageing issues and promote and organize services for superannuated workers.

In the year, 2009, the Indian Parliament passed Maintenance and Welfare of Parents and Senior Citizen Act. This enabling legislation besides making the family legally responsible for care of aged parents and relatives; made express provision for model old age homes in each district to care for the poor and destitute elderly. This provision did not get implemented due to paucity of funds and land.

Meanwhile, market forces have responded to the effective need for old age homes in the country and many homes and retirement communities have mushroomed. These homes are ranging from individual initiatives in small apartments to large scale specialized projects in cities like Jaipur, Delhi, Bengaluru, Pune, Hyderabad and Chennai. These services are completely unregulated from the point of view of special needs of older persons. Those started by individuals and voluntary organisations are only regulated by other municipal and care services by laws.

If we examine the voluntary organisations that were given grant by the central government under IPOP, we find that in the period from 2008 to 2016, 774 voluntary organisations were given grant to undertake 1653 various age care projects. This data needs to be examined thoroughly to understand the kind of services provided to the older persons in the country along with the impact of these projects on their lives.

HelpAge India: In Service of Elderly for Four Decades

Visionary Founding Fathers

It is important to understand and appreciate the role of HelpAge India in old age care in India. In the genesis, it is important to mention the contribution of the few visionaries who set up the organisation in an era where age care was unheard of. The First Of The Founding Fathers, Mr. Samson A. Daniel, Secretary of the Delhi Christian Friend in Need Society, who was helping the Society build an old age home in Fatehpur Beri, Delhi, could envision a future where large number of the elderly would need care. While building the Home, the Society could muster resources only for the ground floor of the Home, but work stopped because of lack of funds for the first floor that was to house the ladies. He had to run from pillar to post to get a sponsor. He realized that two hurdles were challenging him: lack of awareness and lack of funds. While searching for sponsors he heard that Mr. Cecil Jackson-Cole, a pioneer of modern charitable giving was visiting India in 1974, he decided to turn to him for help.

Mr. Jackson-Cole had played a key role in the founding voluntary organisations like Oxfam, ActionAid. He was of the view that voluntary organisation could no longer function as traditional charities which were based on complete trust. Donors just handed over money to the charities and assumed that the money would be well spent. He was convinced that voluntary organisations should be structured and function like any other professional entities if they were to make any significant impact in the modern society. So, Mr. Daniel did not get a simple cheque from Mr. Jackson-Cole but training to raise funds. This remains the core competence of the organisation even now. Mr. Daniel put theory into practice by organising a fundraising event at Queen Mary School, Delhi in the mid-seventies for the construction of the Society's long-awaited ladies wing. No less than Rs 8000 was raised by the end of the day!

Both Daniel and Jackson-Cole realized that this was just the beginning. To tackle the issues concerning elderly in future an organisation dedicated to their cause had to be established. Mr. Jackson – Cole's wanted the Indian organisation to follow the model of Help the Aged, UK. He also realized that this organisation could not depend on the funds from the United Kingdom, but raise it from local sources. HelpAge India came into being in 1978 with Jackson-Cole as its first President.

HelpAge India commenced its operations from a tiny office in Himalaya House, Kasturba Gandhi Marg in Central Delhi in 1978, functioning out of two cramped rooms with a staff of 30 people. Though the office was registered with the Government of India, it functioned as a branch of HelpAge International, UK. Indeed, its first meeting was held in Dower Street, London!

Daniel a pioneer in the art of fund raising in India also joined HelpAge India and started sponsored walks (events where school children walked for a cause and in the process raised funds for it). Raising funds from schools was the idea of Mr. John F Pearson, a Trustee of HelpAge India. They approached top schools first and were astonished by the overwhelming response which seemed nothing short of a miracle. Mr. Daniel maintained his links with the organisation in an honorary capacity till 1986.

With Philip Jackson, one of the founder members of HelpAge International, on board in 1978 as HelpAge India's first Chief Executive, it was decided that the organisation would function in partnership with various community-based and voluntary organisations (NGOs) to implement appropriate programmes for the benefit of elderly. The official organisational policy stipulated that HelpAge India would play the role of a catalyst in the welfare of the elderly. It would fund other and smaller NGOs. The main task assigned to the staff was to raise funds and they would be operating mainly from their own homes. Staff salaries were fixed at Rs 1000 a month and they were provided bicycles for field work.

The year 1980 saw the advent of an individual who was to become an integral part of HelpAge story and its driving force. Mr. Madan Mohan Sabharwal, who had a successful career in the corporate world, began to focus his attention and his skills for promoting the cause of the aged. Interestingly, he was rather reluctant to join the organisation when he was invited to do so in 1980 by the then President of HelpAge for the simple reason that he could not devote adequate attention and time to the organisation. They persuaded him only to give an hour every day. He is quoted as saying, "So I had to agree, 'little realising that this would become my consuming passion". In due course of time, he took over the reins as President of HelpAge India's Governing in 1986–87 succeeding Mr. Pearson.

Mr. Sabharwal's career included being Chairman of several corporations including Dunlop India Ltd., Shalimar Paints, Needle Industries (India) Pvt. Ltd., Britannia Industries and Bata India. For him, working for a small organisation like HelpAge India, which was doing work for poor elderly was a new experience and his challenge was colossal, to turn it into a pan India body. Being the meticulous man that he was, he started by attending lectures and workshops to better understand how the charity organisations functioned and also about the issues concerning the elderly.

He always maintained that in a society whose fabric is changing as fast as India's, the elderly need to be taken care of more than ever before. It was this belief that finally led him to continue to be the crusader for the cause and the organisation. He tapped his social and professional contacts to help both. He wanted to raise funds for direct intervention programmes for the poor and disadvantaged elderly and raise general awareness about ageing and aged in India. He continued to be associated with HelpAge India till his last with same alacrity.

Initial Efforts of HelpAge India

In 1979, a year after its inception, more than two lakh children participated in the first sponsored walk—a unique combination of fund and awareness generation—one of the earliest initiatives to involve students and bring the cause of the elderly home to their parents. In 1982, school students of Delhi participated in walks to collect funds for HelpAge India's first medicare programme: the Mobile Medicare Unit (MMU). HelpAge India's first Mobile Medicare Unit was inaugurated in March that year for Delhi and Faridabad areas. Around the same time, the local community in Madangir Colony in the Capital made available a room where the service was temporarily centred. With this modest Unit, HelpAge India crossed the threshold of the most important and robust programme for health care of disadvantaged older persons. Mobile Units were designed to service those older persons who could not seek or reach the standard stationary medical units that were the order of the day. It was targeted at the rural and urban poor who for various reasons were excluded from getting health care services, hence also known as "Reaching the Unreached".

The spread across the country in an effort to provide quality health care to older people via the Mobile Medicare Unit necessitated the use of a symbol. Added to this was the need for visibility. The then CEO, Mr. Nigel who was from advertising background played major role in designing the logo for HelpAge India.

As HelpAge India was expanding its operations in the country, new needs of the older persons were coming to light. Thus, a new programme was born in 1983 known as Adopt-a-Gran, the programme called Support-a-Gran today was modelled on a similar concept propagated by Help the Aged, UK. This programme was designed to look after the basic needs of the destitute elderly except housing. The donors/ sponsors were supporting the basket of goods for the included elderly for their lifetime. The Little Sisters of the Poor, a Chennai-based organisation, was the first partner chosen to implement Adopt-a-Gran. The programme has since then, touched the lives of thousands. The following case study will illustrate the usefulness of this programme.

Ramlal, a 70 years mill worker survived a near fatal accident that severely injured his leg. Constant dizzy spells led to brain surgery. He tried to earn a living by running small tea stall; but, his deteriorating physical condition—increasing age, poor hearing and eyesight—made it difficult for him to continue. Under deep debt due to expenditure on seven leg surgeries and need for constant medication, with approximately Rs 2000 monthly expense on medicines, etc. life became unliveable for him. The main earner was now his wife Makati, who earned barely enough to keep body and soul together by selling vegetables. The enrolment of Ramlal in HelpAge India's Support-a-Grandparent programme with regular supply of monthly ration and money brought much needed support for him and his family.

The next logical step in ensuring income security for the disadvantaged older persons was to design and implement income generation programme by giving micro credit to the elderly. The core principle remained what was the cardinal rule for HelpAge, i.e. cost effective and benefiting the elderly. In the year 1991–1992, HelpAge India launched this programme aimed at involving elderly persons in income generation through the revival and upgradation of traditional crafts, cottage industries and animal husbandry units. The major thrust of the programme was that of organising the elderly as a group and increasing their participation in individual and group-based income generating activities. It was an end to end programme with elderly involved in all the steps from procurement to production to selling of the product. Small-scale enterprises were set up like candle making in Bhopal and carpet-weaving in Bhadoi. There were other enterprises like vermi-composting, horticulture, garland making, flower selling, tea shops, etc.

HelpAge India conducted a nationwide survey to assess the quality of life of elderly beneficiaries covered under its various welfare programmes. The findings of the survey led HelpAge India to shift from pure welfare to development-oriented work. It is for this reason that HelpAge India added the Micro-Credit Programme to its growing portfolio in 1999.

HelpAge India also made effort to address the next most important concern of the elderly, viz shelter. The first ever such project that HelpAge India took up was the old age home in Fatehpur Beri in Delhi. In the initial years, HelpAge supported through grants more than 40 old age homes including homes like the Little Sisters of the Poor and the SahayaIllam, both in erstwhile Madras, which benefitted from one of the organisation's most successful sponsored walks.

Next Leap: Sagacious Mix of Old and New

Old age brings with it many problems, of these, health is the most important as it directly impinges on quality of life of older persons. In a country like India the size of population and a low pace of economic growth worsens the situation. According to estimates, for an effective health care structure, the Government needs to earmark at least over 6% of Gross Domestic Product (GDP) on public health system but the allocation has been much less. Thus, there is a huge gap between the need and what is actually given. In 1981 there were 44 million older persons in India. Today there are about 100 million older persons and the figure is likely to cross 177 million by the year 2025. Of these, 90% belong to unorganized sector, which means no social security cover in old age. About one third of these live below the poverty line and another one third just above the poverty line, thereby about 66% of the older persons are in a vulnerable situation without adequate food, clothing and shelter. In the absence of State's medical facilities, private practitioners, including quacks, thrive and charge heavily from innocent and uneducated poor older people.

The government health services are generally based on Primary Health Centres (PHCs) but inaccessibility to and inadequacies of most of these PHCs have limited their utility. Moreover, the distance from the place of stay of poor elderly and compulsions like absence of someone to take the elderly to Primary Health Centre or to a doctor, pose a major deterrent. In the absence of State's medical facilities, private practitioners, including quacks, thrive and charge heavily from innocent and uneducated poor older people. In short, the basic medical services, which should be their right, are either not available to them or are unaffordable.

Nearly 36 years ago, HelpAge India (HI) recognized the need to reach older people who could not access health facilities those living in urban slums, resettlement colonies and peripheral villages, are mainly engaged in the unorganized sector of the economy. These people are daily wage earners and cannot afford to miss out on work to take family members to hospitals or dispensaries. As part of a major programme called Reaching the Unreached, HI has been providing poor older people with basic health services in their community. These MMUs not only meet essential health care needs but also raise awareness among older people and others of the importance of maintaining good health in old age.

The professionals touring in the medical vans provide:

- Preventive health care and counselling
- Medical check-ups
- Medication to treat the most common ailments.

Each van is equipped with medicines and equipment to diagnose and treat the most common ailments. These include viral diseases, diabetes, blood pressure and arthritis. Each unit has a manager/social worker who organizes the visits and the shifts. Besides a driver, each shift consists of a doctor, a pharmacist. Geriatrics is not a field of specialisation that is generally available in India—although there are some local initiatives to train medical students. Instead, older, experienced doctors are recruited for the work.

All staff members receive training to familiarize them with the most common ailments affecting older people and sensitize them to older people's needs. Staff members are also required to abide by a specific code of conduct in their work. HI has a regular system for monitoring and evaluating the performance of each unit against precise targets.

The medical vans visit each area regularly, usually once a week at the same time. In order to provide a comprehensive service, HI has secured agreements both with the hospitals in the areas visited by the medical vans and with pharmaceutical companies to provide medicines. The pharmaceutical companies provide HI with a range of common medicines at a discounted rate, which enables the units to provide these free to patients. People needing more help, for example, X-Rays and a range of basic diagnostic tests, eye tests and dental examinations are sent to a local hospital for free investigation and treatment.

The staff members keep detailed records of each person attending the unit. Patients are also provided with a registration card recording their case history. Medicines are usually provided for a week at a time to ensure that patients attend again at the unit's next visit and thus receive continuous treatment. The staff is generally able to cater for almost 90% of the health problems presented to them. The remaining 10% are dealt with through referral to hospitals.

This programme has received financial support from the corporate sector in India and NRI organisations. They have generously provided money for covering the capital cost of the Units. However, the major issue has been that of finding sources to fund the annual operational cost.

From the modest beginning of a mobile dispensary with one doctor, one pharmacist and social worker, in many areas, it has adopted a more advanced model of providing additional services like pathological test facilities and physiotherapy services. It has also built networks and partnerships with tertiary care units and provide referral services.

Mobile Health Care Units not only work to provide health care services during normal times; but play a crucial role in disaster affected areas. Within 24 h of the catastrophe in Gujarat 4 MMUs manned with surgeons and paramedics reached the affected area. At 12 noon on 26th January 2001, the first HI MMU reached Ahmedabad and was extricating a child out of Shri Narayan School. During the initial phase, MMU infrastructure was used not only for providing medical care but also for distribution of about 1,00,000 potable water pouches and also water sterilization kits and food packets to the affected people. These MMUs mainly targeted the interior villages those un-reached by other agencies. 60 surgeries were performed by the MMU staff in near field conditions. For about 45 days two MMUs were working on the project of provision of artificial limbs to the people in cooperation with other NGOs. In other words, MMUs perform a wide array of useful activities in times of emergency and help not only the older persons but all those who are affected. The entire programme was conducted with cooperation from the State Government and Central Ministry of Social Justice and Empowerment and other agencies like HelpAge International, DFID, DEC. Four MMUs continued to work in the area till the end of November 2001. A total number of about 72,000 people of all age groups benefited from MMU operation in the area up to 31st December 2001. MMUs perform a wide array of useful activities in times of emergency and help not only the older persons but all those who are affected.

This programme has proved to be one of our most successful programmes in health security. It has demonstrated that positive role, sincere efforts of NGOs, can play to supplement the efforts of governments in the field of health. It not only provides preventive health care for older persons but also sensitize older persons and the community to the issue of healthy ageing. Besides, in times of emergency, it could expand its activities to cover an area much beyond health care for older persons. It is a novel experiment that could be emulated in resource-deficient countries. However, to be really successful requires wholehearted support of other actors in society like the corporates, who could come forward to finance these ventures.

Mobile Medicare Unit programme made steady headway, with new MMUs being regularly added to the fleet. In 1996 the programme saw a quantum jump mainly because of the extraordinary response from the sponsored walks in the schools. The Best example to illustrate the response is that in the year 1998–1999 just one school in Chennai collected as much as Rs 5.04 lakh!

It made steady headway and from the modest beginning of mobile dispensary with one doctor, one pharmacist and social worker, in many areas, it has adopted a more advanced model of providing additional services like pathological test facilities and physiotherapy services. It has also built networks and partnerships with tertiary care units and provide referral services.

Mobile Health care programme was unique at the time it was launched. For the first time, health care services reached the door steps of the urban poor elderly in resettlement colonies. As mentioned today it has expanded throughout the length and breadth of the country. The model has been standardized and scaled up, both in terms of external and internal processes. To provide best services to the poor elderly medical team is duly certified, generic drugs are procured through a centralized system from certified manufacturers and proper inventory is maintained to control delivery and weeding out expired drugs. A web-based, multiple sites, direct upload facility is sued for monitoring and reviewing field operations, patient registrations, treatments and disease patterns.

HelpAge's MMU units are spread across Andhra Pradesh, Bihar, Chandigarh, Chhattisgarh, Delhi (NCR), Goa, Gujarat, Himachal Pradesh, Jammu & Kashmir, Jharkhand, Karnataka, Maharashtra, Madhya Pradesh, Assam, Tripura, Odisha, Puducherry, Punjab, Rajasthan, Tamil Nadu, Uttar Pradesh and West Bengal. Besides providing primary health care, some MMUs also provide additional support such as counselling, physiotherapy, yoga, shelter assistance and organize health camps.

Normally, each MMU works six days a week from 9 am to 5 pm. It covers a cluster of 10–15 community sites/villages on a weekly schedule averaging 200 km per week. This means that each MMU targets at reaching medical services to 100–150 patients per day in remote rural locations and around 200 patients in urban areas.

In fact, the partnership between ONGC and HelpAge India was one of the biggest ever in the history of both organisations. The pan India health care programme for the elderly called Varisthajan Swasthya Seva Abhiyaan was launched across 20 locations via HelpAge's MMUs. Asian Paints and Bharat Electronics (BEL) also came forward to support the MMU programme in a big way,

To function effectively, the MMU initiative requires a huge amount of medical supplies, Pharmaceutical major Pfizer Limited (India) stepped in to help HelpAge's MMU operations and CIPLA, another pharmaceutical giant, came forward to lend a hand. In 2000–2001, they donated Rs 38 lakh worth of medicines to assist the then existing 20 MMUs, benefiting four lakh elderly persons. In 2002–03, HelpAge received nearly Rs 1 crore worth of medicines from CIPLA, which helped treat thousands of older people. Help for the MMU unit has also come from Ranbaxy, Bharat Heavy Electricals Ltd. (BHEL), GAIL (India) Ltd., the GMR group, KPMG as well the Department of Science and Technology, Ministry of Social Justice and Empowerment and the Uttarakhand State Government.

The Limca Book of Records in the year 2008 recognized it as the largest mobile health care network for the elderly in Asia.

Mobile Health Care programme made steady headway and reached a record of 154 Units in financial year 2017–18 with the total treatment of 27.69 lakh in and at the moment there are 160 Units in 24 States and Union Territories, covering 2483 locations in 131 Districts. Most of these Units are supported by corporate Donors through their CSR initiative and Public Sector Units and a few are supported by philanthropists.

Each Mobile Health care Unit is designed to provide primary health care services for the poor at their doorsteps who are economically and socially backwards. The current services are:

- **Free treatment**: The doctor examines patients and, based on available equipment, clinically diagnoses them and prescribes medicines. Where required, the patients are referred to pathological laboratories for detailed investigation/secondary/tertiary health care service providers for specialist treatment and care.
- **Free medicines**: The Units stocks medicines for all common ailments occurring in the community. These medicines are issued to the patients free of cost by the pharmacist on the basis of the prescription. The pharmacist also explains the dosage of medicines and their side effects, if any, to the patients.
- **Basic diagnostics**: The Unit is equipped with basic diagnostic equipment such as stethoscope, BP apparatus, thermometer, weighing machine, etc. for checking the vital signs. In addition, there is a 'glucometer' for blood sugar testing.
- **Home visits by doctor (in case of bedridden patients/patients unable to reach MHU)**: The doctor and the paramedic team conduct weekly visits to the houses of bedridden elders who otherwise cannot approach or be brought to the vehicle. The doctor and paramedic team examines & clinically diagnose the problems presented by the elder patient or caregivers and prescribes medicines and advice the patient and their caregivers.
- **Counselling for patients, elders, family members and caretakers**: The counsellor and the doctor provide necessary advice and counselling to patients and caretakers on various ailments and home care. The project team also conducts regular counselling sessions on various aspects for healthy ageing, i.e. (a) diet and nutrition; (c) weight reduction; (b) regular exercise; (d) smoking; (e) alcohol; (f) social activities. By adopting a healthier lifestyle, the risk of a whole range of diseases can be reduced.
- **Community awareness on the rights of the elderly**: Every person has the right to freedom and respect and the right to be treated fairly by others. A positive,

supportive and caring attitude by family, friends, caretakers and the community will help people to continue as integral, respected and valued members of society.

- **Creating awareness in the community** especially among the younger generation will help to sensitize them on the various aspects of taking care of the aged and in long term and preparing them for their old age.
- **Preventive Health Awareness Programme with IEC Materials and Sanitation Awareness Programme** MHU Team aware community to take preventive measures of the prevailing diseases within the area.
- **Referral linkage with local health providers**: The team promotes initiate linkages with private as well as government health care facilities so as to ensure that the required services would be available on demand. The linkage between the HelpAge India beneficiaries and these identified institutions would ensure accessibility and affordability of the services.
- **Linkage with Govt. schemes and programmes**: This initiative aims to increase awareness among the elderly poor about various social security, food security and Health security schemes and thus enabling them to advocate/demand their rights. We realize that elderly people need support to avail these schemes. The MHU plays a facilitating role in linking them with the local and district administration and also collecting the information from the government offices and disseminating this information to the concerned/eligible beneficiaries thus improving their access to social welfare schemes.
- **Linkages for Cataract Operation**: The team helps elders to get cataract detection and operation from recognized Hospitals.
- **Regular Health Camps/Multi-speciality Health camps**: Team organizes regular Health camps in the surrounding area of sites and specialized health camps to meet the requirement of community for the specific checkup from specialist medical consultants.

Mobile Health Care Units address the problems of lack of affordability, accessibility and availability of basic essential health care to people living in backward regions. The programme fulfils a vital need in the lives of the beneficiaries. Mobile health care Units as a highly effective means of delivery of health services.

Other Health care Programmes

Health care continued to be one of the most urgent concerns of the poor elderly besides income security. As HelpAge India's primary target group is poor, health assumes even more important for them. Most of them do not have any social security in old age and have to work to make two ends meet. As is well known that ability to earn decreases with age particularly the low and unskilled poor workers; but they are compelled and condemned to do hard labour to earn. Secondly, most of them are so poor that they do not have enough to pay for their treatment; poor families are generally reluctant to spend on the health care of elderly. So, health care continues to be one of the top priorities of the HelpAge India in its programme kitty. MHUs provide general care but other important components are ophthalmic care and physiotherapy. Cataract operation restores vision and physiotherapy helps them being mobile. Both interventions help maintain independence and dignity of the individual.

With the Mobile medicare Units beginning, to consolidate their specialized services, a concentrated effort was put into spreading the reach of physiotherapy facilities.

Physiotherapy

Practical field experience and data released by NSSO drew the attention of the Organisation to another important health concern of the elderly population, i.e. mobility. So, a decision was taken to start physiotherapy centres in urban areas, to start with, for providing services to the affected elderly. Physiotherapy is the treatment with physical modalities like heat, cold, mille ampere electric current and with therapeutic exercises for physical wellbeing. The physiological changes result in reduction of muscle power and tone, reduced range of motion and bone density. Symptoms include general weakness faulty body postures, decrease in cardiopulmonary endurance and reduced exercise tolerance. Apart from these, conditions like back pain, shoulder pain and other musculoskeletal conditions, paralysis and other neurological conditions which are common in geriatrics can be managed by physiotherapy.

From 2008, HelpAge India started services in Delhi—NCR and Himachal Pradesh. In Delhi, 35 old age homes with 700 elderly were selected for this service. In Himachal Pradesh, the total target persons for the year was 1000 including one old age home with 30 people and 6 rural villages and one urban community. The success and results achieved during the pilots conducted in Delhi—NCR and Himachal Pradesh, encouraged the Organisation to extend this service activity to Dehradun in Uttarakhand.

The broad objectives of this programme were to

- To carry out physiotherapy need assessment of all residents of Old Age Home and adjacent community members and to provide treatments to those in need of physiotherapy;
- To train care-givers/volunteers in age care;
- To provide basic health and physiotherapy equipment and infrastructure at Old age Home and adjacent community;
- To form an Elder Care Committee in the rural centres.

Over the years, the physiotherapy centres became operational in West Bengal, Madhya Pradesh, Assam, Bihar, Odisha, Chandigarh, Puducherry, Andhra Pradesh, Uttar Pradesh, Jammu and Kashmir besides Himachal Pradesh, Uttarakhand, Delhi—NCR, Kerala and Tamil Nadu where initial centres were opened. From 8000 treatments in 2008, the number of treatments has reached 1.6 lakhs. Here, the story of Sitaram is an example of how physiotherapy can actually change the quality of life.

A 68-year-old daily wage labourer, Sitaram migrated to Guwahati, Assam, in search of a job and now lives in Bamunimaidan's Baikuntha Nagar. A stone-cutter, he had lifted heavy weights all his life. As he grew older, he began to suffer from severe hypertension and weakness and developed a chronic backache. He turned to a walking stick for support; but, the pain grew worse with the daily climb to his hillside dwelling. His wife helped by doing an odd job in neighbour's homes but this wasn't enough for the couple to survive. He was unable to afford special medication. He then heard about HelpAge India's physiotherapy centre and became one of the first to avail of its services. He is now a regular visitor and his health has seen a remarkable improvement. Today, he walks without the aid of a stick and is urging the elders of his community to avail of the centre's services.

Palliative Care

Under this programme, patients and their families are cared for by a team of trained professionals when the patient's disease is no longer responsive to curative treatment and life expectancy is relatively short. A pilot project of three years duration was developed in partnership With the Indian Association of Palliative Care and institute of Palliative Medicine, Kozhikode and funded by HelpAge India, Help the Aged and Help the Hospices, (UK). The project started in Kerala had a 'demonstrate' module in Cuddalore, Tamil Nadu. Nearly 600 health care professionals were trained in Palliative Care, along with HelpAge India's MMU staff. These community managed Palliative Care projects were operational in 52 villages spread across the districts of Cuddalore and Nagapattinam in Tamil Nadu and Kollam in Kerala. The Elders Self Help Groups formed by the organisation manages 14 sub-centres providing professional medical care, home care and assistance to chronically ill and bedridden patients.

Support-a-Gran (SaGP)

For the destitute elders, HelpAge India came up with Adopt-a-Gran in 1983—a programme that quickly became the high point in the lives of many older people. The destitute elderly being serviced through this programme grew to 30,586 in 24 states and support coming from individuals and companies.

The story of 81-year-old Chandrabhaga is a heartening example of how this programme has changed lives. Chandrabhaga had three sons and a daughter—but constant quarrels among her family members forced her to leave home and find work as domestic help. Age, however, caught up with her. She lost her job—her only means of livelihood till Support-a-Gran took her under its wing. Kandi Devi is also one of the many beneficiaries of the SaGP programme. Her family lived a few miles away but did not bother about her as she was old, sick and could neither walk upright nor work or cook a meal for herself. Today as a recipient of the SaGP project, she gets access to free primary medical consultations, free medication as well as food support.

Old Age Homes

Poverty and destitution compel many older persons to live on streets. As mentioned earlier one of the first projects of HelpAge India was Home in Fatehpur Beri in Delhi. HelpAge India in its initial years continued to support old age homes established and managed by charitable organisations. However, in the year 2004, after the Indian Ocean Tsunami, it established a model old age home for the victims in Cuddalore. The organisation has been working towards transforming old age homes into composite shelters which goes beyond dwelling place. Its design and management principles are based on equity, dignity, independence, participation, care and self-fulfilment of the residents. At the moment, HelpAge India is running five old age homes in Punjab, West Bengal and Tamil Nadu.

Elders for Elders: With the lifespan of the elderly on the rise, HelpAge India looked to provide seniors not only with care and shelter but also with more productive means of livelihood. This is the philosophy that drives Elder Self Help Groups (ESHGs), started to help senior citizens work for themselves and for their own betterment—a motive summed up under the principle of 'Elders for Elders'.

A case in point is that of Veera, a village located 45 kms from Anjar, near the Gulf of Kutch in Gujarat. It was here that HelpAge India formed the Ashapura Vridh Mahila Bachat Mandal (Ashapura Savings Association of Older Women), self-help group (SHG) comprising 13 members, under a post-earthquake reconstruction project. To start with, members' attendance was very low and savings were irregular. Constant counselling and formal training for concept clarity and effective leadership helped members of the group understand the benefits of being organized and maintaining their own records to ensure financial security. The group was taken on a trip to Dwarka where they met another women's group working on rights-based issues. This visit supported HelpAge's efforts to broaden the agenda of the group and encouraged group members to address issues other than savings and credit.

Remotely located, Veera tacked even basic facilities like drinking water, health and education. Although there was a pipeline running through it, the water supply was erratic. Constant drought had compounded matters and the women had to walk anywhere between five and 10 kms to fetch water. Neither the villagers nor the sarpanch (village head) was bothered about the problem. So it took a while before this issue was brought up at one of the SHG meetings. The members were slightly hesitant in the beginning but, remembering their experiences during their trip to Dwarka they decided to tackle the problem. With some help, they prepared an application and each member put her thumb impression on it.

This effort by an SHG of older women motivated others and soon the whole village signed up. The sarpanch himself submitted the application to the authorities. During a women's meeting, Benaben, the president of this group, shared her experience with the others. "The district official was taken aback by the confidence of our member. He requested us not to approach the block office and promised to solve our problem. Within two days, two water tankers arrived with drinking water and they have been coming regularly since then. Our water woes are now a thing of the past." Benaben says the group members never believed they would be able to take such an initiative. "Today, it is proven that if we are united and determined, we can achieve the desired results."

Elderly in Disaster Affected Areas

In another pioneering effort HelpAge India, in 1980, set up a disaster rescue and relief unit under the supervision of a senior retired army officer. The unit was trained and equipped for swift and effective relief measures in the face of natural disasters. Its abilities were tested in a post flood situation in districts in Uttar Pradesh. The unit did commendable work without any help from the local administration in many remote villages Sitapur and Jaunpur districts. However, this seed Unit realized its potential in the twenty-first century when natural disasters affected the country in unprecedented manner in terms of intensity, expanse and frequency to require a full-fledged Unit manned by trained professionals. HelpAge India rushed in to help the elderly along with the community in all natural disaster situations from Orissa Super-cyclone in the year 2000 to flash floods in Uttarakhand in 2013. The underlying assumption was that the specific concerns of the elderly affected by the disasters were being overlooked while designing and implementing the post disaster relief and rehabilitation packages. In the immediate relief operations, HelpAge India provided help to all in the community by way of medical intervention, food and survival kits. However, rehabilitation and disaster risk reduction are specifically focused on older persons. It is not restricted to providing support but also building the capacity of the older persons in disaster prone areas to be active participants in the process.

Orissa Cyclone Relief and Rehabilitation

A super cyclone struck Orissa on 29th October 1999. A total population of 1.25 crore was estimated to be affected by the cyclone, i.e. more than one third of the total population and geographical area of the state was affected by this twister. Besides livestock and houses, thousands of hectares of paddy and non-paddy crops were destroyed by high-speed winds, floods, soil-erosion, saline inundation and sand cast. It not only destroyed the standing crops but also the agricultural land. The total loss was estimated to be around 20 billion rupees. This calamity brought unimaginable suffering and miseries to the population. Although the cyclone affected everyone, the vulnerable segments of the population, i.e. children, women and older persons suffered the most.

HelpAge India holds the view that the older persons were disadvantaged because of lack of access (social political physical), invisibility and marginalization. Moreover, they had to shoulder the responsibility of looking after the survivors. Therefore, the team worked on the Relief and Rehabilitation project which was financially supported by DISASTER EMERGENCY COMMITTEE (DEC) through HelpAge International in the state from 4th November 1999 to 10th May 2000 with a budget of Rs. 29,381,440 with the following aims:

(a) To reduce the risk of illness and death among the families of 5000 older persons in the cyclone affected districts of Orissa.
(b) To provide food security, shelter and essential items for 4100 older persons in the project area, for 130 days.

The programme was implemented in two different phases. The effort in the initial phase was to provide immediate aid like food items, polythene sheets for temporary shelter and blankets to the victims. It covered families of 5000 older persons in six affected districts viz. Jagatsinghpur, Cuttack, Keonjhar, Dhenkanal, Jajpur and Puri In the second phase the efforts were more focused. A detailed survey was conducted to identify the beneficiaries and their specific needs. A participatory approach was adopted and the older persons were asked to identify their requirements and programme was planned accordingly.

The ration size was calculated as per WHO guidelines considering average family size, of 5 persons in each household. Thus intervention by HelpAge India ensured provision of food to 25,000 people in the initial phase. The items distributed to each older person included good quality rice, pulses, iodized salt, edible oil, a blanket and a polythene sheet for temporary shelter arrangements. Besides, two Mobile Medicare Units were deployed in the region to provide preventive and curative medicine as well as water purification tablets to the affected population.

The second phase was designed as a targeted feeding programme; its coverage was exclusively for older persons. This targeted feeding was initially designed for 90 days, along with provision of household utensils and support for house repairing for 4100 older persons from 134 villages.

The beneficiaries were provided with 45 kg rice, 6 kg pulses, 2 L edible oil, 2 kg iodized salt, household articles worth Rs. 625 and cash support of Rs. 2500/- to each one. Later, additional food for 40 days was provided for all the 4100 beneficiaries bringing the overall coverage of feeding to be of 130 days.

This programme may seem like a drop in the ocean but it certainly made a difference to the lives of the older persons and their dependents in the areas covered. The intervention brought material and non-material benefits. The food items provided not only provided food security but the money saved could be later used to purchase other items like seeds. It added to the dignity of the older and at times brought families closer to them and gave them the confidence to participate in decision making in the family. These older persons were no longer a burden but an asset.

In response to the needs assessment, HelpAge India selected seven partner agencies that were associated through its various ongoing projects. Our team worked in close coordination with the seven partner organisations—National Youth service Action and Social Development Research Institute (NYSASDRI), Friends' Association for Rural Reconstruction (FARR), Young Men's Christian Association (YMCA), UtkalSevakSamaj (USS), AnchalikaKunjeswariSanskrutikaSansad (AKSS), People's Cultural Centre (PECVC), People's Forum (PF). Feeling of mutual trust and fraternity existed among all the partner agencies throughout the implementation of the programme. The partner agencies reported that they experienced a behavioural change among the younger generations to the cause and care of the older persons in their operational area. They also admit that various training, interaction, joint planning, meetings and the logistical support provided to them by HelpAge India has greatly enhanced their capacity for future disaster management.

During packaging, due care was given to pack the right quantity and in the right manner to avoid any pilferage during transportation and distribution. The re-packed relief goods were then properly loaded, recorded and then transported to the distribution sites mainly by mini trucks. For quick delivery of the relief goods, the items to be given during relief and—rehabilitation were standardized and each agency adopted the same procedure. This helped to implement the relief and rehabilitation programme effectively and efficiently. Each agency, during its planning phase, had identified, distribution points where volunteers and supervisory staff were available to organize the village community with the local authorities to supervize the distribution. The selected beneficiaries were given a distribution slip at least one day before the distribution by the field workers of the agency, clearly indicating the date and place of distribution. The signature or thumb impressions of the beneficiaries were taken on the distribution register or sheet maintained by the agency. HelpAge India's staff participated and facilitated the procurement, packaging, transportation and distribution of all the commodities.

A very effective monitoring system was devised to ensure proper distribution of the commodities. During the Second Phase, all the agencies established their camp offices in the affected areas and the volunteers visited individual households to enquire about the pace of implementation of various components of the relief programme. An end use check format was developed and distributed among the partner agencies to keep a watch on their consumption pattern of food commodities and the progress of household repair. Each agency was asked to do a 10% end use check to understand the way the beneficiaries utilising the commodities.

HelpAge India's efforts to sensitize the international donor agencies and local NGOs to the cause of the older persons were also successful. A vulnerability check list was circulated in the UN meetings, prepared by HelpAge International, which provided indicators to access the health, social, basic needs and mobility aspects of older persons in emergencies. One of the key decisions was that vulnerable older persons, who could not be included in food for work programmes, should be included in the targeted feeding programme implemented by HelpAge India. The Government and the International NGOs did concur with the fact that vulnerable older persons need to be provided with food to meet their immediate needs.

The secret of effective disaster management lies largely in effective preparedness. In order to train volunteers for future HelpAge India organized a one-day training workshop. Representatives of all the seven partner agencies participated in it. Mr. Jagadanand, an authority on disaster preparedness and management in Orissa was the main resources person. Ms. Kwan Li of CONCERN facilitated the group work of the members and helped in the compilation of the group work. This workshop helped the participating agencies to understand the concept and strategies of disaster preparedness.

The broad area touched upon by Mr. Jagadanand included elements of preparedness planning, pre-disaster planning steps, scope of disaster related action, disaster management and development, relief administration and capacity building for coping mechanism towards disaster reduction, disaster management and development, assessment, disaster preparedness framework, common problems in disaster preparedness, recent trends in disaster preparedness and role of NGOs. Ms. Kwan Li shared with the participants the community-based disaster preparedness plan developed by DEC member agencies. The workshop was short but informative and a capacity building process for the partners.

It was a great learning experience for all the members of our Organisation. They learnt how to tackle exigencies of procurement, transportation and distribution of aid material and community behaviour. Their practical experience coupled with the knowledge of the experts invited for the workshop will be a storehouse of knowledge to be used in future programmes.

Gujarat Earthquake

Devastating earthquake caused extensive damage to human life and property in Gujarat in January 2001. Four districts of the state, namely, Kachchh, Rajkot, Surendranagar and Jamnagar suffered major losses. People and administration took some time to get out of this sudden and terrible shock. After an emergency meeting at HelpAge India's Head Office, the team swung into action. Besides dedication, it was equipped with experience of dealing with disaster situations after cyclone in Orissa. HI concentrated on three districts of Gujarat, i.e. Kachchh, Surendranagar and Rajkot comprising of the *talukas* Bhuj and Anjar in Kachchh district, Morbi in Rajkot district and the *talukas* of Limdi and Wadhvan in Surendranagar district. This has a geographical coverage of 43 villages.

The initial reaction was to provide services for immediate needs of quake victims such as medical aid, food, shelter, etc. This was provided to many people irrespective of age. However, in the second phase efforts were made to provide benefits to older people, many of whom were left without any care-givers and many with the additional responsibility of taking care of surviving children.

The main objective of the relief and rehabilitation programme was to reduce the risk of illness, malnutrition and death among the older persons and their families in the affected districts. The specific objective of the project was to restore stable living conditions of 7500 vulnerable older persons and their family members.

All the four partner agencies were given adequate training to select the beneficiaries. The selection of the target group for the programme intervention is primarily selected on the following criteria:

1. Those above the age of 60.
2. Below the poverty line.
3. Sick and abandoned.
4. Widows.
5. Without any extended family for support.
6. Disabled.
7. Those who had lost their earnings.
8. With house severely damaged.

The main objective of the relief and rehabilitation programme was to reduce the risk of illness, malnutrition and death among the older persons and their families in the affected districts. The specific objective of the project was to restore stable living conditions among 7500 vulnerable older persons and their family members.

The target groups identified were from those villages, which were inaccessible to the relief services provided by different agencies, socio-economically backwards and had suffered severe damage in the earthquake.

HelpAge selected four project partners with the logistic capacity to manage relief operations. The initial relief programme was designed to provide immediate food supplies for a 60 day period, household utensils, blankets and polythene sheets. The food package included wheat, rice, *dal,* oil, salt and *bajara* and targeted 7500 older persons and their families.

Six MMUs, each with a team of a doctor, a pharmacist, a programme officer and a driver operated. The medical intervention by HelpAge Mobile Medicare Units concentrated in *Bhuj, Anjar, Bhachau* and *Rapar* in *Kachchh* district. 221 villages were covered and a total of 35,472 patients were treated. On average, during the first five days of the emergency, one hundred and fifty patients per day were provided with medical assistance and referral services in *Kachchh* district. The MMUs provided preventive medicines, antibiotics, water purification tablets, oral dehydration solutions, together with orthopaedic treatment and psychosocial support, in collaboration with partner agencies. Where necessary they referred patients to other agencies such as Medicines Sans Frontiers (MSF). Special attention was paid to the needs of older patients, who not only suffered physical injuries but also were found to be suffering from high anxiety, depression and fear.

The emergency aid packages addressed primarily food and shelter needs. In the worst affected villages, most of the houses had been completely destroyed or seriously damaged. People were living in flimsy shelters hurriedly constructed from whatever was easily available. Older people had not received any tents and were living in the open fields or in makeshift shelters made of plastic sheets and sacks and old clothes. These were vulnerable to wind and dust and it was difficult to cook inside them.

Older people had two main difficulties as far as food and nutrition were concerned. One, they depended on others for cooking their food and second, they preferred to eat traditional food, i.e. *bajriratlo,* garlic, onion, chillies and vegetables. When these were not available they tend not to eat enough. The food distributions took account of older people's compromized digestive systems and their desire for familiar food.

After the immediate relief operation, the focus was shifted to midterm and long-term rehabilitation of the earthquake victims. The long-term needs identified were strong and earthquake proof houses and livelihood support. To meet the said needs, HelpAge implemented Disaster Emergency Committee supported Income Generation and House Rebuilding Programme, with the aim to restore the living conditions of earthquake affected older persons through the reconstruction of housing and livelihood support.

Shelter is one of the most basic necessities in human life, as it influences the quality of life. HI action plan for house reconstruction support to elderly people is explained in the chart. After conducting a workshop with the programme partners, a detailed strategy for the implementation of the shelter programme was finalized. The following strategic decisions were taken with the consultation of the programme partners:

- Support for rebuilding of the house was given to those who had been supported under Emergency Relief Programme.
- Only those villages were taken up where the destruction was about 70–80%.
- The programme partners finalized the structure of the houses after a thorough survey, considering the physical environment of the area.
- Only house building materials were provided.
- All the houses were constructed with the participation of the village community and older persons.
- HI provided material for construction but the beneficiaries provided labour to rebuild houses.
- The quake-resistant houses were built based on a mix of modem and traditional technology.
- The houses constructed were culturally acceptable.
- The houses were constructed on those lands, where the beneficiaries had authentic land records. For relocation of the older people, proper documents were collected from the concerned authority. If the relocation was done on the community land, a proper land record was obtained from the concerned '*talhati*'.

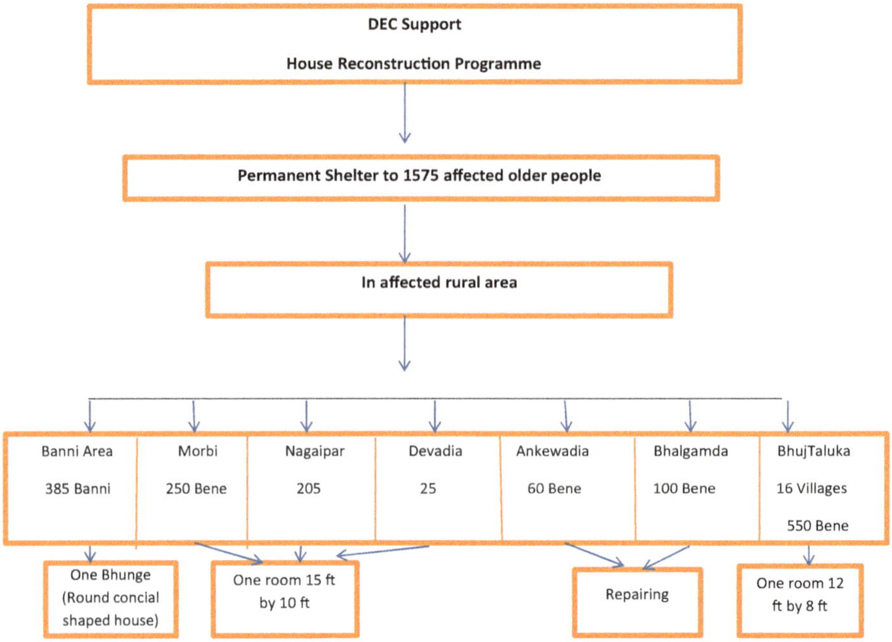

For the implementation of the shelter programme, all agencies appointed required staff at their local office and appointed village level facilitators. A village committee, which included one NGO representative, was formed. This committee identified the beneficiaries to be supported for house reconstruction. This was again verified by meeting individual beneficiaries selected for housing support programme by HI field staff and Programme Manager to ensure that all proposed beneficiaries met all eligibility criteria. Widows, handicapped and those who are left alone were given priority. Group discussions were held with the beneficiaries to finalize the design and type of house to be built. As a result, the house design developed was socially and culturally accepted by the beneficiaries. The appointed engineers and architects of the agencies further worked on same design developed in partnership with beneficiaries and community members to make it earthquake and cyclone resistant.

In the Banni area of Kachchh district, people live in traditional houses called "*Bhunga*" (conical shape house) in their local language. The material used to construct a traditional "*Bhunga*" cost around Rs. 60,000. One of the innovations included designs developed for earthquake and cyclone resistant low cost *Bhungas*.

In this '*Bhunga*' the wall was constructed in casting situ RCC and the whole structure was supported by the friction between wall and soil as well as support by the bearing of base. The construction style being monolithic and lightweight had rare chance of getting structurally disintegrated and collapsing due to heavy jolts of earthquake or cyclone. Use of this technology reduced the expenditure by about half costing about Rs. 20,000.

As a result of devastation, many older people lost their livelihood support and were left in economic distress. Hence, they were perceived as disabled, unproductive and burden on family. HI implemented the Income Generation Support Programme with the aim to change this negative stereotyped image and to establish more balanced view of both their needs and capacities. These programmes had impact on the lives of the older persons and raised their income status. The following objectives were set to be achieved at the end of the programme:

- Ensure economic security;
- Revive the traditional occupations;
- Organize older people into small groups;
- Enhance the dignity of the elderly in the family;
- Involve older persons in the holistic development of their village.

Transition from relief phase to rehabilitation phase had been marked by the change of operational strategy. More development-oriented approach was taken for the implementation of the Income Generation Programme. After identification of a beneficiary the agency identified some income generating trades, which could be undertaken by the beneficiary, or any member of the extended family. Then an analysis was done to find out the viability and sustainability of the income generation activity identified. Equal care was taken to find out the viability of the trade to raise the economic status of the beneficiary. Procurement plans of supportive material for income generation and its distribution were prepared by each agency. There was no cash transaction from the agency to the beneficiaries but support was there in terms of technical instruments to the older persons.

All the partner agencies would continue to follow up on income generation activities and ensure that the benefit of the programme goes to the needy elderly. Bank account is opened in the name of the beneficiary, who needs support of family members. Every month the family member who is supported by the income generation activity has to deposit a part of the income earned in the beneficiary's bank account. The agencies and HI field staff would regularly monitor it.

HelpAge Mobile Medicare Unit (MMU) teams and project staff conducted a rapid needs assessment in the most-affected areas of Kachchh. At the early stage, a strategy was designed for the MMUs to collect baseline information in the villages they were visiting. MMU staff gained an overview of needs and recorded information. The project officers who travelled with the vans were trained social workers and were, therefore, able to win trust and talk to older people in remote villages.

This rapid assessment was conducted in 72 villages of Bhachau *taluka,* 33 villages of Bhuj taluka, 6 villages of Anjar taluka and 30 villages of Rapar taluka. In addition, a more detailed rapid needs assessment was carried out to complete the initial assessment under a senior professor from the University of Baroda. The needs assessment took place in 15 villages (samples) to assess the immediate needs following the immediate onset of the emergency and to reinforce current and future intervention in meeting the needs of older people and their families.

This rapid needs assessment was carried out using participatory tools; case studies focus group discussion representing categories of vulnerability and semi structured interviews involving the team of HelpAge India and its partner NGO staff, who were from the local areas and familiar with local language and customs. Structured interviews with NGO leaders operating in the quake-hit areas were conducted. The entire support programme was built on focus group discussions, semi-structured interviews with the affected people and the leaders in the affected areas.

HelpAge staff on the ground was dedicated, motivated and worked round the clock in very difficult conditions. This was a tremendous effort with strong collaboration between HI and the four partner agencies. Strong working collaboration had been established between HelpAge International and HelpAge India's relief team.

The partner agencies were provided with practical training in participatory needs assessment as well as mechanisms for implementation of immediate relief assistance and distribution with emphasis on inclusion and participation of older people in needs assessment, planning and distribution.

Before the start of the programme, the Programme Advisers visited each of the partner agencies to develop the strategy and the implementation plan. Monitoring tools were developed and explained in detail to the implementing personnel of the partner agencies. Emphasis was given to the selection of beneficiaries. HelpAge also set up quality control procedures for procurement of commodities. Each of the partner agencies, before purchasing commodities had to get approval from HelpAge Programme Advisers. Packaging of food commodities was done after bulk breaking for packaging in smaller packages, which were easily carried by older persons. During packaging, emphasis was laid on cleanliness and ensuring that correct amount of commodity was packed. The procurement of all items was made in India.

The monitoring system implemented and emphasized, both the process as well as the outputs. The reports were prepared by the agency and forwarded to *Bhuj* field office through the respective field monitors based in the block and who supported the partner agencies. The field monitors visited the project areas to provide support and ensure adequate implementation (i.e., plan, timeline, etc.). Participatory approach was crucial to monitoring and for the community to have a sense of ownership. The progress of the implementation of the programme was documented and shared with partner agencies for transparency.

Monitoring being an important key for the success of the programme, a clear strategy was formulated for the same. A three-tier system for programme monitoring was adopted. The first level of the monitoring would be done by the older person group as well as by the facilitators of the partner agency. The field monitors of HelpAge India did the second level of monitoring. A monitoring format was developed and used for the above purpose. Monitoring reports were compiled and necessary instructions regarding the progress of the programme were forwarded to the partner agencies. The relief manager and the project coordinator did the third level of monitoring. Their role was to guide both the partners and the field officer to run the programme smoothly.

HelpAge India's Mobile Medicare Units were used after the Gujarat earthquake to provide immediate emergency care in rural communities. However, an assessment of the emergency response in Gujarat suggests that MMUs can play an effective role in emergency relief. The MMUs proved to be a very useful rapid response mechanism, reaching inaccessible areas fast to establish contact and map the scale of need. The main challenge was rapid mobilisation, which, in this case, was achieved. Although the MMU s is not part of a specialized emergency service, the staff had been able to improvize and adapt.

Overall HelpAge MMU's intervention was very timely, with a good logistic and supportive infrastructure to attend to patients at their doorsteps. The overall coverage in rural villages was an achievement, which at critical times was very much needed by these communities.

Besides direct medical intervention, HelpAge Mobile teams coordinated with other INGOs/NGOs such as MSF, Red Cross, Purna Clinic, Government Health Mobile Teams and Local level paramedic teams for referring cases, which needed immediate attention. During the reporting period, a total of 158 cases, which required immediate attention were referred to and followed up with the respective agencies for holistic health care. HelpAge medical teams, with hired surgeons, directly conducted 131 orthopaedic surgeries during the first three months. This team also helped patients who were in need of other aids and appliances by coordinating with the orthopaedic unit set up by the Ministry of Social Justice and Empowerment at *Bhachau.* Many of the handicapped persons received devices like callipers, wheelchairs, artificial limbs and other supportive appliances, which were needed by the patients. Overall HelpAge MMU s' intervention was very timely, with a good logistic and supportive infrastructure to attend to patients at their doorsteps. The overall coverage in rural villages was an achievement, which at critical times was very much needed by these communities. The outreach of the programme reached a high level where repeated visits were conducted to meet the needs of the affected people.

Food commodities to 7500 older people and their families provided them with security that helped them on relief to the rehabilitation continuum. This as per the analysis available provided them with a net saving of approximately Rs. 2500.

The timely distribution of relief items helped revive older people's livelihoods. Older people felt respected and empowered as they received all the items for distribution themselves and put them to use directly. Dignity is the most important aspect, which older persons and especially those affected by disaster would like to have restored.

There have been observations made that the capacities of older persons having substantial dry rations and a provision of immediate food to meet the daily needs, led to an increased decision-making capacity and brought back members of the families who had earlier left the older persons to care for themselves. It was observed that in all the areas where HelpAge relief and rehabilitation programme was implemented, older people were enjoying enhanced respect and security from their family members and from the community as a whole.

This experience has proved that the response to emergencies can best emerge if there is a proper planning process between the implementing partners and its staff to show the logistics of supporting a particular activity.

The NGOs that HelpAge partnered with were very popular among the community they were working with. This is one of the reasons why these agencies had the support of the community either by their earlier presence or through their short-term association during the earthquake. This was important as it enhanced the delivery mechanism of relief items, which somehow had failed during the government's distribution of relief commodities and other agencies that had attempted to do direct deliveries.

It was also an opportunity for learning about the need for the local staple food, which was slightly different from that which had been listed in the original planning. The national and international level agencies distributing relief items mostly included foreign food items, which were locally acceptable.

The participatory approaches adopted in the process of planning needs identification and intervention went a long way in ensuring that the objectives of the programmes were met. Consulting older people about their needs has been a key to HelpAge's immediate response. Listening to them had been a crucial assessment tool in determining their need as well as in ensuring that immediate relief items provided were adequate. Each of the partner agencies visited the villages and carried out a needs assessment and discussed targeting criteria and then each of the partners came back to the villages to discuss the distribution process and participation.

People participated in the distribution helping those who could not carry their parcels. Participation is essential to understanding local needs and customs. It is also important to involve beneficiaries in the planning, implementation and monitoring of the programme to ensure its relevance and effectiveness.

A year and a half after the disaster struck, almost all the agencies involved in the relief and rehabilitation work withdrew. HelpAge, in consultation with—the people in the villages, where it was conducting rehabilitation work, felt that it was also important to prepare the community for any future disaster. That was the beginning of a three months training programme titled "Community-Based Disaster Preparedness". The aim of the training was to protect people and prevent further human casualties during earthquakes/cyclones and train the community to take proactive role in times of any disaster.

Effective disaster management entirely depends on the preparedness and the warning system; emergency relief operations and rehabilitation and reconstruction. Preparedness is crucial in disaster management and includes planning. Preparedness and mitigation is the key to rapid identification of frail or isolated older people during an emergency, reducing its impacts on them and supporting their rapid recovery afterwards.

Effective disaster management entirely depends on the preparedness and the warning system; emergency relief operations, rehabilitation and reconstruction. In order to draw upon a viable community-based disaster preparedness strategy various components were highlighted, for better outcomes as a result of appropriate preparedness on the part of the community. The disaster preparedness programme had to be acceptable to the community. The training programme made efforts to make the community aware of their vulnerabilities and to build their capacity towards coping with natural and (hu)manmade disasters. Sixty villages were trained in the entire duration of the training; in rescue operations, evacuation and first aid, mapping of vulnerable spots and making of a contingency plan in case of a mishap. Young and old, men and women, flocked around the training team (5 teams in all, with 5 members each) to listen with interest and learn from them the techniques of disaster mitigation. The training team in turn learnt a lot from the experiences of the locals learning in one village and imparting another. Few of the important aspects of this kind of training were that the people now had a checklist on things that had to be done or interventions that had to be followed in case of a disaster.

Each village formed its own crisis management team comprising volunteers for each aspect of disaster mitigation that they were being trained in. The elders of the village formed an advisory team to guide these volunteers who would look after the rescue operations in case a need arose. At the end of the training, each village was given a survival kit—a first-aid box, set of ropes meant for rescue operations, a shelter and a fire extinguisher.

The Indian Ocean Tsunami

Nearly 900.000 elderly people were affected by the tsunami, which devastated the states of Tamil Nadu, Andhra Pradesh and Kerala. Indeed, close to 30% of the dead and missing were estimated to be senior citizens, rendered vulnerable because of their frailty and often lack of physical mobility. To address their needs, HelpAge India in coordination with HelpAge International and Help the Aged, UK, put in place a Tsunami Rehabilitation Programme, the mandate of which was three-pronged: provide sustainable livelihood, social protection and disaster preparedness and advocacy.

With these objectives in mind, HelpAge started work. Older Fishermen were provided with catamarans and solar lights. This helped them employ people who use his catamaran to help them fish. The organisation gave small grants of money to villagers to enable them to make handicrafts which they could then sell. Many agars had no idea of how to make such goods until they struck, wiping away previous means of livelihood and leaving them with no choice but to pursue new work for survival. One such admirable example was 68-year-old Dhanalakshmi. She learnt the art of weaving baskets and was subsequently given a grant of Rs 5000 by HelpAge India to buy the raw material. In addition, she joined a self-help group that the organisation set up and learnt how to save some money every month.

Villagers who used to work on the land before the tsunami struck also benefited from HelpAge's desalination and de-sanding programmes. The case of 70-year-old Pattammal is a good example. Before the tsunami, Pattammal was working in a salt pan in Vedaranyam and was paid daily wage of Rs 40—earning an average of Rs 800 a month. She had, in addition, three acres of agricultural land and a few cows and goats, which also gave her some income. Her husband was a fisherman and supplemented her income with his own. And then, after Tsunami the land was silted and became uncultivable. HelpAge India helped her to de-sand her land. Later, she also became a member of HelpAge's self-help group *Sudhanthiram*, meaning 'Independence', through which she has learnt how to save.

Earthquake, Kashmir

Measuring 7.4 on the Richter scale, with its epicentre in Muzaffarabad, Pakistan, the earthquake ravaged Jammu and Kashmir, destroying households and public infrastructure and killing humans and livestock with deadly equality.

HelpAge India was among the first NGOs on the scene. The earthquake of October 2005 brought it face to face with a population suffering tremendous loss and limited response. The response to this crisis had to be planned close in coordination with district and regional organisations as well as the military. The army played a vital role in getting the resources together for such a gargantuan task. It was a tougher challenge than the ones hitherto faced by the Organisation. Along with the rugged mountain terrain, approaching winter and bad weather made the work unimaginably difficult more so in remote villages like Dulanja.

Months after the tremors were felt, relief was yet to reach the tiny spot of Dulanja, located some two-and-a-half hours from Sarai which was then the last motorable point in Uri. Connected to the Muzaffarabad highway only by a rickety rope trolley which could take two people at a time further restricted by the visiting time because of its nearness to the Line of Control, Dulanja was left behind as rescue work in other areas proceeded. It was not until April that two doctors and pharmacists from HelpAge India were able to visit the village and set up a medical camp for its 350 inhabitants.

Winter was fast setting in and need for shelter along with basic ration and medicines were most urgently required for the affected older persons and their families. Working with local contractor semi-permanent insulated houses was constructed before the harsh winter.

Medical Relief was provided to nearly 8 villages along with food and non-food packages. HelpAge also tried to expand the local MMU service to Uri region, by developing a volunteer system in collaboration with the medical colleges of Jammu and Srinagar. People from the area were appointed to work for the local MMU after rigorous induction and orientation programmes. This effort was supposed to revive the declining primary health services in the area. The unit eventually treated more than 500 victims providing free medicines and holding medical camps in remote villages.

HelpAge India put in place quick and easy cash transfer systems along with the provision of dry rations that were distributed among affected villagers and their families. The grim fact was that the earthquake had destroyed almost every available food stock so a square meal was a dream for most families in remote villages. Help in far-flung areas was in the form of rice, sugar, milk powder, tea, candles and matches, which were distributed along with winter packages of clothes and bukharis (traditional stove, which can be used to cook and to heat rooms).

In addition, HelpAge worked to restore the crushed livelihood opportunities in consultation with the committees which included the villagers and the headman/woman whereby older people would be the direct beneficiaries of programmes that facilitated new means of livelihood. These committees were spread across villages, thereby creating a network of community and rehabilitation workers.

But the going was hard and often, tough. The economy of the state took plunged, so did the morale of the villagers. This was when HelpAge India's experience in implementing disaster relief operations in different situations came in useful. The organisation's staff well equipped to deal with such adverse conditions developed an understanding and empathy with the people. Staff members worked with local communities to train, especially women, in disaster preparedness, prevention and management. Confronting formidable obstacles, natural, social and political, HelpAge India made a notable impact in the midst of the devastation and the cold Himalayan winter of 2005.

Floods

Floods in 2007 created havoc in Uttar Pradesh, Assam and Bihar, resulting in heavy loss of lives and livestock, crops and property. The poor were the worst hot like always because of the scarcity of dry ground and houses, no food and drinking water along with a fear of epidemics made life miserable. HelpAge India's team got into action to provide facilities to these flood-affected states supported by ECHO (European Commission Humanitarian Aid Office), Cordaid and HelpAge International.

In 2008, floods hit Bihar once more causing substantial loss of life and property to more than four million people especially in the north Bihar districts of Supaul, Araria, Madhepura, Saharsa and Purnea. HelpAge India responded immediately with medical and other relief measures to remote villages targeting the elders, women, children and the disabled.

Since then, HelpAge has continued its work in the area through health care, social protection and disaster risk reduction programmes in addition to special programmes for the community volunteers. MMUs were pressed into service in order to further improve access to primary and emergency medicare; establishing physiotherapy centres and forming Elder Self Help Groups (ESHGs), which led to reducing the financial dependency of elders on their children for minor expenses.

Cloudburst, Leh, Jammu & Kashmir

Tragedy struck in Leh on a day in August 2011. An unexpected cloudburst caused massive flash floods which left an estimated 1000 people dead and over 500 missing. The devastating floods caused landslides and damaged agricultural land, livestock and property. HelpAge India was the first NGO to respond with its MMUs, treating nearly 2500 patients.

Flash Floods, Uttarakhand

HelpAge launched a major relief programme in the first week of the disaster itself. Its staff and volunteers tracked over mud and landslides braving incessant rains and worked in 99 villages in affected districts: Rudraprayag, Chamoli and Uttarkashi. It started with primary emergency medical care through 3 Mobile Medicare Units. The distribution of emergency family food packages, tarpaulins and blankets for the remotest villages which were totally cut off and had not received any relief. HelpAge moved 84 tonnes of relief material and distributed it in selected villages during June/July 2013. 3800 families were given relief packages to last them for a fortnight. In addition, more than 4500 people received medical care through HelpAge India Mobile Medicare Units operating in the affected three districts. Later many useful initiatives were taken in Rudraparyag and Chamoli in terms of stationary health care unit, skill development and installations of renewable sources of energy.

Kerala Floods

HelpAge India made similar attempts in Kerala ravaged by the floods in 2018. Emergency Medical Camps in Wayanad district with its local eHealth Centre, Nadavayal team started operation on 10th August 2018. Later, five more Existing MHUs from neighbouring states were relocated for Wayanad, Vizhinjam for Pathanamthitta districts for emergency medical camps. 94 camps were conducted in the 4 affected districts to provide 6479 treatments.

3790 families, 2940 in Wayanad and 850 in Idukki were provided flood relief kits with 33 food and non-food items which were expected to last them two weeks. The distribution was conducted through 14 g panchayats in 39 locations.

Helplines

By the early twenty-first century, the situation in India had changed from a society that took pride in respecting and caring for the elders to a society where more and more elderly were facing neglect and violence at home. The upper caste, upper-class protection bubble for the elderly had been punctured. Cases of abuse were getting reported in public domain, something that was unheard of in India. HelpAge India faced these issues of familial neglect and abandonment in Chennai, where in the year 2004, with the initiative of the Police Commissioner the first helpline was started for the benefit of older persons.

People like 70-year-old Lakshmi, a widow from Ekkaduthangal, Chennai neglected by her only son Raja and abandoned on the road after her failing health. Unable to afford medical attention, her condition worsened and she was left squirming in pain after she had a severe fall. A well-wisher called HelpAge's Elder Helpline service and social workers rushed to the spot. Lakshmi was immediately shifted to KMC Hospital and doctors confirmed a fracture. After treatment, she was able to move again. She was admitted to a local charitable old age home to spend the last days of her life with dignity and care.

To ensure that senior citizens like Lakshmi found immediate help the Chennai helpline was manned by a social worker and a psychologist. The same situation was experienced in many other big cities in the country and gradually HelpAge India established helplines in 23 state capitals. It also got a toll free number that was accessible from anywhere in the country. The Helpline programme has expanded its scope of work and now is equipped to deal with all kinds of services ranging from information queries to rescue and rehabilitation to counselling on issues like family dispute, legal and police assistance in case of violence and or abuse.

The helpline service that covers 26 cities in 21 states is operated by trained helpline counsellors supported by social work professionals, volunteers, students and interns. The helplines have proved to be a boon for thousands of elders across the country.

Advocacy Initiatives

The PACS Initiative

With India recording a rise in the demographics of the elderly and rural to urban migration, many elderly people were and are still, left without any clear idea of their rights. This thought was behind the formation of the HelpAge India led Poorest Areas Civil Society Programme (PACS), supported by the Department for International Development. The programme was implemented in three states Uttar Pradesh, Madhya Pradesh and Jharkhand. This basically underlined the need for social protection, calling for the inclusion of the elderly into the mainstream of society, rather than relegating them to the fringes. It was mainly focused on the rural poor elderly. It was designed to create awareness among the elderly and the community about the rights of older persons. The older persons along with the community were mobilised to demand better implementation of the schemes and policies meant for the benefit of the older persons. It also encouraged youth to be involved in the process and help spared the massage and build the capacity.

Student Action for Value Education (SAVE)

When HelpAge started with the school education-cum-fund-raising programme as their major fund-raising effort, resource mobilisation was of paramount importance. Elite schools were chosen as the mainstay of the resource mobilisation activity because of their positive responses to HelpAge India's attempts to give to charities through students. However, as mentioned above the social context in the twenty-first century had changed and now it was not just the older persons in poor families that required support, elderly in middle and upper class families also felt marginalized and neglected. A ray of hope was seen in the young children who could be sensitised to the plight of the elderly and expected to care for them and also influence their parents to do so.

HelpAge began a formal and structured programme of value education on age care in schools across the country in 2008. A multi-pronged approach was adopted. It targeted the teachers and the principals of the schools at one level; at another, it tried to persuade the state education departments to include age care in the curriculum and also in the syllabus text books wherever possible. The school children who were the main target group of this programme were encouraged to take a pledge to respect and care for the elderly. The students of the member schools form SAVE committees within their own schools headed by the principal and guided by teachers, these committees chalked got plans for the implementation of the programme within the school and the community outside. The aim of these committees was to spread awareness about SAVE's three core values. They also work to further various other age-care programmes either in partnership with HelpAge India or on their own.

HelpAge India has been advocating for inclusion of value education on elder role in society in school curriculum. This effort has now started yielding results with states of Uttarakhand, Andhra Pradesh, Uttar Pradesh and Punjab have initiated action for this addition in their state education curriculum.

HUG (Help Unite Generations) Programme

A related initiative to deal with isolation faced by the elderly with involvement of youth was HUG. As society progresses to nuclear families, the elders are left mostly alone without the companionship of family and young children. This situation can lead to a state of depression among some elders. It aims to alleviate any sense of isolation among elders by enthusing youth volunteers to engage with elders by keeping in touch through telephone calls and occasional face to face meetings. The volunteers are required to enquire about his/her health and chat about news and events. The elder is given the volunteers phone number so that he/she can contact the volunteer anytime, especially at times of emergency.

Policy Advocacy

Mr. M. M. Sabharwal understood the importance of sensitizing the government to mainstream the concerns of ageing population in India, way back in the 90s. HelpAge India collaborated with the Ministry of Social Justice and Empowerment to conduct regional and national level seminars that formed the basis of National Policy on Older Persons (NPOP). It again collaborated with the Ministry in 2004 to involve all stakeholders in an attempt to develop a plan of action for effective implementation of NPOP. Mr. Sabharwal was later appointed as a member of the Review Committee set up by the Ministry in 2009 to recommend changes to the NPOP. The Committee under the Chairpersonship of Dr. Mrs. Mohini Giri presented its recommendations to the Ministry in March 2010. The state offices of HelpAge India also try and sensitise respective governments to adopt a specific state policy on older persons to give a direction to implementing elderly friendly policies and schemes.

Working with Elderly

HelpAge India recognizes the potential of the elderly and is involving them in various activities. It was also recognized that when they come together they can form a powerful advocacy voice. HelpAge actively works with Senior Citizens Associations (SCAs) to help them better understand elders' issues and mobilize support for improvement. The organisation began to advocate policies to ensure that seniors could work for and participate in their own rights' movement.

Senior Citizens Associations (SCAs) were brought to organize programmes and workshops in various of the country that would benefit the aged: Healthy Heart Drives. Reverse Mortgage than Physiotherapy Care. Seminars are organized by HelpAge in conjunction with Senior Citizens Associations (SCAs) across the country on National Policy on Older Persons, Maintenance & Welfare of the Parents and Senior Citizens Act (2007), reverse mortgage and many more such topics. As a result of these seminars, the Government in various states is initiating action for speedy formulation/implementation of state policies on older persons and implementation of the Maintenance & Welfare Act. Senior citizens are now feeling empowered to raise their voices and take action on issues concerning them.

Today HelpAge is working with more than 2000 SCAs across India and the numbers are growing. HelpAge India has been encouraging seniors to come together under the aegis of SCAs and persuading them to form federations at the state level. Federations in 4 States, Delhi, Uttarakhand, West Bengal aria Uttar Pradesh have been formed through efforts of HelpAge India. In several states including Orissa and Rajasthan, this work is in process.

The People Behind the Organisation

HelpAge India's history of four decades is an illustrious journey of a pioneering organisation set up by visionaries and taken forward by passionate humanists. The organisation responded to the changing needs and concerns of the ageing population in the country and expanded its programmes based on that. Its inclusive approach, both in terms of including the ever-growing and changing concerns of the elderly and the segments and sections of society who could collaborate to help the elderly is the key to its glorious march. Sensitivity and concern for the elderly remain the bedrock on which this approach flourished. It is an example for other age care organisations to emulate. The basic issues of income, health and emotional security are universal and will continue to be so, but how these needs are felt by the different segments of the ageing population and how response to these needs are made more effective and efficient is the challenge that voluntary organisations need to be conscious about.

Population ageing is going to be a major issue in the coming decades, simply due to the staggering numbers, increasing longevity and decreasing birth rate. The need for age care will be felt by one and all at some point in their lives. The scope is vast and ever expanding; there is a need for voluntary organisations to respond adequately.

Chapter 14
Empowerment of the Elderly

Kiran Puri

Abstract With the increasing number of elderly every year and the disappearance or reduction of joint family systems in India, it has become imperative to have policies, programmes and workshops to empower and educate the elderly from an early age; so that they can look after themselves, for as long as they live or for the maximum years of their lives. The government departments and many NGOs have announced adult education, professional training and personalized learning programmes for seniors on dementia, computers, smartphones and digital literacy, hobbies like art, craft, dance and music, courses on learning of languages like English, German, French and Spanish and long and short distance online e-learning programmes which also include vocational skill development as well as access to enrolment in graduation and post graduation courses. These initiatives are helping senior citizens in upgrading their knowledge and enabling them to be in tune with modern devices and upcoming technology. The skill development and professional classes are opening up new options of re-employment and earning money and thus making them economically independent. It is helping them in fostering respect for themselves, gaining confidence in their potential, adding happiness, satisfaction and contentment to their lives. All this would definitely lead to the reduction of dependence and their chances of becoming victims of neglect and abuse in old age. It would definitely help in adding life to years and not just years to life. This article reflects on different empowering strategies for older men and women taking place in the country.

Keywords Empowerment · Objective · Approach · National state assistance · Retirement homes · Medical facilities · Pension schemes

The population of senior citizens in India has been steadily rising. From 1.98 crore in 1951 to it has risen to 10.38 crores in 2011. The projections indicate that this trend would continue and the number of 60+ in India will increase to 14.3 crores by 2021and then further rise up to 17.3 crores in 2026. (Ministry of Social Justice and Empowerment) By 2050 this number will be more than 300 million and every fifth Indian person would be an older person as people are living longer nowadays.

K. Puri (✉)
Director, Development Welfare and Research Foundation (DWRF), New Delhi, India

M. K. Shankardass (ed.), *Gerontological Concerns and Responses in India*,
https://doi.org/10.1007/978-981-16-4764-2_14

This has resulted because of improvements in health and medical care as well as the aspiration of people to limit family size. On the one hand, it calls for celebration but on the other side, it poses challenges to be taken care of. The society today is facing challenges to take care of the physical and mental health of the elderly so that the elderly live a healthy, safe and comfortable life free of abuse. Due to a lack of empowerment, the elderly are reluctant to seek help or enforce their rights (both statutory and otherwise). Thus the empowerment of the elderly is really essential.

However, a lot of effort has been made to develop a model of health and social care in tune with the changing need and times. It may be an opportunity for more innovation in health system development, though it is a major challenge.

The elderly face a greater burden of ailments (which the National Sample Survey Organisation defines as illness, sickness, injury and poisoning) compared to other age groups (see National Sample Survey Organisation, 2006, Fig. 1), across genders and residential locations. Multiple chronic diseases afflict the elderly like chronic bronchitis, circulatory diseases, anaemia, hypertension, chest pain from cardiovascular illness, kidney problems, digestive disorders, vision problems, diabetes, rheumatism, depression and cancers. It is very important to mention that there is a definite need to emphasise the fact that disease and disability are not part of old age and help must be sought to address the health problems. The concept of Active and Healthy ageing needs to be promoted among the elderly, which includes preventive, curative and rehabilitative aspects of health.

Traditional Norms and Values

The traditional norms and values of the Indian society laid stress on showing respect and providing care for the aged. However, in recent times, society is witnessing a gradual but definite decline of the joint family system, As a result of which a large number of parents are being neglected by their families exposing them to lack of emotional, physical and financial support. There are cases of occurrences of emotional, psychological or financial abuse, neglect and abandonment of elders.

This clearly indicates that ageing needs to be addressed very seriously and the elderly should be empowered so that they develop the potential of dealing with untoward situations and circumstances which might crop up in their old age.

Active and Healthy Lives

Active management and control of one's social setting is an essential basis for physical and psychological wellbeing. Population ageing has profound implications on many facets of human life. An ageing population will affect everything from individuals, economies, communities, labour markets, national and international life, to health and social care. It poses unique challenges to every society. Apart from this some other facts which cannot be ignored are the increasing proportion of older women and more widows than widowers. This prospect requires a better understanding of the implications and possibilities posed by population ageing as well as the situation of older persons themselves. When people live longer they need more care and also income security to lead a dignified life. In this type of scenario, it has become imperative to have policies, to ensure healthy lives and promote wellbeing of the elderly, to safeguard the elderly from abuse and neglect, to conduct programmes and workshops to empower them, to keep their minds alert and engaged, so they learn daily and pick up an additional degree/certificate to further enhance their calibre and potential soon after they retire; so that they can look after themselves, for as long as they live or for the maximum years of their lives.

The Main Objective

The main objective of the ministry of social justice and empowerment is to provide facilities, concessions and relief to senior citizens by taking care of basic necessities of life like shelter, health care, education, food, medical care and welfare, financial security, protection of life, property and entertainment opportunities so that the elderly age well. To improve life support for capacity building of State/UT Governments/Non-Governmental Organisations (NGOs)/Panchayati Raj Institutions (PRIs)/local bodies and the community at large.

Steps in this direction have been taken continuously by the government. First in 1999 came the national policy of elderly, then 'The Maintenance and Welfare Bill of 2007 'and now the king 'Ministry of Social Justice & Empowerment ' has come out with 'The Maintenance and Welfare of Parents and Senior Citizens of 2018 ' to amend the 'Maintenance and Welfare of Senior Citizens Act, 2007.'

'The Maintenance and Welfare of Parents and Senior Citizens of 2018'

'The Maintenance and Welfare of Parents and Senior Citizens of 2018 ' are under consideration but major amendments proposed in the existing Maintenance and Welfare of Parents and Senior Citizens Act, 2007 comprise, removal of maximum ceiling of maintenance allowance; extension of right to appeal to the respondents also; extension of benefit of revocation of transfer of property to parents also; reckoning of time limit for disposal of applications by the Tribunal from the date of receipt of application. Codification of such rights and providing a mechanism for enforcement has resulted in a sense of entitlement among elders. Rights conferred by law and specifically under the MWPS Act have encouraged elders to seek relief in courts/tribunals or assistance of helplines to protect their statutory rights.

Approach

Assistance under the scheme will be given to the Implementing Agencies such as State/UT Governments/Panchayati Raj Institutions/local bodies and eligible Non-Governmental/Voluntary Organisations for the following purposes:

1. Programmes catering to the basic needs of Senior Citizens particularly food, shelter and health care to the destitute elderly.
2. Programmes to build and strengthen intergenerational relationships particularly between children/youth and Senior Citizens, through Regional Resource and Training Centres (RRTCs).
3. Programmes for encouraging Active and Productive Ageing, through (RRTCs)
4. Programmes for proving Institutional as well as Non- Institutional Care/Services to Senior Citizens.
5. Research, Advocacy and Awareness building programmes in the field of Ageing through (RRTCs)
6. Any other programmes in the best interest of Senior Citizens.
7. NGO Portal Integrated Programme for Senior Citizens
8. A Central Sector Scheme to improve the quality of life of the Senior Citizens (Revised as on 01.04.2018)
9. An integrated Programme for older people. NGO wise Grants in Aid released during 2015–16 under the scheme integrated Programme for Older Persons
10. State wise amount released a number of projects assisted and beneficiaries covered during 2015–16. The policy stipulates that the State Government will take affirmative action to provide comprehensive facilities to render relief to senior citizens to improve their quality of life.

As people live longer they need more care and also income to lead a dignified life. Most of the elderly become vulnerable due to their reduction in earnings.

Major Reasons Which Lead to Low Income in Old Age

1. A large informal employment sector.
2. Low female work participation rates.
3. Their preference is to invest in their children who are perceived to be the source of old age security.
4. Sometimes low income at old age can also be attributed to inability to work during younger ages due to sickness and as a result of that long period of unemployment.

The Need for Retirement Plans

Retirement plan ensures that people live with pride and without compromising on their standard of living during advancing years. When people and families are not able to make arrangements for the care of the elderly, their needs must be provided for by society/state, either in cash or kind (through social insurance and social assistance schemes). In this type of scenario, it has become imperative for the Central government and the states to have policies to promote wellbeing of the elderly and to ensure their healthy lives. To start measures like pensions, to provide social security for the elderly especially when their children and families are not in a position financially to take care or support their expenses.

National Social Assistance Programme

The National Social Assistance Programme (NSAP was launched on 15th August 1995). The National Social Assistance Programme (NSAP) represented a significant step towards the fulfilment of the Directive Principles in Articles 41 and 42 of the Constitution recognising the concurrent responsibility of the Central and the State Governments in the matter. In particular, Article 41 of the Constitution of India directs the State to provide public assistance to its citizens in case of unemployment, old age, sickness and disablement and in other cases of undeserved want within the limit of its economic capacity and development.

Objectives of National Social Assistance Programme

National Social Assistance Programme is a social security and welfare programme to provide support to aged persons, widows, disabled persons and bereaved families on death of primary breadwinner, belonging to below poverty line household. Besides the central assistance, states/UT contribute an equal amount as their share. "Old Age pension of Rs. 200 per month from Centre reaches 22.318 million people (government data on BPL.

Eligibility and Scale of Assistance

For getting benefits under NSAP the applicant must belong to a Below Poverty Line (BPL) family according to the criteria, prescribed by the Govt. of India. As per the revised eligibility criteria new beneficiaries will be identified from BPL list prepared by the States/UTs as per guidelines issued by the Ministry of Rural Development

(MORD) for the BPL Census 2002. The Identification of eligible beneficiaries will be carried out as per the BPL list required to be prepared in connection with poverty alleviation programme of the ministry of Urban Housing and Poverty Alleviation.

Presently NSAP Comprises of Five Schemes, Namely

1. Indira Gandhi National Old Age Pension Scheme (IGNOAPS) Indira Gandhi
2. National Widow Pension Scheme (IGNWPS 2009)
3. Indira Gandhi National Disability Pension Scheme (IGNDPS 2009)
4. National Family Benefit Scheme (NFBS)
5. Annapurna (2002)

Indira Gandhi National Old Age Pension Scheme

The Ministry of Rural Development of India introduced Indira Gandhi National Old Age Pension Scheme (IGNOAPS) under National Social Assistance Programme (NSAP) in the year 2007. IGNOAPS was also called as National Old Age Pension Scheme (NOAPS) which came into effect from 15th August 1995. Under IGNOAP scheme, it was decided senior citizens of India would receive monthly pensions. Indira Gandhi National Old Age Pension Scheme is a non-contribution pension. It means that the beneficiary does not have to contribute any amount to receive the pension. This scheme provides social assistance for old age persons. The total beneficiaries of the scheme are (34,664,556). (NSAP, 2018, Nov 30).

Eligibility Criteria

The following criteria should be met to obtain Indira Gandhi National Old Age Pension:

The eligible age for IGNOAPS is 60 years.

Monthly Amount

The pension is Rs.200 p.m. for persons between 60 and 79 years.

For persons who are 80 years and above the pension is Rs. 500/per month.

"The National Social Assistance Programme guidelines" clearly state that the central and state contribution should equally match to ensure a decent pension amount to the beneficiaries. The implementation of social pensions is not the same across states. It varies from state to state. Many State Governments have either stopped using the BPL methodology for identifying eligible beneficiaries. People from non—BPL households who are not eligible for social pensions under NSAP are also given pensions under the state pension schemes to increase coverage of social pensions for those living below the poverty line. The maximum pension (including central and state contribution) is Rs. 2000 in states and Union Territories like Kerala, Delhi, Goa, Puducherry, Andaman and Nicobar Islands. It comes through that the states contribute to the social pension schemes largely and many states are running their own schemes since pension is a concurrent list subject. All elderly above the age of 59 and widows whose annual income from all sources is below RS. 24,000 are eligible for the Madhu Pension Scheme in Odisha. The National Population Commission has estimated that India's population of the elderly in the age group of 60 years and above is expected to grow to 173 million in 2026 (NPC, 2018).

Indira Gandhi National Widow Pension Scheme (IGNWPS)

The eligible age is 40 years and the pension is Rs.300 per month. The elderly widows also get that but after attaining the age of 80 years, the beneficiary will get Rs.500/per month.

Indira Gandhi National Disability Pension Scheme (IGNDP):

The eligible age for the pensioner is 18 years and above and the disability level has to be 80%. Disabled Elderly can also get benefit from it. The amount is Rs. 300 per month for the elderly but after attaining the age of 80 years, the beneficiary will get Rs. 500/per month.

Annapurna Scheme

With the Annapurna Scheme, it was decided that 10 kgs of food grains (wheat or rice) are given per month per beneficiary. The scheme aims at providing food security to meet the requirements of those eligible old aged persons who have remained uncovered under the IGNOAPS.

Source (National Social Assistance Programmes 2014–2015).

Pension Parishad Report (2018)

According to civil society organisation Pension Parishad in India Report 2018, 58 million people in India are living without pension or any other form of assistance. The Indira Gandhi National Old Age Pension Scheme (IGNOAPS) has remained unchanged at Rs. 200 per month for over 10 years. The Central government spends as little as 0.04% of the GDP for its flagship Indira Gandhi National Social Assistance (IGNOAPS) programme to ensure income security for the elderly.

"It will cost only about 1.6% of the present-day GDP to ensure 90% of the elderly population a pension of Rs. 2500 per person every month," says economist Prabhat Patnaik. The report, published on September 28, 2018, says that 14 states provide a monthly pension of Rs. 500 per person or less to the elderly and Assam was one of them. The highest pension of Rs. 2000 per month per person is given by states such as Delhi, Goa, Kerala and Andaman & Nicobar Islands. The government has often been criticized for these low pensions. Often the pension parishad has demanded an increase in them as it is felt that such low monthly pensions cannot meet up with the rise in inflation. In fact, it is commonly felt that such meagre amounts are 'an insult to the dignity of the elderly. According to National Social Assistance Programme (NSAP), a welfare programme administered by the Ministry of Rural Development, 80 million elderly people in India are entitled to a pension of Rs. 200 per month. However, even this small amount reaches only about 22.3 million people, says Pension Parishad Coordinator, Nikhil Dey. Taking into account the condition of immense poverty in the country the Indian government should increase the pension amount.

National Pension Scheme (NPS) and Income Tax Benefits (Budget, 2018)

When a person puts money into the National Pension Schemes he gets tax benefits. Finance Minister Arun Jaitley In Budget, 2018, announced to exempt 40% of the total amount payable to the National Pension System (NPS) on closure of an account or when a person opts out of it. In order to provide a level playing field, it is proposed to amend clause (12 A) of section 10 of the Act to extend the said benefit to all subscribers. This will save the elderly from a lot of taxation. With effect from 1st May 2009, NPS has been provided for all citizens of the country including the unorganized sector workers on voluntary basis. The subscriber will be allotted a unique Permanent Retirement Account Number (PRAN). This unique account number will remain the same for the entire life of the subscriber. This unique PRAN can be used from any location in India.

Benefits of NPS

Some of the benefits of the National Pension System (NPS) are as follows

1. **It is transparent**—NPS is a transparent and cost effective system wherein the pension contributions are invested in the pension fund schemes and the employee will be able to know the value of the investment on day to day basis.
2. **It is simple**—All the subscriber has to do is to open an account with his/her nodal office and get a Permanent Retirement Account Number (PRAN).
3. **It is portable**—Each employee is identified by a unique number and has a separate PRAN which remains the same even when the employee gets transferred to any other office.
4. **It is regulated**—NPS is regulated by Pension Fund Regulatory and Development Authority with transparent investment norms & regular monitoring and performance review of fund managers by NPS Trust.

Lakshmi Bai Social Security Pension Scheme

As the Indira Gandhi National Widow Pension Scheme (IGNWPS) only covered widows between the age group of 40–59, the government of Bihar has launched state widow pension schemes covering all widows above the age of 18 years whose annual family income is below Rs. 60,000.

Old Age or Retirement Homes

Old age or retirement homes are becoming a necessity today as people are living longer. Due to emphasis being laid on women liberalisation and emancipation, more women are stepping out of the threshold of the house to work. They are doing a great job as professionals on one side but at the same time, they have to reduce their time as caregivers at home. When age catches up with people, the elderly become demanding and need a lot of care. They need a lot of physical, emotional and psychological support. As people grow older they also become less mobile and if the family does not have time for them they become lonely. They need a lot of intervention programmes and counselling. The largely ignored concept of retirement housing has been slowly witnessing an increased consumer interest across India. With a large number of senior citizens being financially stronger than their earlier generations, the concept of luxury is also being adopted within various retirement home projects. Since India has diverse financial demographics there are a number of options for senior citizens opting to stay in retirement homes. Retirement homes are becoming an answer to the recent set of concerns that are rising up due to lifestyle changes. Retirement homes are a place for living for not only the senior citizens who are unable to stay with their families or are destitute but for even the senior citizens who want to live in a place that can cater to their requirements. Since India, today has diverse financial demographics there are a number of options for senior citizens opting to stay in retirement homes.

There are 728 Old Age Homes in India today. Detailed information of 547 homes is available. Out of these, 325 homes are free of cost while 95 old age homes are on pay and stay basis, 116 homes have both free as well as pay and stay facilities and 11 homes have no information. A total of 278 old age homes all over the country are available for the sick and 101 homes are exclusively for women. Kerala has 124 old age homes which are maximum in any state. (Directory of Old Age Homes in India, Help Age India, 1998).

What Should the 'Retirement or Old Age Homes' Possess

Most of the old age homes which are being built today have special medical facilities for senior citizens such as mobile health care systems, ambulances, nurses and provision of well-balanced meals, attendant service and even travel assistance within the city so that they can live a healthy life. Good services and good behaviour of the staff is mostly an added advantage of these homes because they are trained and paid for it. Thus they specialize in "elder care" which is fulfilment of special needs and requirements that are unique to senior citizens. The elderly can live in these homes without a compromise to their dignity. Many of them are today getting equipped for even rendering services for long and short term ailments with 24 × 7care. They provide not just a living, free from social pressures but that which encompasses assisted living. Proper care is taken to the preparation and service of food which is thus palatable. In many homes, there are nutritionists who recommend the diet plan of each elderly. The elderly in these homes therefore may or may not bother to cook food. Safety is definitely an issue for senior citizens. The steady security in an old age home gives the elderly protection from intruders and helps them live a safe and secure life. Old age homes also provide access to telephones and other forms of communication so that residents may keep in touch with their loved ones. They lay emphasis on social interaction by providing opportunities through a lot of interactive activities. They are in constant company of people of their own age group. The entertainment and library facilities are also available for the sole purpose of the senior citizens. They have exercise and yoga facilities too. These homes also create a family like atmosphere among the residents. Senior citizens experience a sense of security and friendship when they share their joys and sorrows with each other. In old age homes, old people have a lot of free time, so they can utilize it creatively. They have the freedom to pursue and participate in religious activities.

Types of Retirement Homes in India

Senior Citizen Communities
Senior citizen communities or hubs are slowly but surely replacing traditional independent living homes. A large number of builders and developers have jumped into the market offering dedicated senior citizen communities with a host of amenities. Since an old body is quite prone to infections these hubs are usually built in close proximity to hospitals, banks and markets. Such community hubs have a team of in house doctors, for monitoring the health issues of the elderly. A large number of such community homes are built with a joint collaboration between builders and hospital management teams. Most builders offer good discounts for booking options in such communities making it a good option for the elderly. These senior citizen communities provide adequate security around the clock.

Independent Living Home
Independent living homes is an old concept that has been active in Indian society for a long time. Most people save money all along their working days to buy a plot and build a small home to live peacefully after retirement. The downside to such an arrangement is the increasing land prices. With a massive increase in real estate prices, including the rising construction costs, construction of such a house is not quite recommended. Also supervising the daily construction activity is a tough task for senior citizens.

Assisted Living Houses (AL or ALF)
With advancement of age, senior citizens require constant medical attention and aid. If medical care is taken off their mind then they feel more comfortable otherwise that is a big reason for stress for them. The Assisted Living Federation of America (ALFA) defines Assisted Living as a senior living option that combines apartment style housing, organized social interaction and private duty support services as needed. An elderly can also live with an assistant including a family member or a medical nurse or helper. Such assisted living houses are comparatively a newer concept in India but are likely to pick up in the near future. The advantage of having a medical assistant cuts out the travelling time to hospitals, making such homes quite useful for people with medical issues and other disabilities. Health care services are often provided by outside providers who either rent an office in the building or visit the building periodically. Assisted living is designed for individuals who require assistance with everyday activities such as meals, medication management, or physical assistance with bathing, dressing and transportation. Some residents may have memory disorders including Alzheimer's, or they may need help with mobility, incontinence, or other challenges.

Skilled Nursing Facility (SNF)
A (SNF) is defined as an institution or part of an institution that meets criteria for accreditation established by the sections of the Social Security Act. Skilled nursing care includes rehabilitation, psychological counselling, physiotherapist and skilled

medical and nursing procedures and staff. These campuses gather all levels of care onto one property. Generally, the nurses and therapists of the SNF unit provide care as necessary to the AL and IL residents. However, the first priority of the health care staff on the campus is to care for the SNF residents. Often external providers of health care and private duty services are brought in to deliver care to the residents of the IL and AL.

Training Programmes and Activities Carried Out for the Elderly

Empowerment of the Elderly is not only a necessity but urgency. Training programmes and courses would bring a lot of gains to the elderly. Help them to cope with stress, pain and the challenges of everyday life. Deal with disturbing events with grace and composure. These courses would help them to plan their lives better. Give them the confidence to take care of their finances and health. While retirement is taken negatively by many people and a feeling of depression overwhelms them, it should be basically regarded as a period of transition from one phase of life to another. A period of time when people have more free time at hand, to do whatever they want to, like take care of their health, pursue their hobbies and passions which previously they could not do, due to time constraints and also because of the stress and strains of their jobs. They can even take out time to do things which were getting postponed previously.

Many senior citizens register for pursuing their education, post-retirement. There are few benefits of doing such a thing; one is that they keep themselves engaged. They learn daily, their mind is kept alert and they pick up an additional degree/certificate, whichever may be the course. There are many workshops: long and short distance courses announced by the government and the NGOs every year. Options can be checked out and courses taken on, based upon a person's interest and convenience. While in early life and career, an additional degree may not matter but it gives a tremendous amount of self-boost and a great sense of satisfaction in having achieved this when you are a senior citizen. These people also become an inspiration for others.

The Indira Gandhi National Open University

The Indira Gandhi National Open University announces many learning options for all (senior citizens) every year. Lots of senior citizens enrol themselves for these 'Long and Short Distance Courses'and complete them in style too. They choose to pursue their graduation and post-graduation studies in many principles like history, psychology, German, French, B'ed and many other disciplines. There are also courses that can be done online.

The International Longevity Centre-India (ILC- I)

The Longevity Centre-India (ILC) which was set up in 2003 has been working on activities regarding the Elderly. (ILC) is also a member of the Global Alliance of the

International Longevity Centres and as its member enjoys Special NGO Consultative Status with UN ECOSOC. ILC-I is also a Satellite Centre for the SAARC region of the United Nations' International Institute on Ageing, Malta.

With the support of Gharda Chemicals, ILC-I (January 2018-March 2018) had undertaken several programmes for the wellbeing of an important segment of society, namely, the senior citizens over the age of 60 years. One such programme was the 'Mobile Literacy Training Programmes for Senior Citizens'! These Mobile Literacy Training Programmes were half-day workshops meant for those senior citizens who wanted to understand and use mobile phones for more than just telephonic communication purposes.

Since 1997, ILC-I has also been organising international training programmes of UN INIA in Pune, Mumbai and Hyderabad. Anyone interested can join, even the elderly. These courses also help to train people in the field of empowering the elderly by giving them a thorough understanding of ageing issues. Participants are also trained to start thinking on their own and contribute to suggestions for the formulation of policies, which will ensure a high quality of life for older persons, in their own society. (silverinnings.blogspot.com) The programme consists of lectures and the topics dealt include Population ageing: A global perspective; Key concepts in gerontology; Social Economic and Psychological and Health aspects of ageing. These courses thus cover the concerns of the elderly comprehensively.

Pakalveedu at Thiruvananthapuram

Pakalveedu is a daycare centre in Thiruvananthapuram started for old people to spend their daytime by NGO director Fr K J Thomas in 2016. This centre also gives educational training to its members. In the year 2018 as many as 76 inmates, all senior citizens, of Pakalveedu at Poovar got ready to attempt their first literacy exam under Kerala State Literacy Mission's 'Akshara Lakshyam' project. Neglecting their old age issues, the inmates took the third-standard equivalent exam on August 5, 2018.

It all began when Loyola Social Welfare and Charitable Society in Poovar, an NGO for old people, realized that many inmates of its 'Pakalveedu' at Poovar were illiterate. The NGO, in association with the Kerala State Literacy Mission Authority, enrolled them into the 'Akshara Lakshyam' project that focuses on non-formal education. Soon, classes were held once a week every Wednesday.

Their enthusiasm was not hindered by their old age. "Out of 130 students, around 80 were illiterate. The educated ones and the teachers helped to teach and made things simple," said Sunitha Yesudas, pakalveedu, coordinator and teacher. Games and other activities were also included in the class to make the students feel happy. After qualifying the exam, they would join the next phase, the fourth-standard equivalence class.

(Published: 26th July 2018 06:07 AM|Last Updated: 26th July 2018 06:07 a.m).

Senior Citizens in Mumbai (NGO)
The Senior Citizens in Mumbai (NGO) conduct a lot of programmes for the elderly, to keep them busy and engrossed in developing their skills. Many workshops are conducted at nominal charges.

Technology

- Technical courses on Design Thinking & Building Innovative Products.
- Market Research.
- MVP Identification, Ideation & Prototyping.
- KPI Improvement & Investor Pitch Development.

Painting Classes and Workshops

- Finger and Fluid Painting.
- Palette knife Painting.
- Sand Art Painting.
- Acrylic Painting Workshop.
- Water colour Workshop.
- Canvas Painting and Block Painting.

Baking Classes and Workshop

- Eggless Brownies,
- Cookies.
- Cupcakes workshops.

Caligraphy

- Modern Calligraphy.
- Brush Pen Calligraphy.
- Dip Pen Calligraphy.

Embroidery and Beadwork Workshops
Lippan and Mud Mirror Work.

Self-grooming Courses
Professional Makeup Workshop.

Literature Courses
Be Better with Storytelling.

Senior Citizens Council of Delhi

The Senior Citizens Council of Delhi has been working since 2007. It is associated with the Ministry of Social Justice & Empowerment, Govt of India, Social Welfare Department of Delhi Govt, I.C.C.R and Senior Citizens Cell of Delhi Police. The Council is working for the cause and care of the elderly and to protect them from abuse, neglect, injustices and humiliation inflicted on them by their own children. The Council has also created a network of active senior citizens and offers lots of recreational activities and other programmes for the elderly to join in like Computer Training, Yoga & Meditation, Physiotherapy, Indoor Games like CaromBoard, Ludo Snakes & Ladder, Spiritual Discourses, Social & Cultural Activities, Newspapers and Library Books, Free Consultations by Doctors, Health Check-Up Camps, etc. Every effort is being taken to free and protect the elderly from loneliness by organising group visits to Religious & Historical Places in India and abroad. A lot of cultural programmes and fashion shows are also conducted in which both the male and females participate.

Sulabh International
Sulabh International is another non-profit organisation that is working for the cause of widows living in Vrindavan and other ashrams. It also conducts vocational training for the elderly. Sulabh international also has a helpline for widows who need help. As a result of these schemes, the lifestyle of these old and young women has changed. They have understood the value of their lives and many of them have started to live independently, working on various vocational projects. Thus Sulabh International has succeeded in bringing awareness about the concept of active ageing in the minds of these elderly widows.

Local Classes or Workshop in Every City
Today with the continuous growth of the elderly population every city is also taking steps to see that the elderly live a comfortable and dignified life. To empower them to meet the ever increasing demand of the usage of technology in every sphere of life digital workshops or classes are being organized and conducted by a majority of cities for the elderly citizens. Apart from this the various clubs and Community Centres of almost all cities hold activities for the elderly so that they remain busy and do not get lonely. These classes and activities encourage the Elderly to get out and learn with peers. These certificate courses, run by private institutions can also help the seniors to get an earning option if so required.

Agewell Foundation
Agewell Foundation, New Delhi, India, is a not-for-profit NGO that has been working for the welfare and empowerment of older persons of India since 1999. Agewell Foundation gives training to volunteers and senior citizens to empower them. It has set up a network of volunteers spread across India and interacts with older persons on daily basis through its volunteers' network.

Recognising the work being done by Agewell Foundation ECOSOC has granted Special Consultative Status to Agewell Foundation at United Nations since 2011. It is associated with Department of Public Information, United Nations (UN-DPI-NGO). Agewell has also been member of various Working Groups and Steering Committees on Social Sector for three consecutive Five- Year-Plans of Planning Commission of India since 2002.

'Ageing in Place' National Council for Ageing Care

Ageing in Place the National Council For Ageing Care also offers courses in technology like the use of computers, tablets and smartphones which can help seniors to stay connected with their families, friends and communities. Some of the elderly get intimidated by its usage as during their younger days they had never got a chance to use technology at their workplace. This would especially be useful for the senior citizens who wish to live independently and stay in their own homes in old age.

Getting digital literacy can induce confidence in the minds of the elderly. They would develop independence and would be able to access information and services online.

Department of School Education and Literacy

Ministry of Human Resource Development conducts a lot of programmes for adults and elderly. Adult Education aims at extending educational options to those adults, who have lost the opportunity and have crossed the age of formal education, but now feel a need for learning of any type, including literacy, basic education, skill development (Vocational Education) and equivalency. With the objective of promoting adult education, a series of programmes have been introduced.

Adult Education Programme

Adult Education Programme to replace Saaksha Bharat Scheme. The government has set the target to raise the overall literacy of the country to 80% and to reduce the gender disparity to 10% by the end of 12th five-year plan. The age is not the criterion.

Government and NGOs

The government departments and many NGOs have announced adult education, professional training and personalized learning programmes for seniors on dementia, computers, smartphones and digital literacy, hobbies like art, craft, dance and music, courses on learning of languages like English, German, French, Spanish and Japanese. Learning these languages would not only make the elderly happy but would also provide earning opportunities if a person is interested. There is a dearth of people who know foreign languages and these skills can be utilized in many ways. Teaching English to foreigner's online, working as translators, etc. are some of the options that can be explored.

The long and short distance online e-learning programmes that also include vocational skill development as well as access to enrolment in graduation and post-graduation courses. All these courses and concepts aim at building empowerment and abilities for an individual to shoulder responsibilities and successfully lead an autonomous life.

There are some foreign Institutes that also hold courses for the empowerment of the elderly:

Creative Retirement Institute (CRI)

There are online courses and most of them are free. The elderly who are educated can make use of these courses for improving their credentials and also improving their knowledge, developing confidence and even making themselves legible for further jobs as lots of companies in the world have their retirement age as 70 years. Learning always gives happiness and peace of mind throughout all stages of life, especially as we grow older.

It makes you more knowledgeable about the current trends. Creative Retirement Institute (CRI), offers a variety of non-credit classes, without giving any homework, or taking exams. They just satisfy the passion for learning. CRI members are eligible for an Edmonds CC EdPass, which gives them access to the college library, gym and other Edmonds CC student services. Classes are held at Edmonds CC, Edmonds Senior Centre, Lynnwood Senior Centre, Fairwinds Brighton Court and Homage Senior Services in Lynnwood.

Institute on Ageing

Institute on Ageing puts an emphasis on continuous learning and throughout the year they offer many opportunities for education.

They believe that awareness and training help you be a more effective and helpful caregiver to loved ones. And while growing older might seem like a common topic, new and innovative ways for helping with the ageing process are always being developed and improved upon.

Institute on Ageing fosters a community that is knowledgeable about the current trends in aiding ageing adults and people with disabilities. They host a number of conferences, talks, workshops and educational sessions that bring new discoveries and techniques to the forefront, for community members, medical experts and psychotherapeutic professionals. These events can also be a great resource for family members, caregivers and older adults themselves. Their IOA experts remain active in the community, both locally and nationally, providing a speaker's bureau of experts to share new and innovative techniques and build a community of knowledge.

Mindfulness-Based Stress Reduction (MBSR)

Mindfulness-Based Stress Reduction (MBSR) is a blend of meditation, body awareness and yoga: learning through practice and study, how your body handles (and can resolve) stress neurologically.

The online MBSR training course 'Palouse Mindfulness' is 100% free, created by a fully certified MBSR instructor and is based on the programme founded by Jon Kabat-Zinn at the University of Massachusetts Medical School.

The ISU3A offers lifelong learning or third age learning programmes. Google Groups allows people to create and participate in online forums and email-based groups with a rich community experience. A person in this group can also share documents, pictures, calendars, invitations and other resources.

University of the People (Uo People)
University of the People is an American non-profit distance learning institution of higher education that offers undergraduate and graduate degree courses that are free and online. They are rigorous academic courses—designed and led by instructors employed and educated at the world's leading institutions—comprise a high-level curriculum that is both practical and well-rounded. In some cases students do not pay for instruction or materials—only a nominal assessment fee has to be paid for each course. Qualified students who cannot afford these modest fees are invited to apply for scholarships. Degree programmes at the associate and bachelor's levels are offered in business administration, computer science and health science, as well as an MBA. All degrees are fully accredited in the United States—a standard held in the highest regard worldwide. Study at your own pace with the flexibility you need to fit a serious education into your busy life. 100% online, you won't find any programme more convenient or accessible. Special opportunities are made available by partner companies and organisations and the dedicated staff at university, who prepare students for the job search, guiding them towards successful employment. So if the Elderly are physically fine, can get re-employed in companies where the retirement age is seventy or else if they are working in a company which allows them to work as long as they can and are physically fit.

Lifelong Learning Institutes (LLIs)
Lifelong Learning Institutes, offer computer, technology and other useful courses for elderly retirees. Two organisations Osher and Elderhostel support approximately 500 (LLI) programmes nationwide.

Senior Net
Senior Net offers instructor-led workshops at 36 learning centres throughout the United States. This organisation conducts basic online computer courses although a fee of $43 has to be paid for membership the first year.

Websites to Learn Technology Courses
GCFLearnFree.org, is a website that can be used by the elderly for learning technology and math. It is supported by the Goodwill Community Foundation.

Another free website that teaches seniors basic computer skills is Tech-Boomers.com.

Many instructors offer quick overviews on computer applications and specifics such as setting up a Facebook account or doing Skype calls with the help of videos on YouTube.

Medical Facilities for the Senior Citizens

The Union Budget of 2018 had many proposals for senior citizens. It announced the increase in deduction limit under section 80D of the income-tax Act under which one would be able to avail benefits for payment of health insurance premiums. The premiums that a person paid towards a health insurance policy would qualify for tax deduction. The Union Budget, 2018 announced this deduction for senior citizens from up to Rs. 30,000 to a maximum of Rs. 50,000. "On an average, senior citizens pay around Rs. 10,000 as premiums but the health insurance cover is insufficient given the rising health care costs and their increased medical attention. Increasing the deduction limit in that sense will encourage senior citizens to buy a higher health insurance policy, which is the need of the hour," said K. G. Krishnamoorthy Rao, managing director and chief executive officer, Future Generali India Insurance Co. Ltd.

This change would be applicable for the financial year 2019. What has also changed is that senior citizens can now claim a deduction of Rs. 50,000 towards medical expenditure, instead of claiming on account of health insurance premiums only. "Currently, senior citizens—who are above 80 years of age—can claim a deduction of up to Rs. 30,000 incurred towards medical expenditure, in case they don't have health insurance. The Budget has increased this to Rs. 50,000 and also allowed the same flexibility to senior citizens. Even individuals who pay premiums for their dependant senior citizens parents can claim the additional deduction on health insurance premium or medical expenditure," said Homi Mistry, partner, Deloitte Haskins and Sells LLP.

Other than increasing the deduction under section 80D of the income-tax Act, the Union Budget has also increased the limit of deduction for medical expenditure for self, spouse, dependant parents, children and siblings in respect of certain critical illnesses like malignant cancers, chronic renal failure, haemophilia and thalassemia—from Rs. 60,000 in case of senior citizens to Rs. 80,000. In case of very aged elderly —to Rs1 lakh for all senior citizens under section 80DDB.

Senior Citizens Need Health Insurance

Over the last few years, the health care costs have been continuously increasing. Old age, many times leads to dependency and brings with it critical illnesses which require a lot of finances to be treated. The senior citizens today find it very difficult to meet the expenses related to comprehensive medical health examinations and hospitalisation which might occur because of serious illnesses. Purchasing a comprehensive health insurance policy is, therefore, a necessity to reduce the financial burden on the elderly as well as on their families. People should be guided to take medical Insurance when they are young as the premium is much higher if taken in old age. In old age the income of the elderly becomes less and so in that eventuality it becomes very difficult for them to pay the premiums.

Some points to be noted before choosing health insurance for senior citizens

- The Insurance policy which continues to give coverage for citizens even after they cross the age of 60 should be opted for.
- A policy with the maximum renewal age should be chosen.
- An insurance policy which offers maximum coverage against a large number of illnesses including pre-existing conditions is more beneficial than others.
- A medical insurance policy, the benefit of which can be availed in maximum number of hospitals Is always regarded more beneficial than others.
- A policy which offers cashless hospitalisation is normally beneficial.

Some other medical facilities and other empowerment of the elderly projects undertaken by the government

Arogya Arunachal Yojna

Arogya Arunachal is a health assurance scheme launched by Prema Khandu the chief minister of the state especially to give financial support to the socially and economically backward tribal population. This allows citizens to avail cashless health services in enlisted hospitals through a web portal. This Chief Minister's Arogya Arunachal Yojna would also be joined with the centre's Ayushman Bharat. The scheme offers health care services up to Rs. 5 lakhs per family. By improving the efficiency of the public health care system the chief minister wants to extend this health care facility to all by 2030.

'Ayushman Bharat National Health Protection Mission'

The Union budget, 2018–19 of the Government of India announced 'The Ayushman Bharat Programme' which aims to carry National Health Protection Scheme 2017, proposals forward. This programme focuses on the health care facilities of the poor and vulnerable to ensure that Indian citizens have access to quality cashless health care services. The entitlement is decided on the basis of deprivation criteria in the Socio-Economic Caste Census (SECC) database. Each family is entitled to be provided with health care services worth Rs. 5 lakh per annum for secondary and tertiary care hospitalisation. These benefits can be utilized by the poor across the country.

National Programme for Health Care of the Elderly (NPHCE)

Under the National Programme for Health Care of the Elderly (NPHCE) during the 12th Five-Year Plan the government has decided to expand and implement activities of tertiary level care, open new Regional Geriatric Centres, set up two National Centres for Ageing one in AIIMS, at Ansari Nagar, New Delhi and another in.

Madras Medical College, Chennai. These centres are equipped with 200 beds and specialize in geriatrics. They support research activities and train people to become experts in the care of the elderly. They also set up special programmes for the elderly population above the age of 75 like yoga therapy. Financial assistance is given for recurring and non recurring activities like drugs and consumables and Human Resources. The human resources for National Centres of Ageing (NCAs) are engaged on contractual basis, especially AYUSH practitioners for interventions for the very old population. Emphasis is given on early diagnosis and screening. A total amount of Rs. 477.49 crores have been earmarked under the Scheme.

Information, Education and Communication (IEC) activities

The National Centres of Ageing also print and distribute pamphlets/booklets in English, Hindi and regional languages of (IEC) Information, Education and Communication materials taking into account scientific evidence on various commonly occurring disease conditions such as coronary disease, stroke, osteoporosis, dementia, tuberculosis, COPD, BPH, cataract, etc. The information is also provided through electronic media.

Rashtriya Vayoshri Yojana

The Department of Social Justice and Empowerment has launched a Central Sector Scheme namely "Rashtriya Vayoshri Yojana" (RVY) on 1st April 2017: Under the Rashtriya Vayoshri Yojana" (RVY) the elderly living below poverty line and suffering from any of the age related disability are entitled to get assisted living devices like walking sticks, elbow crutches, walkers, wheelchairs, artificial dentures and spectacles and hearing aids free of cost. These devices will thus help the poverty stricken elderly to overcome age related disabilities and return normalcy in their life and also help them to carry on with their day to day activities. The Scheme is implemented through the 'Artificial Limbs Manufacturing Corporation (ALIMCO), and the expenditures are met by Senior Citizens' Welfare Fund (SCWF). So far, total 138 distribution camps have been organized across the country under RVY.

Mobile Elderly Project

Selected Regional Geriatric Centres have started the facility of treatment of the elderly through the use of mobile telephones. This is especially useful for the elderly above the age of 75 and for those who want to avoid repeated visits to hospitals. Depending on its feasibility, the programme will be extended to more Regional Geriatric Centres and District hospitals.

Human Resource Development

Looking at the statistics and data of the increasing elderly population, MD in Geriatric Medicine is becoming very popular and is an approved course of the Medical Council of India. Clinical and operational research would also be emphasized.

Lasi Project

The Lasi Report was released by Dr. Harsh Vardhan on January 6th, 2021. The Lasi report is the first scientific data of its kind in India and consists of a national investigation of the health, economic and social determinants of the ageing population in India.

It has carefully kept into account the institutional and cultural characteristics of India and at the same time has collected reliable data on mental health disease, functional health and social and economic wellbeing of elderly population (https://pib.gov.in/PressReleasePage.aspx?PRID=1686552). The facts from this report would help to facilitate further formulation of health care programmes and policies for the health care of the elderly population in India. In addition, LASI has obtained indicators for the four metropolitan cities of India- Delhi, Kolkata, Mumbai and Chennai. The commendable work of the Lasi report can easily be compared with the Health and Retirement Study (HRS) done in the United States and the sister surveys in Asia—such as the Chinese Health and Retirement Longitudinal Study (CHARLS) and the Korean Longitudinal Study of Ageing (KLOSA).

Conclusion

With all these projects being undertaken for the benefit of the elderly and with advances in medical and health care related sciences, people would be able to live not only much longer than in the past but also lead an active healthy life. This would result in improving the quality of life of the elderly which would also reduce the burden of care on the caregivers. The medical insurance schemes when taken wisely would give them solace and reduce the financial stress and strain in their minds of medical expenses. Majority of the elderly reside in their homes with their families and wish to remain there but retirement homes can be another choice if need be. Families provide majority of care to their older relatives. Although this practice is not new, changes in society and lifestyles have made care more complicated. Today home care services are available to help to assist the caregivers at home. The retirement homes give the elderly the facility of doctors and nurses at call. Nurses who help in giving medication, checking temperature, blood pressure, sugar levels and even help patients in bathing, dressing and provide assistance in toileting, feeding and grooming patients. These retirement homes help the patients to get rid of loneliness by conducting a lot of activities and also help them to socialize with other inhabitants of the home. There are services like meals on wheels which help the elderly to order food if they do not want to cook. Updating the elderly in the usage of technology by training them in the usage of devices like computers, smartphones, tablets would help to make their life comfortable because a lot of work is done online today. This would help them to stay in touch with friends and family and especially benefit the old people who wish to live independently. Thus the outcome based training programmes and activities would really help in the endeavour to empower the elderly. Shifting their focus from input based exercise to outcome based potential. Making them financially self-sufficient through policies and pension schemes of the government, so that they can lead a life of dignity and have not succumbed to family or societal abuse. All this would result in increasing their confidence levels which would make them believe in their abilities to move forward in life with a positive attitude of never getting demoralized, stressed or defeated by circumstances or people around them. They would be able to channelize growth by opening up new avenues for themselves to get self-employed. They would always demand their rights and treat old age as the beginning of a second inning in life. They would make a place in the hearts of their near and dear ones as well as friends and relatives with the tremendous treasure of their experiences, maturity and insight into the complexities of life.

References

https://pib.gov.in/PressReleasePage.aspx?PRID=1686552).

https://www.india.gov.in/spotlight/rashtriya-vayoshri-yojana

Agewell Foundation. (2012). *Comprehensive study on the status of older persons-Delhi and NCR.* New Delhi, Available at http://www.agewellfoundation.org/

Ardington, C., Case, A., & Hosegood, V. (2009). Labor supply response to large social transfers: longitudinal evidence from South Africa. *American Economic Journal Applied Economics American Economic Association, 1*(1), 22–48.

Beneficiaries of National Old Age Pension Scheme (NOAPS). (2002–03 to 2014–15). Available at: https://community.data.gov.in/noapsignoaps-beneficiaries-from-2002-03-to-2014-15

Budget. (2018). Available at: https://economictimes.indiatimes.com/ wealth/tax/budget-2018-proposes-to-exempt-40-of-nps-corpus- from-tax-for-non-salaried-subscribers/articleshow/62457515.cms

Government of National Capital Territory of Delhi and UNDP Homeless Survey. (2010). New Delhi.

Government of National Capital territory of Delhi (GNCTD). Approach to the Twelfth Five Year Plan (2013). (2012). Available at: (http://www.delhi.gov.in

Kaushal, N. (03, September 2014). *Ideas for India for more evidence based policy.* National Bureau of Economic Research.

Kaushik, A. (2011). *Active ageing: A study of elderly contributing in urban.* VDM VerlagDr.

Ministry of Health and Family Welfare. Available at: https://mohfw.gov.in/sites/default/files/8072971981455275414.PDF

Senior Citizens Health Insurance. Available at: https://www.bankbazaar.com/insurance/senior-citizen-health- insurance.html?ck=Y%2BziX71XnZjIM9ZwEflsyDYIRL7gaN4W0xhuJSr9Iq61O%2BKI7BUSdfRb9O3UreX%2F&rc=1

The National Social Assistance Programme. (1995). Available at http://nsap.nic.in/

United Nations Population Fund. (2017). Caring for our elders: Early Responses"-India aging report (2017). UNFPA, New Delhi

Vasi, S. (2016). Active aging through volunteerism: A review. *The Journal of Madras School of Social Work,10* (1&2), 61–89.

Chapter 15
Ageing and Armed Conflict: Understanding the Problems of Parents of Disappeared Persons in Kashmir

Saima Farhad and Shazia Manzoor

Abstract Conflict increases vulnerabilities of people. These include insecurities and risks associated with armed violence, which are linked to civilian casualties, injuries, damage to property, fears, instabilities, breakdown of social and institutional support mechanisms as well as economic avenues, etc. Such impacts of the conflict form the most visible contours of life in the armed conflict in Kashmir; the region has seen armed violence since late 1980s. Various studies have pointed out that the effects of the violence, associated with armed conflict, due to its frequency, persistence and spread, have been felt by the whole civilian population. Within this, we observe that a lot of focus, both academic and interventional, is on groups like orphans, widows and half widows, people with injuries, etc. However, the group of aged people affected by violence in Kashmir has hardly been given any attention. The challenges which are linked to ageing, including issues related to health, financial and emotive insecurities, etc. are amplified for this group due to the impact associated with the conflict context. This may include loss, often sudden, of a family member to violence, damage to property, livelihood insecurities, fears and social changes associated with conflict, etc. The aged population in Kashmir stands as a witness to the conflict and has struggled with the breakdown of the social milieu; they negotiate their life with not just the violence of the present, but also the memory and experience of the 'normal' before the armed conflict. Within this group, our particular focus in this paper is on the elderly parents of the disappeared persons in Kashmir. In the conflict toll on civilian population in Kashmir, disappearances stand out as a unique issue—even though there is no absolute clarity on the total number of disappeared, most report put it at more than 8000. The parents of the disappeared struggle with not just the loss of a young family member but also struggle with an emotive pain where there is no closure; they bear the emotive pain of 'not knowing' which is often associated with a hope of return. Associated with this are issues which may include loss of an earning member of the family often the only one, taking up financial and social responsibilities, dealing with structures of the conflict, etc. Through this paper, we aim to understand the problems and challenges faced by the aged parents of the disappeared persons in Kashmir and seek to identify processes and mechanisms of

S. Farhad (✉) · S. Manzoor
Department of Social Work, University of Kashmir, Srinagar, Jammu and Kashmir, India

M. K. Shankardass (ed.), *Gerontological Concerns and Responses in India*,
https://doi.org/10.1007/978-981-16-4764-2_15

intervention. Such a study will not just aid the understanding of this sub-group but will relate to aged populations affected by contexts like armed conflict, etc.

Keywords Kashmir · Armed conflict · Disappeared young people · Aged people · Elderly parents · Challenges and negotiations · Interventions

Introduction

The most profound impacts of the armed conflict in Kashmir have been borne by the civilian population. These include high civilian casualties, damage to property, fears, economic loss, etc. Within the civilian population, a few groups stand out as regards this conflict impact; these include widows, half widows, orphans, internally displaced migrants, etc. For these groups, conflict introduces new marginalities and compounds pre-existing problems. This compounding of vulnerabilities also holds true for other marginal groups, including the elderly population affected by armed conflict—a group which does not get the same attention.

In such a context, normal everyday problems linked to economic, demographic and developmental changes, get linked to the instabilities and the breakdown of the conflict context. Placed such, problems which exist elsewhere in India, like issues linked to livelihood insecurities, health care, education, disasters, marginality of women, etc. may often be aggravated. A distinct example is that of half widows in Kashmir, which is linked to disappearances in Kashmir. Estimates by civil society groups put the number of disappeared at 8000 and the number of half widows is estimated to be more than 1500 (APDP, 2011). Defined as a woman whose husband is missing, a half widow can't remarry due to religious proscription for the lack of suitable proof of husband's death (Qutab, 2012). Introduced into grave economic insecurities due to the loss of the earning family member, the suffering of the half widow is aggravated by pre-existing religious and cultural norms, the absence of formal support, as well as the search for the disappeared husband in police stations, prisons, army camps, hospitals, graveyards in distant villages, etc. (Bashir, 2010). Placed such, the life of a half widow has been referred to as one which remains in a 'state of perpetual limbo' (APDP, 2011) or trapped in a form of 'permanent liminality' (D'Souza, 2016).

Linked to the problem of disappearances is the case of aged parents of the disappeared. They form a distinct sub-group of the larger group of elderly population affected directly by violence; this larger group includes elderly who have suffered a civilian casualty in the family, injuries due to violence, damage to residential property/livelihood, forced migration, etc. For this larger group, the problems associated with the conflict context merge with issues linked to ageing, but the elderly parents of the disappeared have to contend with persistent grief of 'not knowing' which is intensified with false hope of return of the disappeared. References to this group are not uncommon in media reportage on Kashmir; this often concerns reports of silent protests by parents seeking whereabouts of their children (Bedi, 2017), or the death 'without a closure' of elderly lonely parents still waiting for any news of disappeared son (Jaleel, 2009).

Kashmir Conflict and Impact on Civilian Population

Before we set out to discuss the challenges faced by the elderly parents of the disappeared, we will attempt to give a brief description of the conflict context and its associated violence. The break into armed conflict in the Kashmir valley, in the state of Jammu and Kashmir in India, is largely traced to 1987 election malpractices. Following this, the political dissent in the region, aided by external factors, converted into an armed insurgency. The result of this insurgency and counter-insurgency is a massive militarization of Kashmir; it is often located as one of the most militarized regions in the world. As a result of this, the social world in Kashmir has had to deal with unprecedented loss of life, trauma and suffering; the number of causalities alone is more than 43,000; this includes more than 5000 security personnel (police, army and paramilitary), more than 20,000 militants (local and non-local) and more than 16,000 civilians (Maqbool & Muzaffar, 2012). As most of the fighting took place in inhabited areas, civilians casualties have remained high; the civilian casualties linked to armed violence peaked in 1995 and 1996 with more than 1000 civilians killed each year (Rashid, 2017). The number has decreased substantially thereafter, but there have been increases since 2017 (Jain, 2018). A significant conflict toll in the Kashmir conflict relates to disappearances; rights bodies estimate the number to be more than 8000 (APDP, 2011). Linked to this, is the presence of thousands of unmarked graves in Kashmir; the J&K State Human Rights Commission gave orders to investigate and conduct DNA tests for over 2000 unmarked graves in 2017 (Ehsan, 2017).

The conflict tolls are not just limited to casualty figures and disappeared. More than 100,000 people (mostly Hindus, but also Sikhs and some Muslims), pursuant to targeted violence based on religious or political affiliation, had to flee the Kashmir valley. Among these migrants, the majority was that of Kashmiri Pandits, as more than 90% of the community fled from the valley to other places in India (Datta, 2016). Many people, mostly Muslims, fled in the opposite direction to areas controlled by Pakistan (Ahmed, 2010).

Like any armed conflict, women became particular targets and the conflict has been linked to widespread incidence of rape and sexual violation (Dewan, 1994; Kazi, 2009) and in the emergence of category of widows and half widows (Bashir, 2010). While the number of half widows, has been estimated at more than 1500, the number of widows is estimated to be around 20,000 (APDP, 2011). Similarly, the impact on children is particularly pronounced for thousands of children who have been orphaned due to the conflict (George 2011).

It will be very difficult to quantify the number of injuries associated with violence, due to the extent of the spread of the violence. As per a report by Human Rights Watch (HRW), 'Most Kashmiri families have lost a relative, friend, or neighbour in the violence' (HRW, 2006, p. 1). Placed such, this conflict can be located as a setting where armed violence or the threat of violence is persistent; here the entire population of this zone has been witness to various forms of armed violence, detention, torture, or kidnapping (de Jong et al., 2008a) and its effects include high levels of distress, personal vulnerability and mass psychological suffering (de Jong et al., 2008b; Varma, 2012).

Elderly and Armed Conflict

Within these high levels of distress and suffering, we locate the group of elderly population within Kashmir; this population has had to deal with profound effects of the armed conflict. The aged population in Kashmir stands as a witness to the conflict and has struggled with the breakdown of the social milieu; they negotiate their life with not just the violence of the present, but also the memory and experience of the 'normal' before the armed conflict. While as there is hardly any violence that hasn't had a bearing on this group, particular mention is of loss of a family member, damage to property, injury, etc. This group includes the elderly parents and grandparents of those who have died in the conflict; including civilians, security personnel as well as local militants. They also have to bear the consequences of the sufferings of the family members directly affected by violence; this includes elderly parents of widows, half widows, rape victims, orphans, disappeared, or those elderly aged parents who have to deal with injuries to a family member. Associated with this are issues that may include loss of an earning member of the family, taking up of financial and social roles and responsibilities, suffering forced migration from the native place, etc.

We observe that the group of aged people affected by the Kashmir conflict has hardly been given any attention; this follows the larger neglect towards this group on knowledge and research on crises (Karunakara & Stevenson, 2012). In the sparse literature on elderly and armed conflict, we find references to themes like reduced health and mental health outcomes, elderly women health issues, nutritional needs, mortality risks due to traumatic events, heightened social isolation, etc., but there is larger consensus that these areas remain largely unresearched (Hutton, 2008; See Massey et al., 2017; Sibai et al., 2001). This larger in-attention particularly applies to areas where aged populations may be residents of a site of armed conflict.

Our problems for not being able to contextualize the condition of elderly in armed conflicts in literature were compounded by the larger neglect of themes like ageing in Kashmir, particularly within social sciences. Despite the proportion of elderly being around 9.3% of the total population, 9% rural and around 10% for Urban (Census Commissioner G.O.I, 2016), ageing and elderly care have not been a mainstream of academic and policy discussions in Kashmir. It has only entered these domains with the prominence of issues linked to ageing and care at the national level in India. Within this new attention, which is unconnected from the conflict context, the larger problems are identified with regards to health, loneliness, break of traditional support networks and the need for formal support systems (Manzoor & Farhad, 2018; Showkat, 2016). Literature on displacement of elderly populations due to development projects in J&K also identifies loneliness and absence of traditional support (Kumar & Mishra, 2018). We also observe that various reports indicate the prevalence of various psychological distress markers for Kashmir, particularly for the age group above 55 years of age where Post Traumatic Stress Disorder (PTSD), distress and depression was higher compared to lower age groups (MSF, KU, & IMHANS, 2016). These references notwithstanding, ageing, elderly care, particularly the case of elderly affected by conflict remains largely unexplored.

Placed within the larger gap of literature on ageing and conflict, we attempt a study of elderly parents in the Kashmir conflict; for this paper, we limit our inquiries to the parents of disappeared persons. Such a study will not just aid the understanding of this sub-group but will relate to aged populations affected by contexts like armed conflict, etc. We particularly reason this on the argument that the challenges which are linked to ageing, including issues related to health, financial and emotive insecurities, etc. are amplified for this group due to the impact associated with the conflict context. Following this, our paper is an attempt to locate and understand the problems and challenges faced by this group of aged parents of the disappeared persons in Kashmir and we seek to explore questions like, What are the experiences of elderly parents of disappeared? How do they make sense of their loss? And how does the conflict context interact with the problems related to ageing?

Field Work and Emerging Themes: Helplessness, Insecurities and Fears

The study was conceptualized as a qualitative study; the researchers attempted to understand the issues of the elderly parents of the disappeared. Six case studies were conducted in South Kashmir in the months of August and September 2018. For each case, both father and mother of the disappeared son were interviewed together. In two cases, the disappeared was the only son, but they had daughters. In most cases, the disappeared were below 20 years of age, with most studying at school (Secondary and Higher Secondary). There was only one exception; he was 25 years old and used to work in the family medical shop. All of the six were unmarried. The time since disappearance ranges from 20 to 25 years have passed since the disappearance. Interviews were conducted in Kashmiri and translated and transcribed into English. Two research assistants helped with locating the families and interviews.

In all the cases, some similarities emerged as to the way of disappearance; the son was either picked up from home, or the son never returned back after leaving home. In the latter, the import of 'not knowing' is more pronounced than in the former were the parents knew the doors they had to knock for information. Yet, after some time, in both these cases, after failing to get any information, the parents would widen the search, going to villages, camps, police stations, graveyards, etc. This search became the key driver of their lives for a time, after which it became another component of their lived lives, where other concerns linked to livelihood, health and security started getting in the way of the search. Most of the parents were below 60 years of age when their sons disappeared, but all are above 60 now. Their journey into the group of elderly has been mediated by the disappearance of their children. Some continue the search for their sons, some have given it up, but all linger to the hope of return.

This is only an unrepresentative outline of the lives of 12 elderly parents, mothers and fathers and this should not in any way be juxtaposed on their realities, which deal with innumerable complexities, problems and adjustments. From our limited probe into their lives and based on what the participants felt secure to share, we could locate the following key emerging themes;

1. Helplessness and Unsettled Life

All the participants continue to live with anxiety and helplessness, where there has been no closure as regards the fate of their disappeared sons. Starting from the memory of the event, when their sons disappeared, often from front of their eyes, they keep reliving the associated trauma. This leads to a futile search, over the geography of the conflict, taking them out of the security of home, often taking them to places and sites considered ‘dangerous’ and ‘out of bounds’. It is within interactions at these sites, that the participants expressed their helplessness; the idea that they are being denied information by ‘people’ who picked up their sons and not being able to questions back, instead of having to request them, to beg and weep before them in vain. It is as two parents narrate:

> This was not just a struggle but a war between me and the unknown to find my lost son, my lost hope. I spent every penny in finding my son. I roamed around like an insane person. I went to every jail in search of him…wrote letters and applications to various offices and officers. I went to all the graveyards. We went to all the religious places, saints, etc with the hope of finding him one day (Case III. Rehman, Father. 72 years old)
>
> I have three more sons, financially our family is well off but still, his absence pains us. Only a mother can tell u how you feel when you lose your child. Due to disappearance of my son, my husband lost his mental balance, due to which our whole family got devastated. He was *faulaad* (iron), but he is broken now. Initially, I thought that our son must be stuck somewhere and will be returning soon, but he kept us waiting forever. This was the start of miseries and helplessness (Case IV. Dilshada, Mother. 65 years old. Waheed, Father is 69 years old)

This helplessness is located in terms of references to becoming insane during the search, in terms of miseries and continuing pain. In case of the participants we interviewed, we observed that even though they had resumed their normal where they did not let the life stop, the effects of the ‘misery’ brought on by the disappearance kept appearing in multiple ways, compounded by the armed context; the memory of the traumatic event reinforced by every news of a young boy dying in the conflict. Their helplessness and unsettled state remain in search of certainty of closure. The ritual of mourning for loss remains incomplete and these are complicated by feelings of guilt and denial (Blaauw & Lähteenmäki, 2002). Within this state, the elderly parents of the disappeared, struggle with prolonged and aggravated trauma (Pérez-Sales et al., 1999). While this was true of all parents, we could feel that the aged mothers felt the continued effects of the disappearance at a heightened level.

2. Compounded Insecurities: Health and Financial Problems

In all the cases, we observed that the elderly parents associated their health related problems. This was also linked to the financial strain associated with the search. The participants expressed that while as in cases where the son died, people felt a sense of sympathy and could help; in most cases of disappearance no help was forthcoming. It was as if the family was left to their mourning and loss. In a common thread, the participants described that they tried to spend money on formal legal means, but had to stop pursuing it, not only because of the money involved at various levels, but also the larger disregard of the system towards them. As three parents narrate;

> I went door to door, village to village, jail to jail, but he became invisible, how would I have found him? Amid these sufferings we managed to file a case but we unfortunately don't know what happened to that and we were not in a sound financial condition so that we could have spent some amount of money to follow the case. These all sufferings were written in our fate and we failed! Due to neglect, our business has vanished. We are penniless now (Case II. Rashid, Father. 70 years Old)
>
> During my search for my beloved son, I fell down many times which resulted in injuries and damage to my bones. My memory is lost and I don't know what I talk about? (Case II. Haleema, Mother. 67 years Old)
>
> Till now I have spent more than 18 lakhs in order to find him. But now I don't have a penny left. Due to this loss, my health has deteriorated. I have been operated 9 times and my wife is bed ridden. We both (me and my wife) are aged now. We don't have strength to do anything now, even buying medicines is very difficult for us. This is the time when we would have needed our son the most. He would have not only been a support but also he would have supported us financially. His absence is a constant reminder of our helplessness. We had registered a case inhuman rights commission but it yielded no results. I kept searching for him for so long but now I think my son died the death of an unknown. (Case V. Ghulam Mohd, Father. 74 years Old)

For the elderly parents of the disappeared, the disappearance as well, as the associated search, adds layers of adversity, which varies through social and economic status. While as in one case, the parents because of their economic position did not care much about their financial condition, in most cases the families often struggled on this front. This is compounded by the increasing medical expenses on medical ailments, for which the primary cause in their narration is the disappearance itself. In explaining the adversities in their financial condition, the elderly parents also linked financial loss to failure of social networks as well as the apathy of the government and NGOs towards them.

3. Fears, Stigma and Strain in Social Relationships

A prominent theme that emerged from the participants was the heightened feeling of fear and stigma and strain in social relationships. It is as two participants explain:

> I stopped my search due to the fear of *Ikhwan* (counter-insurgents). I felt insecure and my home was already destroyed. I thought that they might kill me and people will tag me as a *Mukhbir* – an informer. I couldn't continue my search. You know, I also had to take care of my daughters. (Case I. Ramzan, Father. 65 years Old)

> We were left over by all our near and dear ones. I can just say that only the wearer knows where the shoe pinches. The disappearance of our youngest son was written in destiny, we were blessed with other children but we are unfortunate enough! They all left us alone. We have no one who'll look after us, No one to whom we'll share our feelings and sufferings. Our children quarrel with us, which adds salt to our wounds. There is a lot of misery in our lives. My husband does all the odd jobs to satisfy the fire of our bellies. He hardly earns 4-5 thousand rupees a month. I lost all the strength and hope (Case VI. Nafeesa, Mother. 68 years Old. Saleem, Father is 71 years old).

These parents did not have the luxury to only live for the disappeared and have to take care of other social responsibilities. Alongside, the larger apathy towards them, they also have to struggle with suspicion due to their travels to police-station and army camps, as well as the fears of reprisal from those threatened by their queries. Alongside this, we see that some of the parents explained a strain in social relationships, even with their other children. Here, feelings of loneliness, which may relate to issues linked to ageing elsewhere interact with the conflict context and aggravate the problems of the elderly.

Conclusions

Based on these interviews, it emerges that the key problems concern the helplessness related to 'not knowing', the associated reliving of grief associated with loss and the associated anxieties. We observed that alongside such helplessness, the elderly parent of the disappeared had to deal with aggravated income insecurities and health problems, as well as loneliness, apathy and strain in social networks. We do not seek to extrapolate these observations, for either the elderly parents of the disappeared, or for the elderly in contexts of armed conflict and understand that these observations form just the tip of the iceberg. Alongside importance of ageing related issues related to poverty, women, health and income insecurity, we realize that there is a crucial need to engage, both quantitatively and qualitatively with elderly and armed conflict. This can inform practices of intervention, which can help to overcome the profound apathy felt by this group.

References

Ahmed, I. (2010). Thousands fled India-controlled Kashmir. Are they better off in Pakistan?—CSMonitor.com. Retrieved November 1, 2018, from https://www.csmonitor.com/World/Asia-South-Central/2010/1013/Thousands-fled-India-controlled-Kashmir.-Are-they-better-off-in-Pakistan

APDP. (2011). *Half Widow, Half Wife*. Retrieved from http://www.jkccs.net/wp-content/uploads/2015/02/Half-Widow-Half-Wife-APDP-report.pdf

Bashir, A. (2010, October 11). Kashmir's half-widows shoulder the burden of a double tragedy. www.Theguardian.com. Retrieved from https://www.theguardian.com/global-development/2010/oct/11/1

Bedi, R. (2017, May 11). The missing: Fury over Kashmir's disappeared men and boys grows amid security clampdown. *The Telegraph*. Retrieved from https://www.telegraph.co.uk/news/2017/05/11/missing-fury-kashmirs-disappeared-men-boys-grows-amid-security/

Blaauw, M., & Lähteenmäki, V. (2002). "Denial and silence" or "acknowledgment and disclosure." *IRRC*, *84*, 848. Retrieved from https://www.icrc.org/eng/assets/files/other/irrc_848_blaauw_virpi.pdf

Census Commissioner G.O.I. (2016). Population composition. In *SRS Statistical Report 2016* (p. 21). Retrieved from http://www.censusindia.gov.in/vital_statistics/SRS_Reports__2016.html

D'Souza, P. (2016). Life-as-lived today: Perpetual (Undesired) Liminality of the Half-widows of Kashmir. *Culture Unbound: Journal of Current Cultural Research*, *8*, 26–42. Retrieved from http://www.cultureunbound.ep.liu.se/v8/a04/cu16v8a04.pdf

Datta, A. (2016). Dealing with dislocation: Migration, place and home among displaced Kashmiri Pandits in Jammu and Kashmir. *Contributions to Indian Sociology, 50*(1), 52–79. https://doi.org/10.1177/0069966715615024

de Jong, K., Ford, N., van de Kam, S., Lokuge, K., Fromm, S., van Galen, R., Reilley, B., & Kleber, R. (2008a). Conflict in the Indian Kashmir Valley I: Exposure to violence. *Conflict and Health*, *2*(10). https://doi.org/10.1186/1752-1505-2-10

de Jong, K., Ford, N., Kam, S. van de, Lokuge, K., Fromm, S., van Galen, R., Reilley, B., & Kleber, R. (2008b). Conflict in the Indian Kashmir Valley II: Psychosocial impact. *Conflict and Health*, *2*(1), 11.https://doi.org/10.1186/1752-1505-2-11

Dewan, R. (1994). 'Humsheera', 'Humsaya': Sisters, neighbours: Women's testimonies from Kashmir. *Economic and Political Weekly, 29*(41), 2654–2658.

Ehsan, M. (2017, November 3). Unmarked graves in Poonch, Rajouri: J&K human rights panel recommends DNA profiling. *The Indian Express*. Retrieved from https://indianexpress.com/article/india/unmarked-graves-in-poonch-rajouri-jk-human-rights-panel-recommends-dna-profiling/

George, A. (2011). State of orphans in the earthly paradise. *Economic and Political Weekly, 46*(10), 19–22.

HRW. (2006). *Everyone Lives in Fear: Patterns of Impunity in Jammu and Kashmir*. Retrieved from https://www.hrw.org/sites/default/files/reports/india0906web.pdf

Hutton, D. (2008). *Older People in Emergencies: Considerations for Action and Policy Development*. WHO. Retrieved from http://www.who.int/ageing/publications/Hutton_report_small.pdf?ua=1

Jain, B. (2018, April 19). 13,796 civilians killed in J&K since start of militancy: MHA. *Times of India*. Retrieved from https://timesofindia.indiatimes.com/india/13796-civilians-killed-in-jk-since-start-of-militancy-mha/articleshow/63820704.cms

Jaleel, M. (2009, October 27). Kashmir's lonely Mother is dead. *Indian Express*. Retrieved from http://archive.indianexpress.com/news/kashmirs-lonely-mother-is-dead/533996/0

Karunakara, U., & Stevenson, F. (2012). Ending neglect of older people in the response to humanitarian emergencies. *PLoS Medicine*, *9*(12), e1001357.https://doi.org/10.1371/journal.pmed.1001357

Kazi, S. (2009). Shopian: War, gender and democracy in Kashmir. *Economic and Political Weekly*, *XLIV*(49), 13–15.

Kumar, S., & Mishra, A. J. (2018). Forced displacement and its impact on older people in Jammu and Kashmir. *Indian Journal of Gerontology*, *32*(3), 306–317. Retrieved from http://www.gerontologyindia.com/pdf/vol-32-3.pdf

Manzoor, S., & Farhad, S. (Eds.). (2018). *Ageing and elderly care*. JK Books.

Maqbool, U., & Muzaffar, I. (2012, July 4). Government puts conflict casualty figure at 43000: Deceased include 16000 civilians, 21449 militants. *Greater Kashmir*. Retrieved from http://www.greaterkashmir.com/news/news/government-puts-conflict-casualty-figure-at-43000/124451.html

Massey, E., Smith, J., & Roberts, B. (2017). Health needs of older populations affected by humanitarian crises in low- and middle-income countries: A systematic review. *Conflict and Health, 11*(1), 29. https://doi.org/10.1186/s13031-017-0133-x

MSF, KU, & IMHANS. (2016). *Muntazar: Kashmir Mental Health Survey 2015*. Retrieved from https://www.msfindia.in/sites/default/files/2016-10/kashmir_mental_health_survey_report_2015_for_web.pdf

Pérez-Sales, P., Durán-Pérez, T., & Bacic Herzfeld, R. (1999). Long-term psychosocial consequences in first-degree relatives of people detained—Disappeared or executed for political reasons in Chile. A study in Mapuce and Non-Mapuce persons. *Psicothema, 12*. Retrieved from https://www.researchgate.net/publication/237511043_Long-term_psychosocial_consequences_in_first_-degree_relatives_of_people_detained_-disappeared_or_executed_for_political_reasons_in_Chile_A_study_in_Mapuce_and_Non-Mapuce_persons

Qutab, S. (2012). Bulletin women victims of armed conflict: Sociological. *Bulletin, 61*(2), 255–278.

Rashid, D. (2017, April 29). 13,000 civilians, 22000 militants killed in Kashmir since 1989: MHA. *Greater Kashmir*. Retrieved from https://www.greaterkashmir.com/news/kashmir/13000-civilians-22000-militants-killed-in-kashmir-since-1989-mha/247921.html

Showkat, H. (2016). Need of old age homes: A sociological study in Srinagar District (JK). *International Journal of Research in Sociology and Anthropology (IJRSA), 2*(2), 10–17. https://doi.org/10.20431/2454-8677.0202002

Sibai, A. M., Fletcher, A., & Armenian, H. K. (2001). Variations in the impact of long-term wartime stressors on mortality among the middle-aged and older population in Beirut, Lebanon, 1983–1993. *American Journal of Epidemiology, 154*(2), 128–137. https://doi.org/10.1093/aje/154.2.128

Varma, S. (2012). Where there are only doctors: Counselors as psychiatrists in Indian-Administered Kashmir. *Ethos, 40*(4), 517–535. https://doi.org/10.1111/j.1548-1352.2012.01274.x

Chapter 16
Ageing Related Mental Health Issues in the LGBTQ+ Community

Reetika Dikshit, Pragya Lodha, and Avinash De Sousa

Abstract There is an increasing number of ageing members in the LGBTQ+ community. The present chapter aims to provide a broad overview of various mental health problems that may be noted in the ageing LGBTQ+ community. Depression, anxiety and loneliness are the commonest mental health problems that may be seen in this group. This is coupled with lack of access to health care and hesitation in seeking mental health care. There may also be widespread stigma and discrimination that may be faced by this population from various quarters in society. The chapter also touches upon the need for awareness of dementia in this population. There is an emphasis on training and sensitization of medical students and physicians in the manner in which they must approach patients from the ageing LGBTQ+ community and the language and terminology that must be used. This is combined with a focus on ageing LGBTQ+ caregiving issues, the need for social support and social policy that must include these members. The need for future research in this arena is also stressed.

Keywords LGBTQ+ · Ageing · Depression · Anxiety · Dementia · Mental health

Introduction

There has been an increase in the ageing LGBTQ+ population over the years. In fact, it has been noted that many members belonging to the community may come out at a later stage in life and seek help from a physical or mental health perspective. This is in keeping with the fact that the stigma against the LGBTQ+ community has now reduced and there is an increasing awareness of the normalcy of belonging to the community. There are a number of general and specific mental health issues that

R. Dikshit · A. De Sousa (✉)
Department of Psychiatry, Lokmanya Tilak Municipal Medical College, Mumbai, India

P. Lodha
Clinical Psychologist, Private Practice, Mumbai, India

A. De Sousa
Desousa Foundation, Mumbai, India

M. K. Shankardass (ed.), *Gerontological Concerns and Responses in India*,
https://doi.org/10.1007/978-981-16-4764-2_16

beseech members of the LGBTQ+ community as they age and these issues differ from the normal geriatric population both in epidemiology and mechanism of causation and presentation. The following chapter is aimed at highlighting the various mental health issues faced by the ageing LGBTQ+ community and the various interventions and help available for the same. Few aspects of culture specific issues and need for research and investigation into this specific subset of the community is also discussed. There is an increased need for awareness among the medical fraternity and gerontologists about the specific issues that may be seen in ageing LGBTQ+ populations and this chapter serves as primer for the same.

LGBTQ+ and Ageing Epidemiology

There is no stand-alone documented data for population of the Lesbian, Gay, Bisexual, Transgender Queer (LGBTQ+) community in the world. On average, 8–10% is the prevalence in some countries like India, U.S.A and U.K. Till date, 74 countries recognize the status of LGBTQ+ as being illegal, 72 countries acclaim the same as being a crime and in 12 countries, homosexuality is punishable by death. The status of belonging to the LGBTQ+ community is that of a minority and ageing as a member of the LGBTQ+ community is a doubled edged sword. Lack of census count restricts to reveal an estimate of the geriatric population of the LGBTQ+ community, however, it is well recognized that they face several challenges- the challenges of ageing along with the challenges of belonging to a minority community. As a group, elderly that belong to the LGBTQ+ community experience unique psychosocial, financial and health problems (Choi & Meyer, 2016).

The recorded population of LGBTQ adults above age 60, in the U.S.A is estimated to be between 1.75 and 4 million (Choi & Meyer, 2016). The invisible population is slowly gaining traction, however, the lack of representation in the census remains an epidemiological challenge due to two reasons—the fluidity in gender expression and the stigma of coming out with respect to their sexual orientation and/or gender identity.

LGBTQ+ Populations, Ageing and Depression

Depression is the most common and treatable mental health disorder in geriatric populations. Untreated depression becomes a chronic condition which in turn has effects on quality of life and is plagued with medical disorders as well that may be present that also has an effect on the overall life span of the patient (Chapman et al., 2012). In a large community-based study it has been reported that 29% of LGB older adults (Fredriksen-Goldsen et al., 2013) and 47% of transgender elderly reported a large number of depressive symptoms. Depression is not due to ageing in general but a large number of stressful factors, genetics, biological factors and psychosocial as well as family factors play a role in the genesis of geriatric depression (Fiske et al., 2009). There are a number of factors in the genesis of depression that may be common to the general population as well as the LGBTQ+ community while there are some specific factors intrinsic to the LGBTQ+ community that also exist. Studies worldwide have reported that transgender populations are at a greater risk of depression than the normal population (Clements-Nolle et al., 2001) and the same holds true for suicide attempts (Grant et al., 2011). The specific streessors experienced by LGBTQ+ populations include coming out about their sexual orientation, the stigma faced in a heterosexist society and lack of support from family members and close friends. These put a negative impact on the mental health of LGBTQ+ populations and cause depression. Negative internal representations projected onto themselves by the stigma also contributes in some way (Meyer, 2013). There has been an association between internalized heterosexism and depression in the elderly that belong to the LGBTQ+ community (Fredriksen-Goldsen et al., 2013).

LGBTQ+ Populations, Ageing and Loneliness

Loneliness has been thought to be a major problem and ageism is another factor linked to ageing in general. The intersection of loneliness and mental health for elderly LGBTQ+ populations occur at many points. For example, the presence and diagnosis of HIV have scarred many members of the LGBTQ+ community, especially the elderly and have caused them to lose their friends and support networks. Research findings that elucidate these factors available to elderly LGBTQ+ adults yielded mixed findings. Studies have found that LGBTQ+ elderly have poor social support and even lack support from members of their own community (Fredriksen-Goldsen et al., 2011).

Many research papers have shown elderly LGBTQ+ have better and greater social support than the normal geriatric population and these support groups are devoid of their family members (Lombardi, 1999). Many elder LGBTQ+ adults have an increased risk of social isolation, coupled with poor mental and physical health, presence of cognitive impairment and medical morbidity and mortality than that seen in the general elderly (Cornwell & Waite, 2009). This low social support is linked to poor mental health compared with the normal elderly and social support serve as a resilience factor against threats like stigma, peer victimization and is also associated with positive mental health outcomes (Fredriksen-Goldsen et al., 2011).

Elderly LGBTQ+ adults are more likely to be single than the elderly in the general population and this may have implications for health care, socialization, caregiving when needed and also have financial implications. A recent study reported that being gay and legally married has better mental health benefits (Wight et al., 2012). Elder LGBTQ+ men have less children staying with them than the elderly in the general population and are lonelier as well (Wallace et al., 2011). There are also chances of an increased chance of loss of a partner to HIV in many cases (Cochran & Mays, 2009).

LGBTQ+ Populations, Ageing and Stigma

The stigma of ageing as an LGBTQ+ elderly is two-fold with the intersection of old age and minority community status. It has been severally documented that LGBTQ+ elderly face a plethora of challenges such as physical health, mental health, social status, economic stability in addition to personal challenges (Fredriksen-Goldsen et al., 2017; Teaster et al., 2016). *'Generational differences and lack of legal protection may cause older LGBTQ+ adults to be less open about their sexuality. Social isolation is also a concern because LGBTQ+ older adults are more likely to live alone, more likely to be single and four times less likely to have children than their heterosexual counterparts. More likely, therefore, to face poverty and homelessness and to have poor physical and mental health'* (SAGE, 2011). Sexual issues, racial factors and ethnicity may compound these problems (American Psychological Association, 2017). The elderly LGBTQ+ populations have also been subdued all their lives and now are witnessing the huge sexual upheaval that the community is seeing. There have been huge sexual transformations like the modern notion of homosexuality, the overcoming of social exclusion, the stigma faced by the thought of homosexuality as a medical and psychiatric condition, the rise of the LGBTQ+ rights and multiple pro LGBTQ+ movements, the stigma and treatment availability of HIV, the genesis of LGBTQ+ terminology and multiple sexual and gender based identities along with the normalization and decriminalization of homosexuality and the increasing inclusion of LGBTQ+ community members in social and political matters as well as inclusion at the workplace (Van Wagenen et al., 2013). Being witness to such a transfiguration of the community can lead to heightened emotional and psychological impact, sometimes disillusionment of one's social identity and roles.

Apart from the societal and cultural spheres of stigma faced by the LGBTQ+ elderly, there is a mounted conquest of having access to just health care systems. Apart from equal access to health care, it is a further challenge to find LGBT affirmative health care, in the medical and mental health care systems. There are practitioners who are not fully sensitized about the special needs of the community, may lack training in identifying the unique problems and consequently LGBTQ+ elderly persons are faced with yet another layer of discrimination. Psychologists, mental health professionals and geriatric care services treating older adults should work with elderly LGBTQ+ people and must be aware of their presence and the unique mental health and physical needs that should be integrated into mainstream care.

LGBTQ+ Ageing and Dementia

Dementia is a progressive and irreversible disorder where the symptoms gradually worsen over a number of years and months. It may have mild memory loss in the early stages and slowly these individuals lose their ability to carry out daily social and other tasks and it culminates in being bed ridden and death that ensues. Psychosocial research on ageing is beginning to reflect on elderly LGBTQ+ people and how they may age and encounter the dementia process (McGovern, 2014). However, though literature on dementia is growing in the psychosocial and ad hoc fields, few articles focus on the intersection of dementia in elderly LGBTQ+ populations (Clare, 2003; Gladman et al., 2007; Grossman et al., 2007; Hughes et al., 2011; McGovern, 2010; Persson, 2009; Ryan et al., 2008). The prevalence of Alzheimer's and related dementia is a growing risk among the elderly. The lived experience of an LGBT elderly suffering from Alzheimer's and related dementia is starkly different and doubly stigmatized as opposed to that of an elderly identifying with the heteronormative society.

A common problem with dementia in the elderly LGBTQ+ is the cognitive damage and loss and this is coupled with loss of their LGBTQ+ identity due to being in an old age home where they have to behave as the general population and feel psychologically torn and invisible physically and psychologically (Alzheimer's Society UK, 2012). Dementia is one of the most challenging illnesses for the person and the caregivers with a resulting loss of self, caused by progressive cognitive decline along with disappearance of memories, the lack of capacity to create meaning and abstract and the ability to develop a clear experience of individual and shared identities. Elderly LGBTQ+ people are also more likely to exhibit particular mental health issues that can accelerate how dementia may manifest and impact, like high levels of loneliness and poor social support and marked stigma as they get older (SAGE, 2016).

One of the added difficulties for LGBTQ+ elderly is to have social support and caregiver support. Since they tend to be lonelier, are less likely to have children and may not be necessarily living with their immediate family or biological relatives, care during dementia is an added burden (MAP & SAGE, 2010). There continues to be a rising prevalence of dementia with risk of inadequate care for the LGBTQ+ elderly where in addition, there may also be lack of sensitized professional health care services. Another hurdle that gets added is pervasive absence of memory clinics to rightfully cater to the needs of dementia care. There is a paucity of old age homes for the LGBTQ+ elderly, who may not always be welcomed in heterosexually dominated homes.

LBGTQ+, Ageing and Health care Access

Medical care all over the world in the coming decades will be faced with an increased elderly LGBTQ+ people and the general health concerns faced by these people are the same while there are some distinct medical needs coupled with facing some health care disparities. In order to overcome these health care barriers, physicians and doctors must be trained and aware so that they educate future physicians to treat this population while providing sensitive, high quality and competent care (Cannon et al., 2017). Many health care professionals may harbour their own prejudices and myths related to the LGBTQ+ community and this may cause hindrances in treatment and care. In addition to their mental health problems, older Elderly LGBTQ+ adults have an overall increased risk of disability, smoking and alcohol consumption than the general population. They are also more prone to developing metabolic syndrome and cardiovascular disease (Fredriksen-Goldsen et al., 2014). Even older transgender people are at similar risks for poor physical health, disability and mental health issues compared to non-transgender patients.

> Many older LGBTQ+ individuals are more likely to be single or without children, they are more likely to have a 'chosen family,' or a group of people to whom one is emotionally close and considers 'family,' even though one might not be biologically or legally related. Health care providers and students must be alert to the importance of nonrelatives as a source of support for this community. With these 'chosen families' comes significant differences in caregiving and social support networks in the older LGBT community. (Simone & Appelbaum, 2011)

Specific aspects of ageing and the LGBTQ+ community like sexual disorders, hormonal issues in the transgender populations, menopause and cancer related issues need to be examined. There is a need for training in medical schools and curricula in the language to be used while addressing the community and terms that may be used which shall not be derogatory and demeaning. Students and training doctors must be sensitized to the needs of such a population so that they may seek health care services freely in private and public settings (Snowdon, 2010).

The lack of knowledge and education in health care providers appear to correlate with negative perceptions shared by the elderly LGBTQ+ patient populations. Many have reported concerns about stigma and discrimination as they age. Many feel the fear that doctors may not treat them with dignity and respect. Since there would be a large number of LGBTQ+ elderly in nursing home care in the next 10 years, doctors and health care staff must be educated that this true or imaginary fear of discrimination in such people exists that may cause limited disclosure and even further unmet physical mental health needs (Cohen et al., 2008; Portz et al., 2014).

LGBTQ+ Populations, Ageing and Social Policy

Many social reformists began openly questioning the myths that elderly LGBTQ+ individuals suffer from depression, loneliness and feel sexually undesirable and inadequate. They have always fought against the prevailing societal stereotypes and exhorted that positive management of their identity was effective in providing support to elderly LGBTQ+ populations in promoting successful ageing (Butler & Hope, 1999; Sharp, 1997).

In developing services for elderly LGBTQ+ populations, we must recognize and build on the strengths of these communities. Yet as the elderly LGBTQ+ undergo ageing many do not access services and health care due to past trauma and stigma and current fears of being targeted and fear of victimization. Many have a strong sense of identity and resilience by surviving in many a hostile environment, but this also results in a reluctance to seek help from standard health care systems (Lyons, 2015; Fredriksen-Goldsen, 2016). Innovative strategies are needed to reach the elderly LGBTQ+ populations who face a lack of adequate services, social support and resources and those who are lonely, are needed to make them enter the normal health care system (Fredriksen-Goldsen, 2016).

There is a need for the development of a social policy that will include ageing LGBTQ+ adults. These citizens need to have equal access to health care and insurance rights. They must have equal rights in elder schemes and property. They also must have the right to sound testamentary capacity and to make a valid will. Elderly LGBTQ+ adults may also face discrimination when searching for old age homes and nursing homes and hospital care (Cahill & South, 2002). In a large study, where an elderly LGBTQ+ individual and a heterosexual elder contacted the same senior housing community to determine availability of a home, it was seen that 48% of times, the elderly LGBTQ+ person experienced unfavourable and negative differential treatment for the availability of housing, cost and pricing, financial help, availability of amenities and in the processing of applications (Cahill & South, 2002).

Older LGBTQ+ individuals need to be protected from hate crimes and laws need to be in place. Hate crimes are painful events not because they inflict pain caused by the assault itself, but also the psychological pain associated with social disapproval of the victim's LGBTQ+ status. The pain is caused by the symbolic message to the victim that their group is unwanted, devalued, debased and not liked in society (Herek et al., 1999).

Elderly LGBTQ+ adults have spent their childhoods and adolescence in an environment where homosexuality was considered a mental illness and same-sex sexuality was illegal and criminal and often punished (D'Augelli et al., 2001). Thus, they have faced internalized stigma which is an important concept to explore among elderly LGBTQ+ populations. The effect of internalized homophobia and transphobia on elderly LGBTQ+ people are less known and very few authors have researched this question. Internalized stigma is referring to the internalization of negative societal attitudes about LGBTQ+ people towards the self. For example, internalized transphobia occurs when there is internalization of anti-trans attitudes and beliefs, like the belief that people's gender is congruent with the biological sex assigned at birth and therefore trans individuals are fake. They feel negative about their own gender identity and the whole transgender community in general (Testa et al., 2015). This homophobia and transphobia with the negative ageism leads to ageing related mental health issues in the LGBTQ+ elderly and is associated with depression and other psychiatric disorders (Wight et al., 2015).

The growing population of elderly LGBTQ+ people have experienced an entire range of oppressive institutional stigma and discrimination in their young adulthood and a huge social change to the better understanding and acceptance of LGBTQ+ individuals in their old age. Elderly LGBTQ+ people are largely ignored in social gerontology and sexual research in old age and by legal agencies and multiple stakeholders that cater to these groups (Addis et al., 2009).

LGBTQ+ Ageing and General Mental Health

The journey of LGBTQ+ ageing brings with it unique stressors, some general and some specific to the LGBTQ+ community. Being united as a community does not mean that they would not experience mental health and social challenges. However, as an elder that belongs to the LGBTQ+ community, there are certain stressors that arise as the general community does not accept their sexual identity easily. Elderly LGBTQ+ populations have been largely scarce in geriatric and ageing related mental health research (Institute of Medicine, 2011; Persson, 2009). Studies report that the elder LGBTQ+ participants had significantly poorer physical and mental health, increased physical disability, high incidence of depression and anxiety, more stress than non- LGBTQ+ populations. The findings suggest that these patterns of adverse physical and mental health identified among LGBTQ+ adults in early and middle adulthood persist into old age as well (Conron et al., 2012).

The various issues include stigma and discrimination, homophobia/biphobia/transphobia; rejection from friends and family, outcast by the religious community, bullying, sexual harassment, hate crimes and violence. These traumatic experiences can be long lasting and affect their mental health and physical well-being. Risk factors like internalized stigma, perceived victimization and hate are important predictors of mental health outcomes. Link and Phelan (2006) found that *'being stigmatized is, in itself, a source of chronic stress that negatively affects both physical and mental health'*. The elderly LGBTQ+ are at a higher risk of victimization like verbal and physical threats, harassment by police and law, societal and employment issues and rejection by friends and family. These individuals are at an increased risk for the development of serious psychiatric and mental health related disorders. (Cramer et al., 2012).

The effects of identity concealment cause higher levels of stress and hypervigilance due to a risk of exposure and fear of rejection that can result from concealing their LGBTQ+ identity (Meyer, 2003). Increased rates of smoking and alcohol use are of major concern among elderly LGBTQ+ populations. There is a need for intervention strategies that consider cultural factors that may promote smoking and drinking among the elderly LGBTQ+ people while focusing on long-term management.

LGBTQ+ Ageing and Research Needs

It has been stated that *'a significant impediment to our understanding of ageing within and about LGBT communities in the absence of data; sexual orientation and gender identity have not been included in federal surveys and health records. This dearth is associated with inexact estimates of the size of the LGBT population and a body of research mostly based on small non-probability samples that are collected within select geographic areas'* (Hudson, 2011). There is a need for research to grow in order to better identify the status, needs and challenges faced by the LGBTQ+ elderly that are diverse with the intersection of socio-cultural and demographic variables. There is a need to thus understand better and also propose the required intervention to bridge the gap.

Research into the experience of these individuals also provides an insight into the various challenges such as that of mental health expression and prevalence of mental illnesses in this population. Due to the absence of formal support systems and caused by the stigma and discrimination, elderly LGBTQ+ individuals have struggled to have communities to meet their needs. These efforts have garnered worldwide attention and research has highlighted alternative ways to think about LGBTQ+ ageing, caregiving of these elderly and their acceptance in the community. A better understanding of elderly LGBTQ+ communities is essential for effective and competent medical and health services so that all their needs are met and this also reflects the need to negate maladaptive policies for the elderly (Hudson, 2011). Research can create the niche for developing sound elderly LGBTQ+ policies and programmes that address the effects of stigma and discrimination, psychoeducates the family and accepts the diverse life trajectories that are seen in these communities.

LGBTQ+ Ageing and Support Groups

There is a need for social support and support from their individual families or chosen families when it comes to elderly belonging to the LGBTQ+ community. This is important considering the mental health issues, depression and loneliness faced by the members of the community in addition to the stigma. There has been a surge of support groups for LGBTQ+ elderly and this has led to a lot of help to members where they find people who are unbiased and supportive when they need advice and moral support. There are also a number of online support groups where help can now be sought without the individual having to leave his home.

While there are support groups for the elder LGBTQ+ individuals, there are also support groups for their caregivers. The scarce studies on LGBTQ+ caregiving have pointed to common issues that concern them like managing caregiving responsibilities, the experience of mental, emotional and physical strain, issues with their partner in relationships and experiencing problems related to employment responsibilities (Hash, 2001; Hash & Cramer, 2003; Moore, 2002). Many caregivers also noted positive aspects of caregiving, that gave them the opportunity to show love and maintain a commitment to someone. Support groups are vital for these caregivers as many of their issues are never addressed. Many themes exist that need attention in LGBTQ+ elder caregiving like anticipated and experienced heterosexist and homophobic discrimination in the delivery of health care resources, the management of sound caregiving responsibilities, mental health issues and certain specific aspects of caregiving. Health care providers know very little about caregivers to LGBTQ+ seniors because of the paucity of studies that address the needs and realities of such groups. There is a need for further research on these populations (Brotman et al., 2007).

LGBTQ+ Ageing and the Law

One of the landmark decisions that have overturned the law and legal implications for the LGBTQ+ community was initiated by the American Psychological Association that declined that homosexual orientation was a mental disorder. This was followed by the decriminalisation of LGBTQ+ marriages. The similar has gained popularity in India with decriminalisation of section 377. Ageism within the LGBTQ+ elder community and homophobic tendencies within the mainstream senior community combine to alienate LGBTQ+ elders. This leaves them further vulnerable where neither can they voice their needs and nor the others do so for them. The following section covers the overall laws in brief and not in detail as the implicated laws vary from country to country.

The blanket law (being followed in many countries) focuses on three mainstay aspects- LGBT individuals are recognized as equal to non-LGBT individuals with the allowance of same-sex marriages, workplace anti-discrimination protections and the military's "Don't Ask, Don't Tell" policy (Knauer, 2009). What is essential to realize is that though there may be blanket laws, they differ in implication with socio-demographic diversities. It is clearly identifiable that the needs and challenges of the LGBTQ+ elderly are distinct from their counter majority. Proposals for LGBT equity in ageing must consider the legal fragility of these unique needs and challenges. there is also evidence that there isn't a monolithic LGBTQ+ identity which furthers the challenge.

As the ageing population, differentiation in inequality would lead to higher rates of poverty among all elderly in coming years, LGBTQ+ individuals are even more likely to age into poorer strata. Employment discrimination, lower lifetime social security and insurance benefits and loneliness have left many elderly LGBTQ+ individuals without a pension and many legal tangles and laws have downplayed sound economic benefits to LGBTQ+ elderly (Knauer, 2011).

Anti- LGBTQ+ marriage laws have also meant that many of these individuals have been excluded from the social safety net benefits of marriage and things that protect the financial security of the elderly, making them more vulnerable to economic insecurity. Coverage for medical health care is also a troublesome area with compounded lack of availability of sensitive as well as specialized care (Lannutti, 2005).

In countries like India, coverage for mental health care services for these individuals adds to the trauma of injustice. Housing discriminations and evictions are a further turmoil that LGBTQ+ elderly face, especially the ones who belong to lower economic classes. Advance planning legal documents are critical for LGBTQ+ couples. These documents include wills, financial and other powers of attorney with health care advance directives that have further legal implications for these individuals.

Conclusions

Thus, mental health issues and health care of the ageing LGBTQ+ community is an emerging problem. There are multiple facets that need attention in this regard. First, is the need to tackle the mental health problems of the community like depression, loneliness and other psychological issues. This is coupled with the need for health care professionals and individuals in society to work towards the reduction of stigma and internalized homophobia that may be harboured against and within such groups. There is also a need for training and education among health care professionals on dealing with and managing ageing members of the LGBTQ+ community. The medical profession needs to be trained in the terminology to be used, the unique problems of this group and the various psychosocial issues that may bisect their medical problems. There is a need for social policy for the ageing LGBTQ+ community to be revamped as well with friendlier laws in place that protect them against any discrimination in society. There is also a dearth of research in this group. There is a need for qualitative, quantitative, mixed-model studies and psychopathology research in this unique which shall then pave the way for interventions directed at their specific problems. Research needs to be done in diverse subsets of this population that shall help us understand the challenges of dealing with this population better. There is also a need for us to be sensitive and open to this group and to be certain that they receive no discrimination in health care and with regard to the basic human rights that they deserve.

References

Addis, S., Davies, M., Greene, G., MacBride-Stewart, S., & Shepherd, M. (2009). The health, social care and housing needs of lesbian, gay, bisexual and transgender older people: A review of the literature. *Health and Social Care in the Community, 17*(6), 647–658.

Alzheimer's Society UK. (2012). *Factsheet 480*. Author.

American Psychological Association. (2017). *2017 Annual report of the committee on sexual orientation and gender diversity*.

Brotman, S., Ryan, B., Collins, S., Chamberland, L., Cormier, R., Julien, D., Meyer, E., Peterkin, A., & Richard, B. (2007). Coming out to care: Caregivers of gay and lesbian seniors in Canada. *The Gerontologist, 47*, 490–503.

Butler, S. S., & Hope, B. (1999). Health and well-being for late middle-aged and old lesbians in a rural area. *Journal of Gay & Lesbian Social Services, 9*(4), 27–46.

Cahill, S., & South, K. (2002). Policy issues affecting lesbian, gay, bisexual, and transgender people in retirement. *Generations, 26*(2), 49–56.

Cannon, Y., Speedlin, S., Avera, J., Robertson, D., Ingram, M., & Prado, A. (2017). Transition, connection, disconnection, and social media: Examining the digital lived experiences of transgender individuals. *Journal of LGBT Issues in Counseling, 11*(2), 68–87.

Chapman, R., Wardrop, J., Freeman, P., Zappia, T., Watkins, R., & Shields, L. (2012). A descriptive study of the experiences of lesbian, gay and transgender parents accessing health services for their children. *Journal of Clinical Nursing, 21*(7–8), 1128–1135.

Choi, S. K., & Meyer, I. H. (2016). *LGBT aging: A review of research findings, needs, and policy implications*. The Williams Institute.

Clare, E. (2003). Gawking, gaping, staring. *GLQ: A Journal of Lesbian and Gay Studies, 9*(1), 257–261.

Clements-Nolle, K., Marx, R., Guzman, R., & Katz, M. (2001). HIV prevalence, risk behaviors, health care use, and mental health status of transgender persons: Implications for public health intervention. *American Journal of Public Health, 91*(6), 915–921.

Cochran, S. D., & Mays, V. M. (2009). Burden of psychiatric morbidity among lesbian, gay, and bisexual individuals in the California quality of life survey. *Journal of Abnormal Psychology, 118*(3), 647.

Cohen, J. N., Byers, E. S., & Walsh, L. P. (2008). Factors influencing the sexual relationships of lesbians and gay men. *International Journal of Sexual Health, 20*(3), 162–176.

Conron, K. J., Scott, G., Stowell, G. S., & Landers, S. J. (2012). Transgender health in Massachusetts: Results from a household probability sample of adults. *American Journal of Public Health, 102*(1), 118–122.

Cornwell, E. Y., & Waite, L. J. (2009). Social disconnectedness, perceived isolation, and health among older adults. *Journal of Health and Social Behavior, 50*(1), 31–48.

Cramer, R. J., McNiel, D. E., Holley, S. R., Shumway, M., & Boccellari, A. (2012). Mental health in violent crime victims: Does sexual orientation matter? *Law and Human Behavior, 36*(2), 87–98.

D'Augelli, A. R., Hershberger, S. L., & Pilkington, N. W. (2001). Suicidality patterns and sexual orientation-related factors among lesbian, gay, and bisexual youths. *Suicide and Life-Threatening Behavior, 31*(3), 250–264.

Fiske, A., Wetherell, J. L., & Gatz, M. (2009). Depression in older adults. *Annual Review of Clinical Psychology, 5*, 363–389.

Fredriksen-Goldsen, K. I., Woodford, M. R., Luke, K. P., & Gutiérrez, L. (2011). Support of sexual orientation and gender identity content in social work education: Results from national surveys of US and Anglophone Canadian faculty. *Journal of Social Work Education, 47*(1), 19–35.

Fredriksen-Goldsen, K. I., Kim, H. J., Barkan, S. E., Muraco, A., & Hoy-Ellis, C. P. (2013). Health disparities among lesbian, gay, and bisexual older adults: Results from a population-based study. *American Journal of Public Health, 103*(10), 1802–1809.

Fredriksen-Goldsen, K. I., Hoy-Ellis, C. P., Goldsen, J., Emlet, C. A., & Hooyman, N. R. (2014). Creating a vision for the future: Key competencies and strategies for culturally competent practice with lesbian, gay, bisexual, and transgender (LGBT) older adults in the health and human services. *Journal of Gerontological Social Work, 57*(2–4), 80–107.

Fredriksen-Goldsen, K. I., Kim, H. J., Bryan, A. E., Shiu, C., & Emlet, C. A. (2017). The cascading effects of marginalization and pathways of resilience in attaining good health among LGBT older adults. *The Gerontologist, 57*(Suppl 1), S72–S83.

Gladman, J., Jones, R., Radford, K., Walker, & Rothera, L. (2007). Person-centered dementia services are feasible, but can they be sustained? *Age and Ageing, 36*, 171–176

Grant, J. M., Mottet, L. A., Tanis, J., Harrison, J., Herman, J. L., & Keisling, M. (2011). *Injustice at every turn: A report of the National Transgender Discrimination Survey.* National Center for Transgender Equality and National Gay and Lesbian Task Force.

Grossman, A., D'Augelli, A., & Dragowski, E. (2007). Caregiving and care receiving among older lesbian, gay, and bisexual adults. *Journal of Gay and Lesbian Social Services, 18*, 15–38.

Hash, K. (2001). Preliminary study of caregiving and post-caregiving experiences of older gay men and lesbians. *Journal of Gay and Lesbian Social Services, 14*(4), 87–94.

Hash, K. M., & Cramer, E. P. (2003). Empowering gay and lesbian caregivers and uncovering their unique experiences through the use of qualitative methods. *Journal of Gay and Lesbian Social Services, 15*(1/2), 47–62.

Herek, G. M., Gillis, J. R., & Cogan, J. C. (1999). Psychological sequelae of hate crime victimization among lesbian, gay and bisexual adults. *Journal of Consulting and Clinical Psychology, 67*(6), 945–951.

Hudson, R. B. (2011). Integrating lesbian, gay, bisexual, and transgender older adults into aging policy and practice. *Public Policy and Aging Report, 21*(3), 1–2.

Hughes, D., Harold, R., & Boyer, J. (2011). Awareness and LGBT aging issues among service network providers. *Journal of Gerontological Social Work, 54*, 659–677.

Institute of Medicine. (2011). *The health of lesbian, gay, bisexual, and transgender (LGBT) people: Building a foundation for better understanding*. National Academies Press.

Knauer, N. J. (2009). LGBT elder law: Toward equity in aging. *Harvard Journal of Law and Gender, 32*, 1–54.

Knauer, N. J. (2011). Gen silent: Advocating for LGBT elders. *Elder Law Journal, 19*, 289–348.

Lannutti, P. J. (2005). For better or worse: Exploring the meanings of same-sex marriage within the lesbian, gay, bisexual and transgendered community. *Journal of Social and Personal Relationships, 22*(1), 5–18.

Services and Advocacy for Gay, Lesbian, Bisexual and Transgender Elders—SAGE. (2011). *The aging and health report—Disparities and resilience among lesbian, gay, bisexual, and transgender older adults.*

Services and Advocacy for Gay, Lesbian, Bisexual and Transgender Elders—SAGE. (2016). *Improving the quality of services and supports offered to LGBT older adults by aging network providers—A training manual.*

Link, B. G., & Phelan, J. C. (2006). Stigma and its public health implications. *Lancet, 367*, 528–529.

Lombardi, E. L. (1999). Integration within a transgender social network and its effect upon members' social and political activity. *Journal of Homosexuality, 37*(1), 109–126.

Lyons, A. R. (2015). Resilience in lesbians and gay men: A review and key findings from a nationwide Australian survey. *International Review of Psychiatry, 27*(5), 435–443.

McGovern, J. (2014). The forgotten: Dementia and the aging LGBT community. *Journal of Gerontological Social Work, 57*(8), 845–857.

Meyer, I. H. (2013). Prejudice, social stress, and mental health in lesbian, gay, and bisexual populations: Conceptual issues and research evidence. *Psychological Bulletin, 129*(5), 674–697.

Moore, W. R. (2002). Connecting care providers through a telephone support group. *Journal of Gay and Lesbian Social Services, 14*(3), 23–41.

Persson, D. I. (2009). Unique challenges of transgender aging: Implications from the literature. *Journal of Gerontological Social Work, 52*(6), 633–646.

Portz, J. D., Retrum, J. H., Wright, L. A., Boggs, J. M., Wilkins, S., Grimm, C., Gilchrist, K., & Gozansky, W. S. (2014). Assessing capacity for providing culturally competent services to LGBT older adults. *Journal of Gerontological Social Work, 57*(2–4), 305-321.

Ryan, T., Nolan, M., Reid, D., & Enderby, P. (2008). Using the senses framework to achieve relationship-centred dementia care services. *Dementia, 7*(1), 71–93.

Sharp, J. (1997). Beyond exposé analysis: Hybridity, social memory and identity politics. *Journal of Contemporary African Studies, 15*(1), 7–21.

Simone, M. D., & Appelbaum, M. J. (2011). Addressing the needs of older lesbian, gay, bisexual, and transgender adults. *Clinical Geriatrics, 19*(2), 38–44.

Snowdon, S. (2010). The medical school curriculum and LGBT health concerns. *Virtual Mentor, 12*(8), 638–643.

Teaster, P. B., White, J. T., & Kim, S. (2016). Sexual minority status and aging. In *Handbook of LGBT elders* (pp. 27–42). Springer.

Testa, R. J., Habarth, J., Peta, J., Balsam, K., & Bockting, W. (2015). Development of the gender minority stress and resilience measure. *Psychology of Sexual Orientation and Gender Diversity, 2*, 65–77.

Van Wagenen, A., Driskell, J., & Bradford, J. (2013). "I'm still raring to go": Successful aging among lesbian, gay, bisexual, and transgender older adults. *Journal of Aging Studies, 27*(1), 1–14.

Wallace, S. P., Cochran, S. D., Durazo, E. M., & Ford, C. L. (2011). The health of aging lesbian, gay and bisexual adults in California. *Policy Brief (UCLA Center for Health Policy Research), 1*, 1–8.

Wight, R. G., LeBlanc, A. J., de Vries, B., & Detels, R. (2012). Stress and mental health among midlife and older gay-identified men. *American Journal of Public Health, 102*, 503–510.

Wight, R. G., Le Blanc, A. J., Meyer, I. H., & Harig, F. A. (2015). Internalized gay ageism, mattering, and depressive symptoms among midlife and older gay-identified men. *Social Science and Medicine, 147*, 200–208.

Chapter 17
Ageing Among a Marginalized Scheduled Tribe: An Anthropological Perspective

Chandana Sarmah

Abstract The process of demographic ageing is taking place at a rapid rate in India. Ageing of populations will have implications even among small marginalized communities living in different parts of the country. From the point of view of an individual, a person ages within a social and cultural context. The social structure and organisation of a society determine how the given society views older people and the ageing process. Not much is known about ageing among marginalized communities of North east India or their needs. The present paper looks at ageing among a marginalized scheduled tribe of Assam from an anthropological perspective. It takes into consideration the social, economic and health aspects of ageing of 508 elderly Karbis of Morigaon district in Assam. The study is a cross-sectional one and the individuals who have attained 60 years of age have been taken into the sample. Interviews with a structured schedule has been used to collect the data during the year 2016. The dominant joint family structure among the Karbis provides social support and care for the elderly. Filial piety plays a determining role in co-residence of at least one adult child and his family with elderly parents. So long as their physical conditions permit, the elderly continue to be involved in the traditional occupation of rice cultivation. The household income from agriculture is their main source of financial support. However, the Karbis are ignorant of their health condition. Prevalence of morbidity is apparently low. Preventive measures for health promotion and consultations with medical practitioners are found to be very limited. Prevalence of under nutrition is around 29% but the elderly persons remain functionally independent.

Keywords Ageing · Karbis · Social support · Health condition · Functional independence

C. Sarmah (✉)
Department of Anthropolgy, Gauhati University, Guwahati, Assam, India
e-mail: chandanasarmah@gauhati.ac.in

M. K. Shankardass (ed.), *Gerontological Concerns and Responses in India*,
https://doi.org/10.1007/978-981-16-4764-2_17

Introduction

India is undergoing the process of demographic ageing, as is evident from the census records of rising proportion of elderly population to the total population. During the last few decades of the twentieth century, the process has accelerated at a rapid rate. Among the developed countries of the world, the process has been a gradual one and among them, there was the advantage of economic affluence to support this growing section in terms of state sponsored health care and social security. Increase in the proportion of elderly population has both social and biological implications. In developing countries like India, the phenomenal rate of growth of ageing population is associated with unpreparedness to meet the needs of this growing section.

Moreover, there is diversity within the country in terms of socio-economic condition, social support and care for elderly, health condition, access and availability of health care services, awareness level, etc. This is true for all sections of society including the elderly. The government of India has designed a number of welfare schemes for elderly persons covering almost all areas of need. But the reach of these programmes to the grass root level differs from region to region and largely because of the operation of some of the above-mentioned aspects. The Indian Ageing Report (2017) by UNFPA identifies four basic features of India's elderly. They are feminization of ageing or a sex ratio favouring women in the elderly category, ruralisation or concentration of the elderly in rural areas, more 80 + women and impact of migration of the younger generation on the elderly population. Considering the vast diversity of our country, there is bound to be regional variation or community specific variation with regard to these factors. In order to have a clear understanding of the actual requirements of the elderly from different regions, there is an urgent need for empirical research about community level requirements. This study, therefore, is an attempt to understand the social, economic and health aspects of ageing among a marginalized scheduled tribe of Assam from an anthropological perspective.

The study is among the Karbis, who predominantly live in KarbiAnglong hill district and the adjoining districts of Nagaon, Morigaon and Kamrup. The present study has been conducted within the geographic jurisdiction of Morigaon district as a part of an ICSSR sponsored project. When we look at ageing from the point of view of an individual or society, it can be said that an individual ages in a social and cultural context. The socio-cultural factors or forces provide the overall context in which an individual develops (Cavanaugh & Fields, 2006). Core beliefs of communities are shaped by the prevalent culture which determines the social setting as well the status and living conditions for people of all ages belonging to the community. Roles, functions and social relationships of members are organized through the social institutions. They in turn formulate social life and ensure social integration or isolation. The culture and traditions of society likewise, determine how the given society views older people and the ageing process.

Studies on ageing among the various tribes, castes and communities living in the North Eastern part of India from an anthropological perspective are relatively few. The ethnicity of a particular group plays an important role in the ageing process due to the shared beliefs and practices of the group. As can be pointed out an individual grows old within a social context. This is reflected in their roles, expected social behaviour and cultural practices. The socio-cultural difference among the various populations living in the North Eastern region of India maybe give rise to differences in the ageing process of the groups. A brief review of the research on ageing among the different communities of the region is given hereafter. Sarmah and Choudhury (2011) in their study on the problems of the elderly and their care look into the problems of the elderly of the Assamese community living in the urban context of Guwahati. In addition to dealing with the age related biological decline, the elderly have to deal with the changes arising out of rapid urbanisation and related socio-cultural changes. Consequently the elderly have to deal with a number of conflicting situations. Declining health, loneliness and inability to utilize their time fruitfully are some of the problems faced by the urban community living elderly. Migration of their children compels the elderly to either live alone or with only their spouse. This limits the amount of care that adult children can provide to their ageing parents. Deterioration of health conditions prevents them gradually from remaining active.

Das and Sarmah (2017) studied the nutritional status and blood pressure among the ageing Tiwas, a scheduled tribe, living in the Morigaon district, Assam. Under nutrition was found to be prevalent 26.15% male and 34.85% female ageing Tiwas. 19.23% males and 14.39% females are overweight. Prevalence of underweight is significantly associated with age, sex, economic condition in both the gender and with marital status in females. Hypertension is prevalent among 16.54% Tiwa males and 21.37% Tiwas women. Age and nutritional status have a greater influence on the occurrence of hypertension among the ageing Tiwas compared to other social factors. The traditional culture prevalent among the tribes ensures social support for elderly people. Sarmah and Das (2017) in their study on socio-economic condition and social support among the ageing Tiwas found that the dominant joint family structure is the primary source of support for elderly people. The Tiwas are educationally and economically backwards. A very positive aspect of elderly support in society is that no ageing person was found to be living alone. The Tiwas follow the tradition of having a resident son-in-law in case a couple does not have a son. This system of residence ensures both social support and care for elderly.

In rural areas, women are particularly vulnerable as their roles and duties are non remunerative. They are involved primarily in care giving roles and activities relating to keeping of the household. As such when they grow old they become financially dependent on others for support and care. This has been found in a study on ageing among the Meetei women of Assam and Manipur (Devi & Bagga, 2006). The Meetei women of Manipur have more number and intensity of health complaints as compared to Meetei women of Assam. This may be due to their better socio-economic condition and access to improved health facilities. The study also looked into the morphological age change. Linear measurements, body weight, BMI, appendicular circumference decreased significantly with age in both groups.

Material and Methodology

Morigaon is one of the 32 districts of Assam. It has five revenue circles and its headquarter is in Marigaon town. Data for the study has been collected from 20 villages belonging to the five revenue circles of Laharighat, Mayong, Morigaon, Mikirbheta and Bhurgaon. 11 of the studied villages are homogenous, inhabited by people belonging only to the Karbi community. The remaining 9 villages are heterogeneous. These villages comprise people from other tribes like Tiwa, Boro, Assamese, Koch Rajbangshi and Ahom.

The sample of the study consists of 508 Karbi elderly persons. Among them, 253 (49.80%) are male and 255 (50.20%) are female elderly. The inclusive criterion of the sample is the age of sixty years. All people belonging to this age group from the 20 villages have been included in the study. Though determining age among a semi-literate group with no written records is a difficulty, yet various reconfirming procedures like age of children, age at marriage and other important social events have been used to confirm the age. Their exact chronological age may slightly vary but the broader age group has been correctly assessed. Contact with the villagers was made through the administrative head, i.e. the village *gaonbura* and other senior responsible persons of the villages. The objective and methodology were explained to them and informed verbal consent was obtained. After this, the individuals were selected and only when they consented to be part of the study, data were collected. The respondents were mostly happy and willing to be part of the study.

The demographic data have been collected through a household survey schedule. For the data on biological, economic and social aspects of ageing, a structured schedule pertaining to the objectives has been prepared. Nutritional status of the elderly has been assessed from the Body Mass Index (BMI) calculated from the anthropometric measurements of weight and height. Height has been measured using anthropometric rod and weight with a weighing scale. The data have been collected during the year 2016 as part of an ICSSR sponsored study of ageing among two communities of Marigaon district of Assam.

The People

The Karbis are an ethnic group of Assam. They belong to the Indo–Mongoloid family and linguistically they belong to the Tibeto–Burman group of languages. The Karbis were earlier known as *Mikirs,* but now they prefer to call themselves Karbi. They are also sometimes referred to as *Arleng. Arleng* in the Karbi language literally means 'a man'.

The social organisation of the Karbis is based on clan structure. Clans are strictly exogamous and violation of this customary rule in marriage leads to ex-communication. Clans in Karbi language are called *Kur.* Karbi social organisation has five clans and a number of sub-clans. They use their clan names as titles or surnames. The five clans of the Karbis are *Terang, Teron, Enghee, Ingti* and *Timung*.

The Karbis of Marigaon district primarily follows the traditional occupation of wet rice cultivation. Some of them are involved in other small business ventures like running shops, selling vegetables, firewood, etc. A few are also engaged in animal husbandries like poultry, piggery and fishing. Stone cutting, basketry, weaving are some traditional activities that are used for economic gain, etc. The Karbi religion is based on animism and supernaturalism. After being acculturated with the Assamese population, they have started worshipping different Hindu deities.

The staple food of the Karbis is rice which they generally eat with vegetables and fish. Fish is consumed regularly all through the year. They preserve fish by drying and it is a preferred delicacy. Rice beer which is known as '*Hor*' among them is prepared and consumed by them regularly. It is also a significant part of their religious, social and cultural life. The Karbi women weave their own clothes. They use bright colours and weave artistic designs on both male and female garments. They have a unique collection of traditional ornaments. The women's dress includes a lower and upper garment is known as *Pini* and *Pekok*. The men wear *Arlenachoi* and *Seleng*. Now-a-days, both the males and females wear the currently convenient dresses for everyday use and wear their traditional garments occassionally.

Ageing Among the Karbis

In the present study, ageing has been examined from the social, economic and biological aspects of elderly persons. The social aspects include their age sex distribution, educational level, marital status, social support from their living arrangement and the activity status of the elderly. The economic aspect includes their occupational pattern, independent income of elderly, source of financial support from family and continuing involvement in traditional occupation as contributors to the family income. Health aspects have been looked into from morbidity, treatment of diseases, preventive measures for healthy ageing and healthy eating examined from nutritional status.

Social Aspects

According to Krishnaswamy and Shanthi (2010) an adequate system of social support is integral for optimal health in old age. Traditional societies generally have a natural system of social support. This support emerges from their social structure and organisation. This ensures support for all sections of their members including the aged and disabled. Protection and social security to older persons are provided in explicit rules of co-residence and inheritance of family wealth. The aged are very much integrated into the family life and are rarely excluded from the division of labour (Fry, 2013).

Table 1 Distribution of the elderly Karbis in the three broad age groups

Age sex distribution			
Age group	Male	Female	Total
60–69 years	185 (73.12)	215 (84.31)	400 (78.74)
70–79 years	51 (20.16)	29 (11.37)	80 (15.75)
80 + years	17 (6.72)	11 (4.13)	28 (5.51)
Total	253 (100)	255 (100)	508

(Figures in parentheses indicate percentage)

This is found to be largely true among the Karbis of the study. Their experience, knowledge and wealth ensure a high status in society. According to the classical theory of modernisation of Cowgill and Holmes (1972), the elderly occupy a higher status in societies that follow the traditional means of occupation. Moreover, the living arrangement which again in traditional societies means living with at least one adult child is also an indicator of well-being among elderly (Table 1).

To understand the age related changes the elderly persons of the study are categorized into three age groups. On the basis of chronological age, they are young old, middle old and old-old. The young old include elderly between 60 and 69 years and middle old comprises of elderly in the ages between 70 and 79 years. The 80 years are defined as old-old. In the study, most of the elderly Karbis (78.74%) are found to belong to the young old category. There is a decline in the proportion of elderly in the higher ages. Sex difference in the age distribution is observed among the elderly Karbis. 73.12% of the male and 84.31% of the female elderly karbis belong to the young old age group. There is a sharp decline in the proportion of elderly especially among female elderly in the subsequent age group. 20.16% of the male elderly as compared to 11.37% of female elderly belong to the middle old age group. The proportion of elderly surviving to the old-old age category is much lower. 6.72% of the total male elderly and 4.13% of the total female elderly belong to this age group. In the oldest age group, the proportion of men is higher than women. The age distribution shows statistically significant difference at 0.05 level (chi square 9.58, $p = 0.008$, d.f. – 2).

The elderly Karbis are mostly (73.62%) illiterate with illiteracy being much higher among female elderly (Table 2). 40.32% of the elderly Karbi males had some formal education as compared to 12.55% of the elderly females. Male elderly from the young and middle old age group have studied to high school or beyond. In the highest age group, no male has studied to this level. Very few elderly Karbi females have studied to primary level and even fewer beyond that. There is a high amount of gender difference in educational level among the elderly Karbis. The difference is statistically significant at 0.05 level (chi square 52.1, $p = 0.000$, d.f. – 3).

Being married or having a surviving spouse influence well-being as well as quality of life in elderly people. Elderly Karbi men (78.66%) are predominantly found to currently have a surviving spouse. In the 60–69 years age group, 82.16% men have a surviving spouse but the relative figure for women is much lower (56.28%). Their proportions decline in the two subsequent age groups in case of men. Among women,

Table 2 Distribution of the elderly Karbis by their social variables

Educational level

Sex	Illiterate	Primary level	Middle school	High school and above	Total
Male	151 (59.68)	62 (24.51)	11 (4.35)	29 (11.46)	253
Female	223 (87.5)	22 (8.63)	5 (1.96)	5 (1.96)	255

Marital status

Sex	Currently married	Widow/widower	Nevermarried	Total
Male	199 (78.66)	50 (19.76)	4 (1.58)	253
Female	135 (52.94)	114 (44.71)	6 (2.35)	255

Living arrangement

Sex	Living alone	Living with spouse	Nuclear family	With married children	With sibling's family	With son-in-law	Total
Male	4 (1.58)	10 (3.95)	35 (13.85)	196 (77.47)	6 (2.37)	2 (0.79)	253
Female	2 (0.78)	4 (1.57)	32 (12.55)	207 (81.18)	8 (3.14)	2 (0.78)	255

Current activity status

Sex	Continuing with economic activity	Social activity	Actively involved with household activity	Limited household activity	Only personal care activity	Total
Male	175 (69.17)	13 (5.14)	34 (13.44)	25 (9.88)	6 (2.37)	253
Female	148 (58.04)	3 (1.18)	32 (12.55)	66 (25.88)	6 (2.35)	255

(Figures in parentheses indicate percentage)

the proportion of currently married women declines in the subsequent age group but increases in the oldest age group. 19.76% are widowers and their proportion shows a positive relation with increase in age. 44.71% of the Karbi women no longer have a surviving spouse and their frequency increases from the young old age group to the middle old age group. But the proportion of such women decline in the oldest age group. 1.58% of the Karbi men have never married. They are all found to belong to the young old age category. 2.35% of the elderly women have remained unmarried and they belong to the young old and middle old age group. The gender difference in marital status is statistically significant (chi square 37.6, $p = 0.000$, d.f. – 2).

Social support for the elderly Karbis emerges from their living arrangement or with whom they live. Elderly people in Karbi society are rarely found to be living alone or with just their spouses. Adult children set up independent homes after marriage but one adult child and his/her family continue to live with elderly parents. This is done out of filial piety and is seen to be the custom among them. Sometimes elderly parents relocate to their children's homes within the village. Thus, joint

Table 3 Distribution of the elderly Karbis according to their economic condition

Current occupational pattern					
Sex	Agriculture	Wage earning	Petty trade and service	No longer working	Total
Male	178 (70.36)	3 (1.19)	3 (1.19)	69 (27.27)	253
Female	153 (60.0)	11 (4.31)	2 (0.78)	89 (34.90)	255
Independent income					
Sex	No independent income	Annual income up to INR15,000	Income higher than INR 15,000	Total	
Male	232 (91.70)	9 (3.55)	12 (4.75)	253	
Female	234 (91.76)	15 (5.88)	6 (2.35)	255	
Source of financial support					
Sex	Independent income	Household income	Support from adult children	Spouse/relative	Total
Male	21 (8.30)	176 (69.57)	54 (21.34)	2 (0.79)	253
Female	21 (8.24)	145 (56.86)	78 (30.59)	11 (4.31)	255

(Figures in parentheses indicate percentage)

family is the predominant family type among elderly individuals. The Karbis have a system of patrilocal residence and even elderly persons prefer to stay with sons. However, elderly persons were found to be living with married daughters under special circumstances. Individuals who have remained unmarried or have lost their spouse live with their sibling's family in ancestral homes. This ensures support for elderly who do not have children or spouses. Nuclear families are found among elderly whose adult children have not yet entered into matrimony. There is not much gender difference in the living arrangement of the elderly.

The daily routine of the elderly persons has been looked into to assess their level of activity within and outside the household. 69.17% of men, mainly from the young old and middle old age categories are still involved in agriculture and contribute to the family earning. 17.65% of the men from the oldest age group are still economically active. 68.37% of the women from the young old age are involved in agriculture but the proportions decline to 3.45% in the subsequent age group. None of the women in the oldest age group is involved in economic activity. 5.14% men and 1.18% of women are involved in social activity. Even when the elderly are not actively involved in agricultural work, they do not stay idle. But continue to be occupied with work that does not require their constant involvement. They take care of the kitchen garden look after domestic animals and other matters relating to the running of the household. 13.44% are involved in household activities and also look after the kitchen garden and domestic animals. The men who are able to perform these activities are highest in the middle old age group but decline in the next decade. In the young old age group, their proportion in this category of work is less as they are still actively involved in agricultural work. 9.88% are involved in only household work indicating a limitation inability. Their proportion shows association with age in the oldest age group 41.18% of the men are able to do only household work.

When we look into the daily routine of the female Karbi elderly, we find that 58.04% still are involved in agricultural activities. They belong to the young old age group and from the next decade involvement in economic activity becomes much less. 13.44% of elderly women are involved in household activities and also are involved in taking care of domestic animals but in the oldest age category, none of the elderly women is found to be able to do this work also. The women of the middle old group mostly are involved in this kind of activity. Social convention generally calls for higher participation of men in social activities and as such relatively lesser number of women in the older ages are found to be involved in social activity. 25.88% of the women are involved only in limited household activities and no other work. 65.52% of women from the middle old age group belong to this category. Their proportion is relatively less in the young old age group as in this age group women can perform other activities as well. The remaining 2.35% of the women are no longer able to do any other work other than their personal care activities. The women of the very old age group mostly belong to this category (Fig. 17.1).

The analysis of the daily routine of the elderly gives an idea of the ability to remain physically active or functionally independent. From the examination of their daily routine, it can be said that the elderly remain active as long as their physical conditions allow them to. When they are no longer able to perform hard labour they shift to work which exerts less burden. They continue to be involved in the family division of labour and contribute to the family. Women become unable to be involved in work from an earlier age than men. Moreover, their proportions are higher than in all age groups. There is significant difference between the sexes in their ability to remain active (chi square 27.0, $p = 0.000$, d.f. 4). The elderly, however, can maintain their functional independence.

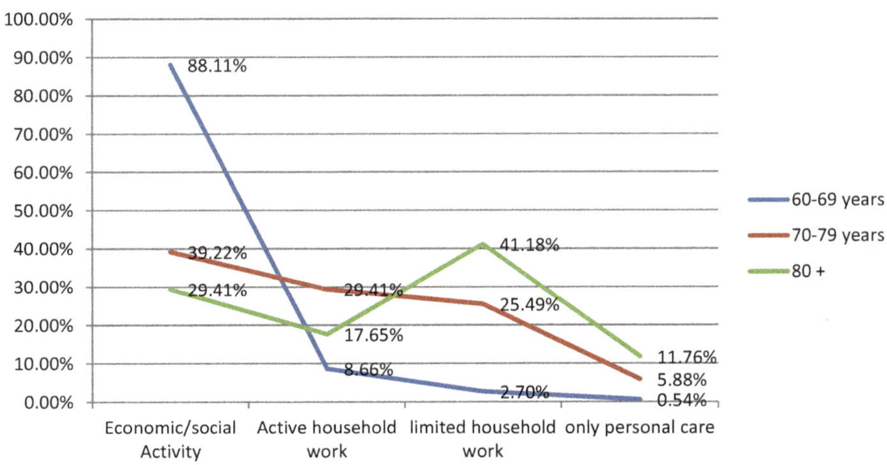

Fig. 17.1 Activity status of the elderly Karbis by their age group

The sex ratio of the elderly Karbis is 99 males per 100 females. But when the sex ratio is calculated in the different age groups, the findings are 86 males per 100 females in the young old age group. In the 70–79 years age group it is 175 males per 100 females. It is 154 males per 100 females in the oldest age group. In the higher ages, the sex ratio among the Karbis of Morigaon district is favourable to the males. Similarly, with regard to the other social aspects like education, marital status, activity status, the gender difference is significant and favourable towards males. No significant difference is found in case of living arrangements.

Economic Aspect

The traditional system of agriculture, which is the primary occupation of the Karbis of Marigaon district, ensures both social contact and physical activity for elderly. Elderly persons, both male and female continue to be involved in agriculture as long as their physical conditions and ability permits them. Though both males and females are equally involved in agriculture there is a basic gender division of labour. Men plough the land while women plant and transplant the seedlings. Harvesting is done by both men and women. With increase in age, the amount and level of contribution to agriculture gradually decline among elderly. They prefer to continue till physical incapacitation sets in.

70.36% of elderly males are still found to be doing agricultural work. With increase in age, the proportion of people involved in agricultural work gradually declines. The elderly persons continue to work as long as they are physically capable. 88.11% of the men from the young old age group are working as cultivators, which declines to 23.53% in the middle old and further to 17.65% in the old-old age category. Proportion of elderly men involved in other wage earning activities (1.19%) such as rock cutting, carpentry and daily labourer. Shop keeping, fishery, piggery and poultry are mostly the types of petty trade followed by the elderly Karbi men. Engagement in service is found to be negligible. 27.27% of the elderly men are not able to be involved in any economic activity any longer due to their age or their physical condition. In the young old age category, their proportion is 10.27% which increased to 70.59% in the middle old age category and to 82.35% in the old-old age category.

The women elderly of Karbi society discontinue their active involvement in agricultural fields relatively earlier than men. 70.23% of the women in the young old age group still work in fields and this proportion declines sharply to 6.97% in the next decade.

This shows that women become incapable to work in agricultural activities beyond the young old age category. In the old-old age group, no women are involved in economic activity. A small proportion of elderly of the young old age group is involved in wage earning (4.31%) such as daily labourer. Petty trade (0.78%) among elderly women of Karbi society are in the form of producing and selling of local beer, selling of poultry, pigs which they rear.

To have an understanding of whether the elderly Karbis have economic independence, an attempt has been made to assess the level of independent income among them. 91.70% male and 91.76% female elderly of the Karbi community do not have independent earning. Even when elderly persons are involved in agriculture it does not generate monetary income. The agricultural produce is generally the family earning and it is used for consumption purposes. Agricultural produce may be sold only to meet family emergencies. A very small percentage of the elderly people were found to have independent income. The sources of income for the elderly Karbi men are making art and craft work (bamboo and cane work) and wage earning. Those who were in service have pension to support them. Among the elderly Karbi women, the main source of monetary earning is from pension of spouse or wage earning.3.55% of the elderly males and 5.88% of elderly females have earnings less than 15,000/– per year. 4.75% males earn more than 15,000/– while the corresponding figure for elderly women is 2.35%.

Financial independence is practically non-existence among elderly Karbis of Marigaon district. Those who are involved in some trade have some amount of financial independence. Others are dependent on the household/family income. They become dependent on their basic needs of clothes, food and medicine. However, feelings of deprivation do not appear as they are mostly dependent on the family or household income. The household income mainly comes from agriculture, where the elderly may have earlier contributed or still continue to contribute. There is thus, a kind of unspoken right over subsequent agricultural produce among the elderly. Moreover, the social organisation also ensures support through the clan and village organisation for elderly who are unable to be economically active. An attempt has been made to look into the main source of support for the elderly person. Elderly Karbis of the study responded that adult male children are their main source of financial support. Married daughters are also primary sources of financial support according to some of the elderly. If an elderly person does not have children to support them, other relatives generally support them. 69.57% of elderly men and 56.86% of elderly women responded that their basic needs are taken care of from the household income. 21.34% men and 30.59% women depend on adult children for support. In the study some of the elderly men and women, though their proportion is low are dependent on other relatives for support. A similar proportion of elderly men and women have independent income. More men reported being dependent on the household income and more women are dependent on adult children or any other relative. The gender difference with regard to source of financial support is statistically significant (chi square 13.6, $p = 0.004$ d.f. 3) at 0.05 level with dependence being higher among elderly women.

Health Aspect

Health as per the accepted definition is defined not merely as absence of diseases but as a state of complete social, mental and physical well-being. Health is the outcome of interaction of an individual's genetic and environmental factors. Among the environmental factors which influence health, nutrition is significant as it is a modifiable determinant. Ageing, health and nutrition are inextricably related. The social and psychological aspects have additional interaction with health, especially among elderly people. Moreover, food and nutrition needs of people are determined by the ecology in which they live as well as their culture and socio-economic condition. Ecology determines the type of food available. Culture and socio-economic condition dictate what and how food is to be consumed. Proper nutrition as a part of an active, healthy lifestyle is a key to successful ageing (Krishnaswamy & Shanthi, 2010) (Table 4).

Awareness about their disease conditions among the elderly Karbis is low. They deal with their ailments through the management of symptoms. Actual cause of the ailment generally remains unidentified. Health among them is defined from the perspective of functionality. A person is considered healthy as long as he/she is able to perform his or her role in the family and society. Disease prevalence can be understood from acute and chronic conditions. Acute conditions were considered from the last fifteen days recall period. Prevalence of acute conditions among the elderly was found to be negligible. Thus, for this present discussion only chronic conditions have been taken into account.

Table 4 Distribution of the elderly Karbis by their morbid condition

Age group	60–69 years		70–79 years		80 + years		Total	
Disease condition	Male	Female	Male	Female	Male	Female	Male	Female
No chronic ailment	124 (67.03)	165 (76.74)	19 (37.25)	11 (37.93)	5 (29.41)	6 (54.55)	148 (58.50)	182 (71.37)
High blood pressure	19 (10.27)	10 (4.65)	5 (9.80)	–	4 (23.53)	1 (9.09)	28 (11.07)	11 (4.31)
Diseases of digestive system	10 (5.41)	13 (6.05)	5 (9.80)	5 (17.24)	2 (11.76)	1 (9.09)	17 (6.72)	19 (7.45)
Body pain	25 (13.51)	17 (7.91)	13 (25.49)	9 (31.03)	3 (17.65)	1 (9.09)	41 (16.21)	27 (10.59)
Diseases relating to respiratory tract	1 (0.54)	5 (2.33)	3 (5.88)	1 (3.45)	2 (11.76)	–	6 (2.37)	6 (2.35)
Diabetes	–	–	2 (3.92)	–	–	–	2 (0.79)	–
Weakness	2 (1.08)	2 (0.93)	1 (1.96)	1 (3.45)	1 (5.88)	–	4 (1.58)	3 (1.18)
Others	4 (2.16)	3 (1.40)	3 (5.88)	2 (6.90)	–	2 (18.18)	7 (2.77)	7 (2.75)
Total	185 (100)	215 (100)	51 (100)	29 (100)	17 (100)	11 (100)	253	255

(Figures in parentheses indicate percentage)

Prevalence of chronic conditions is also less. 58.50% elderly males and 71.37% elderly females did not reportedly have any chronic health problem. High blood pressure, which has been diagnosed by a doctor, is prevalent among 11.07% elderly males and 4.31% elderly females. But in most cases, doctor's prescriptions have not been completed followed. Elderly mostly report ailments which they can identify such as digestive disorders or body pain. 6.72% of the elderly males and 7.45% of the elderly females reported having digestive disorders. Body pain is found to be prevalent among higher proportion of the elderly. 16.21% males and 10.59% females reported suffering regularly from body pain. 2.37% male and 2.35% female elderly reported having disorders related to the respiratory tract. As identification of diabetes needs clinical test and diagnosis by a doctor, prevalence of this disease has been reported to be low (0.79% in only males). Co-morbidity has also been found. Body pain has been reported along with digestive disorders, high blood pressure or respiratory diseases. As the frequency of such individuals is low they have been all placed in the category—others for the study. Consultation with doctors is less due to various causes and is generally done when their traditional management system fails to give them relief. Health conditions may as such remain under reported.

Treatment of diseases may be taken as an indicator of awareness of the health conditions and the necessity of attending to them. As has been mentioned earlier one of the aspects of health that has been looked into is prevention. Precaution for diseases as well as management of conditions falls under the concept of prevention. Prevention may be primary, secondary as well as tertiary. Primary prevention is the avoidance of tobacco, etc. which is not found to be the case in the community. Smoking and drinking of locally brewed rice beer are culturally accepted customs among the Karbis. Rice beer forms an important part of their socio-cultural life and religious practices. Secondary prevention is the screening for diseases for early detection. This is also practically absent among them. Even when a disease condition was identified, only 25% consulted a doctor. Others depended on home remedies or purchased tablets in consultation with the pharmacists. Some of the elderly among them also remain without treatment. Tertiary prevention is the acceptance of treatment for diseases. Treatment or completely following the prescription for disease conditions is not found to be taken seriously. This may be because of their socio-economic condition or the lack of awareness about the need to follow prescribed medication. Among the elderly Karbis prevention is practically absent as avoidance and screening for disease is not prevalent. Consultation is found to be very less (Table 5).

Healthy eating has been examined from their nutritional status. The nutritional status has been assessed from their Body Mass Index and classified according to the WHO classification for adult Asian population. 29.78% of the elderly are found to be under weight. 31.62% male and 27.56% female are underweight. 62.52% of the elderly are found to have normal nutritional status. Prevalence of overweight is among 7.89% of the elderly.

The distribution of underweight elderly in the three age groups show that there is an increase in proportion of both male and female elderly from the young old to the middle old age group. However, in the oldest age group, the proportions come down. Most of the overweight individuals are from the young old age group. In the young

Table 5 Distribution of the elderly Karbis by their nutritional status

Nutritional status on the basis of BMI					
Age group	Sex	Underweight	Normal	Overweight	Total
60–69 years	Male	42 (22.70)	128 (69.19)	15 (8.11)	185 (73.12)
	Female	48 (22.33)	144 (66.98)	23 (10.70)	215 (84.65)
70–79 years	Male	31 (60.78)	19 (37.25)	1 (1.96)	51 (20.16)
	Female	17 (58.62)	12 (41.38)	–	29 (11.42)
80 + years	Male	7 (41.18)	9 (52.94)	1 (5.88)	17 (6.72)
	Female	5 (50)	5 (50)	–	1 (3.94)
Total	Male	80 (31.62)	156 (61.66)	17 (6.72)	253
	Female	70 (27.56)	161 (63.39)	23 (9.06)	254

(Figures in parentheses indicate percentage)

old age group, malnutrition is around 22.5%, which increases to 60% in the middle old age group. In the oldest age group, 44.44% of the elderly are underweight. The chi square test has been done for assessing variation in nutritional status between elderly men and women. There is no significant difference in the prevalence of nutritional status (chi square 6.20 $p = 0.045$ d.f. 2) and in the occurrence of under nutrition (chi square 4.40 $p = 0.111$ d.f. 2).

Conclusion

From the findings of the study, it can be concluded that feminization of ageing may not be the case in this micro study among the Karbis. The sex ratio for the 60 + age group is 99 males per 100 females. But when the sex ratio is calculated for the three age groups it is found to be 86/100 in the young old, 175/100 in the middle old and 154/100 in the old age group. In the older age groups, the number of males is found to be higher than females. The social aspects of ageing are very positive among this marginalized scheduled tribe of Assam. The family is the main source of social and financial support. Filial piety is determining aspect of family structure. At least one adult child continues to live with ageing parents. The proportion of elderly who are living alone or with only their spouse, are low. Even those who have remained unmarried generally stay attached with their sibling's family. Educationally they are backward, which may be a reason for their lack of awareness. Gender difference is found with regard to certain aspects like education, marital status, financial support, etc. Women tend to become physically incapable sooner than men as can be seen from their involvement in agriculture or household chores. But elderly continue to remain active as per their physical ability. As for their financial condition, complete dependence on household income may make the elderly vulnerable. In this situation the needs of the elderly have to compete with the more demanding needs of the younger generation.

This also has an impact on their health related issues. The health condition of the tribal elderly may be enhanced through improvement of the public health service facilities and making them more accessible. Implementation of the schemes assured by the Government for elderly people through the public health facilities may go a long way in providing much needed health support. Moreover, awareness needs to be created among both the elderly as well as the younger generation about the special needs of the elderly and the aspect that every health problem is not an outcome of ageing and can be modified with life style changes.

Acknowledgements The data for the study have been collected as part of an ICSSR, New Delhi sponsored project.

References

Caring for our Elders: Early Response, Indian Ageing Report. (2017). United Nations Population Fund, 55 Lodi Estate, New Delhi 110003.

Cavanaugh, J.C. & Fields, F.B. (2006). *Adult Development and ageing* (5th ed.). USA Wadsworth Thompson Learning Inc.

Cowgill, D. O., & Holmes, L. D. (1972). *Ageing and modernization.* Appleton-Century-Crafts.

Das, B. & Sarmah, C. (2017). Nutritional status and blood pressure among the ageing Tiwas of Morigaon District, Assam. In R. Khongsdier & S. Sengupta (Eds.), *People of North East India: Bio-cultural dimensions.* Kalpaz Publication.

Devi, S. D., & Bagga, A. (2006). *Ageing in women: A study in North East India.* Mittal Publication.

Fry, C. L. (2013). Social anthropology and ageing. In D. Dannefer & C. Philipson (Eds.), *The Sage handbook of social gerontology.* Sage Publication Ltd. London.

Krishnaswamy, B., & Shanthi, G. S. (2010). Health promotion and protection. In S.I. Rajan & C. S. Johnson (Eds.), Ageing and health, Rawat Publication.

Sarmah, C., & Choudhury, B. (2011). Problems of elderly and their care. *Journal of Human Ecology, 36*(2), 145–151.

Sarmah, C. & Das, B. (2017). Socio-economic condition and social support among the ageing Tiwas of Assam. In S. Irudaya Rajan & G. Balgopal (Eds.), *Elderly care in India: Societal and state response.* Springer Nature Singapore Pte. Ltd.

Chapter 18
Policy, Programs and Future Directions for Ageing Population

Vinod Kumar

Abstract India is home to about 110 million aged persons who account for 8.6% of total India's population and represent country's fastest growing segment. Projections estimate 55% increase in general population from year 2000 to 2050 while 60 + and 80 + persons will increase by 325% and 700% respectively in this period. 2/3rd of India's aged are rural and 1/3rd are poor. Average social parameters for India's aged indicate a 43.5% literacy rate, 14.2 as old age dependency and 5.2% living alone. Health parameters like life expectancy at age 60, physical immobility and chronic disease prevalence among the aged are 17 years, 7.8% and 45% respectively. A sizable proportion of aged persons perceive their health as poor and complain of some recent ailment. Recognizing diverse needs of such vast population, the Indian Government launched a National Policy of Older Persons (NPOP) in 1999 addressing several issues including their health and socio-economic security. Although the policy highlights the role of many non-state actors including NGOs and the aged persons themselves, it is heavily weighted in favour of delivering programs through strengthening its already existing inter-sectorial infrastructure. An inter-ministerial Committee and a National Council for Older Persons (NCOP) were constituted for its implementation. However, in the absence of clear time bound Plans of Action and proper budgetary provision, implementation of the policy has remained slow. Inadequate reach of services to rural end users, failure to harness the benefits of new and emerging Indian economic order and changing socio-demographic scenarios are other limiting factors. In 2010, the Government constituted a Committee to review this policy with emphasis on 4 major areas namely the oldest old, Female elderly, rural elderly and harnessing the technological advances. Currently, many Ministries are involved in implementing various components of NPOP but there are 4 core Ministries which provide large chunk of services and these are Ministry of Health & Family Welfare (MOHFW), Ministry of Social Justice & Empowerment (MOSJE), Ministry of Rural Development (MORD) and Ministry of Panchayat Raj (MOPR). This paper provides insight into various national programs and services for aged persons in India. A brief description of activities running in Indian States and Union Territories with specific examples of India's smallest state, the capital city of Delhi has been included. Towards

V. Kumar (✉)
Emeritus President, Alzheimer's & Related Disorders Society of India, Delhi, India

M. K. Shankardass (ed.), *Gerontological Concerns and Responses in India*,
https://doi.org/10.1007/978-981-16-4764-2_18

the end, future directions with proposals for innovation to serve the aged better have been provided. **National Programs** described below include National Social Assistance Programme (NSAP), Integrated Programme for Older Persons (IPOP), National Programme for the Health Care of the Elderly (NPHCE), Maintenance and Welfare of Parents and Senior Citizens (MPWSC) Act of 2007, Rashtriya Swasthya Bima Yojna, a health insurance scheme and other programs. **NSAP (MORD)** was launched in 1995 and among other schemes; it includes Indira Gandhi National Old Age Pension Scheme (IGNOAPS) and Annapurna Scheme. It was revised in 2014. The Programme provides a pension of Rs.200/- per month for 60 + aged persons and Rs.500/- for 80 + belonging to BPL (below poverty line) category. As of 2013–2014, there were 21 million beneficiaries under IGNOAPS with more than half a million rupees as expenditure. Recent figures under NSAP stand at about 32 million beneficiaries. Shortcomings of NSAP include low awareness of programme, inadequate pension amount, difficulties in beneficiary identification and need for complex administrative machinery. Under Annapurna Scheme, 10 kg of food grains is given monthly to those eligible aged persons who have remained uncovered under IGNOAPS. **IPOP (MOSJE)** was launched in 1992 and was revised in 2008 and 2016. It pioneers multiple services including old age homes, day care centres and health in rural and remote areas through NGOs and other Bodies without day to day involvement of the government but its poor awareness and time consuming monitoring of its projects are some of the limitations. **NPHCE (MOHFW)** was launched in 2011 on a pre-existing administrative base of National Health Mission and infrastructure for Non-Communicable diseases and has good financial outlay. However it seems to have multiple objectives on a weak public health structure and slow development, sluggish fund flow and deficiency of services and trained staff are its limitations. **MWPSC ACT (MOSJE)** notified in 2007 is a step towards welfare and dignity of the aged persons and holds children responsible to care for their aged. Its low awareness and slow progress about its health facilities and old age homes are the limitations. **RSBY (MOHFW)** is a PPP model and its new Avtar, National Health Protection Scheme (NHPS) is for providing health insurance for millions of Indian families where aged persons can also get coverage. Rashtriya Vayoshri Yojna is meant to provide physical aids to BPL aged persons for age related disabilities while other national programs covering cancer, diabetes, cardiovascular disease, stroke, blindness, deafness, mental health, oral health, etc. are also available although not exclusive for the aged. Several NGOs in the country also provide services to aged persons at their doorsteps and try to link them with institution based public services. They run programs for their empowerment, shelter, rehabilitation, income generation, social engagement, respite and palliative care and provide health care to those afflicted with cataracts, dementia, cancer and other ailments. **Programs from States and Union Territories** Almost every State supplements IGOAPS old age pension by providing its own pension for their aged. The amount varies. For Delhi, it is Rs.2000/- for 60–70 years old and Rs.2500/- for 70 + . States also participate in various above-mentioned national programs. Delhi's major hospitals provide separate queues, registration counters, OPD rooms, out of turn laboratory test facilities and Sunday special clinics for their aged persons. In addition, Delhi government runs recreation centres, old age homes and security and helpline services with assistance from Police and NGOs. **Future Directions** These include (i) innovating for better convergence and decentralized delivery of multiple services for the end user, (ii) creating strong public private partnerships as substitute for some poorly functioning public services, (iii) harnessing the benefits of statuary provisions from the corporate world for elderly services, (iv) capitalizing on the useful services provided by NGOs and (v) tapping the potentials of the aged persons themselves.

Keywords Aged persons · Policies · National programs · Future directions

Introduction

Ageing persons form the fastest growing segment of population and present unique challenges before the care providers. Unlike the adult population, aged persons are afflicted not only by multiple diseases and disabilities but also frequently suffer from ill health due to normal ageing process itself (Kumar, 2015). This has been depicted alphabetically in Table 18.1. Chronic and lifelong morbidity requiring poly pharmacy among the burgeoning and often socio-economically marginalized geriatric population in developing countries is likely to render old age care quite difficult and complex.

Not only socio-economic but also emotional marginalization of aged persons together with stigma of ageism and elder abuse are often likely to violate their human rights as well. All this and in our fastest growing segment of population leads to a kind of cascading effect that becomes difficult to cope with by policy makers and service providers (Fig. 18.1).

India is home to about 110 million aged persons who account for 8.6% of total India's population and majority of them live in rural areas. Figure 18.2 shows that although this segment of population is rapidly increasing, 80 + individuals are growing the fastest. Thus 80 + individuals will increase by 700% between year 2000 and 2050 compared to 326% increase in 60 + population and only 55% increase in total population during the same period (Draft National Policy on Senior Citizens, 2011).

Table 18.1 Both diseases and ageing cause ill heath

Geriatric diseases	Normal ageing
• Alzheimer's	• Aches and pain
• Brain attack (Stroke)	• Blurred vision
• Cancer	• Constipation
• Diabetes	• Depression
• Essential high BP	• Exhaustion
• Frailty	• Forgetfulness
• Geriatric infections	• Gas in stomach
• Heart disease	• Hearing problems

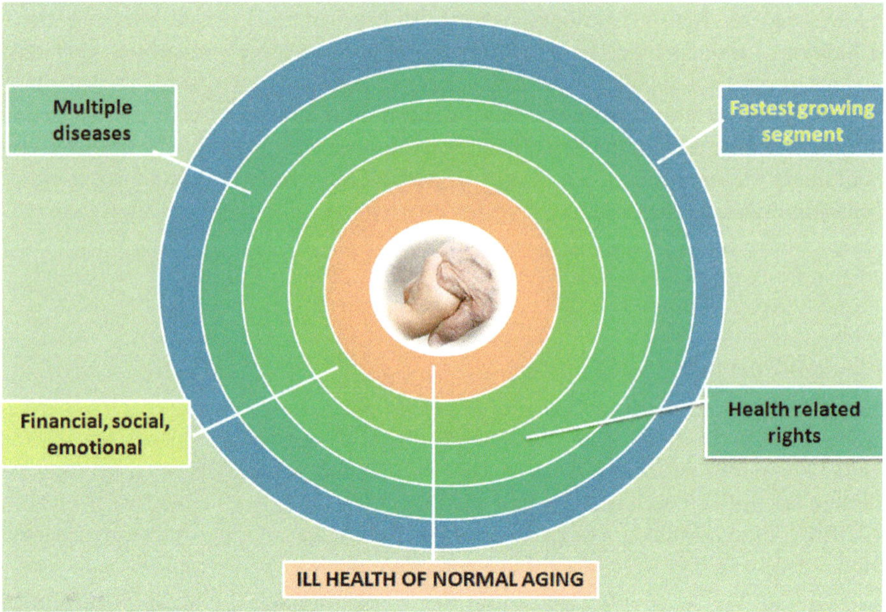

Fig. 18.1 Problem of ageing population

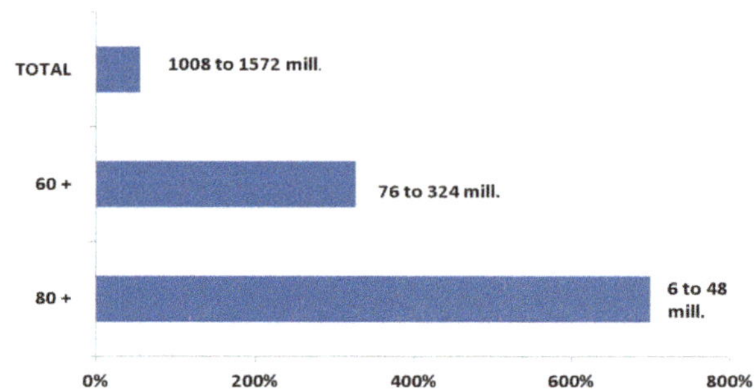

Fig. 18.2 Projected increase in Indian population by age (2000–2050). Draft National Policy on Senior Citizens. *Source* National Policy as reviewed in 2011 (2011)

2/3rd of India's aged are rural and 1/3rd are poor. Like many other countries, they face multiple challenges to their health and social well-being. Their literacy rate, old age dependency and frequency of those living alone are 43.5%, 14.2% and 5.2% respectively. As per Longitudinal Ageing Studies in India (LASI), recent old age dependency has climbed to 19. Health parameters like life expectancy at age 60, physical immobility and chronic disease prevalence among India's aged are about 17 years, 7.8% and 45% respectively. Care for the aged therefore requires a multi-dimensional comprehensive approach. Multiplicity of diseases, disabilities and socio-economic problems in the same individual implies that our 110 million older persons have many hundred million problems to be cared for.

Article 41 of the Constitution of India enshrines that the State shall within the limits of its economic capacity & development, make effective provision for securing the right of public assistance in cases of old age. According to The Hindu Adoption and Maintenance Act, 1956 a Hindu male or female is bound to maintain his or her aged/infirm parents if they are unable to maintain themselves. Himachal Pradesh Maintenance of Parents and Dependents' Act, 2001 also provides for the maintenance of parents, wife and children and for matters connected therewith. Maintenance and Welfare of Parents and Senior Citizens Act, 2007 is a further legal provision that binds children to maintain their parents and failure to do so attracts punishment.

Recognizing diverse needs of such vast population, the Indian Government launched a National Policy of Older Persons (NPOP) in 1999 addressing several issues including their health and socio-economic security. Although the policy highlights the role of many non-state actors including NGOs and the aged persons themselves, it is heavily weighted in favour of delivering programs through strengthening its already existing inter-sectorial infrastructure. An inter-ministerial Committee and a National Council for Older Persons (NCOP) were constituted for its implementation. Important role of Panchayat Raj Institutions was also stressed in its implementation. However, implementation of the policy remained rather slow. Inadequate reach of services to rural end users, failure to harness the benefits of new and emerging Indian economic order and changing socio-demographic scenarios were some of the limiting factors. In 2010, the Government constituted a Committee to review this policy with emphasis on four major areas namely the oldest old (80 +), female elderly, rural elderly and harnessing the technological advances (Draft National Policy on Senior Citizens, 2011). Many suggestions were made during the review of the policy. Currently, several Ministries are involved in implementing various components of National Policy but there are 4 core Ministries that provide large chunks of services and these are Ministry of Social Justice and Empowerment, Ministry of Health and Family Welfare, Ministry of Rural Development and Ministry of Panchayat Raj.

This paper provides insight into various national programs and services for aged persons in India. A brief description of activities running in Indian States and Union Territories by way of a specific example of India's smallest state, the capital of Delhi has been included. Towards the end, future directions with proposals for innovation to serve the aged better have been provided.

National Programs and Services for the Aged

These include National Social Assistance Programme (NSAP), National Programme for the Health Care of the Elderly (NPHCE), Integrated Programme for Older Persons (IPOP), Maintenance and Welfare of Parents and Senior Citizens (MPWSC) Act of 2007, Health insurance scheme, National Initiative on Care of Elderly (NICE), Senior Citizens' Welfare Fund, Rashtriya Vayoshri Yojna (RVY) and some other miscellaneous programs.

(i) National Social Assistance Programme (NSAP)

It was launched by Ministry of Rural Development in 1995. Key principles of NSAP include universal coverage of eligible persons and proactive identification, transparent and people friendly process, regular monthly disbursement of pensions and benefits preferably at the doorsteps, IT based scheme with electronic transfer, robust social audit, key role for local self-government institutions, robust grievance redressal system, automatic convergence and state specific guidelines (National Social Assistance Programme, 2021). In addition to some other schemes like financial assistance to widows and persons with disabilities, NSAP includes Indira Gandhi National Old Age Pension Scheme (IGNOAPS) and Annapurna Scheme. The scheme is revised periodically. IGNOAP provides a monthly pension for 60 + aged persons and an enhanced pension for 80 + belonging to BPL (below poverty line) category. As of now, there are 25 million beneficiaries under IGNOAPS and recent figures under NSAP stand at about 33 million beneficiaries. Shortcomings of NSAP include low awareness of programme, inadequate pension amount, difficulties in beneficiary identification and need for a complex administrative machinery for a diverse and vast country like India. As per Longitudinal Ageing Studies in India (LASI), awareness among 60 + persons is only to the extent of 55% for IGNOAP. It may be mentioned that in addition to the national IGNOAP, most Indian States also provide some old age pension. Under Annapurna Scheme introduced in 2000, 10 kg of food grains is given monthly to those eligible aged persons who have remained uncovered under IGNOAPS but according to LASI, only 12% of 60 + persons are aware of the Annapurna Scheme.

(ii) National Programme for the Health Care for the Elderly (NPHCE)

In spite of constant efforts to strengthen health services for our aged population, it seems some of the health parameters for this segment of population have not shown significant improvement. For instance, as per the 42nd Round of Nation Sample Survey (NSS) in 1986–1987, prevalence of chronic diseases among the aged in India was reported as 45.0% in rural and 44.8% in urban areas (Socio-economic profile of the aged persons, 1987). However, 52nd NSS Round in 1995–1996 recorded a higher figure of 52.7% and 54.5% among rural and urban aged persons in India respectively (The Aged in India, 1998). Building a Knowledge Base on Population Ageing in India (BKPAI) in 2011 also reported 65.8% and 62.1% as the prevalence of chronic diseases in India's rural and urban aged (Pattern of acute & chronic morbidities, care seeking behaviour & financing, 2011). This BKPAI study, however, was carried out only in country's seven selected states having a higher percentage of 60 + population compared to the national average (Pattern of acute & chronic morbidities, care seeking behaviour & financing, 2011). Prevalence of physical immobility among the rural and urban aged also showed a rise, being 5.4% and 5.5% respectively during NSS 42nd round of 1986–1987 (Socio-economic profile of the aged persons, 1987) and 7.7 and 8.4% during NSS 60th Round in 2004 (Morbidity, health care & the condition of the aged, 2004a).

Table 18.2 Strong points of NPHCE

Merits
1. Comprehensive nationwide cover
2. NRHM, NCDs cells, health societies already in place
3. User satisfaction reported in some areas
4. Positive perception about disease screening in some areas

NRHM—National rural health mission; NCDs—Non-communicable diseases

National Programme for the Health Care of Elderly (NPHCE) was launched by Ministry of Health and Welfare in 2010 on a pre-existing administrative base of National Health Mission and that of infrastructure for Non-Communicable diseases and has good financial outlay. It was launched mainly for delivery of accessible, affordable and comprehensive services for India's elderly through existing primary (sub centres and primary health centres), secondary (community health centres and district hospitals) and tertiary health care (regional geriatric centres and national centres on ageing) structure (National Programme for Health Care of the Elderly (NPHCE), 2010). In the 11th plan period, 100 districts of the country had been sanctioned for NPHCE services while in the 12th plan period, 421 districts were sanctioned and as of 2019–2020, all 713 districts have been sanctioned for geriatric primary and secondary care services of OPD, IPD, physiotherapy and laboratory services. So far 20 Regional Geriatric Centres and two National Centres on Ageing for the country have been sanctioned (Status of NPHCE services, 2020). Table 18.2 depicts strong points of NPHCE.

Bhatt et al. (2016) carried out an appraisal of NPHCE in Karnataka and Odisha at primary and secondary facilities levels. Pointing out to its multiple objectives, they felt it was difficult to achieve strides for all the objectives with the current staff strength and facilities. Main areas of concern in the programme implementation were age friendly infrastructure, filling up vacancies, adequate incentives like field allowance for rehabilitation workers from community health centres (CHC), appropriate training, ensuring smooth fund flows, proper monitoring system and all these need to be addressed for improving the programme. In the government's own perspective, NPHCE suffered from slow programme development, non-availability of trained manpower, problems with equipment purchases and problems in submission of quarterly progress reports, financial utilization reports and audited statements (Prakash, 2017), but many of these issues are being addressed.

(iii) **Integrated Programme for Older Persons (IPOP)**

It was launched by Ministry of Social Justice and Empowerment in 1992, renewed or revised in 2008, 2014, 2016 and 2018 and enables NGOs, Panchayat Raj Institutions (PRIs) and other Bodies to obtain support through getting grants-in-aid for their capacity building and providing services to aged persons. Main objective of IPOP is to improve the quality of life of senior citizens by providing basic amenities like shelter, food, medical care and entertainment opportunities and by encouraging

Table 18.3 Merits of IPOP

Merits
1. Provides elderly services in rural and remote areas through a kind of outsourcing
2. No day to day involvement of the government
3. Provides grass root NGOs an opportunity to serve the aged

productive and active ageing. Some of the facilities supported under IPOP are old age homes, day care centres, Mobile medical units, respite care homes, counseling centres, dementia centres, multi-service centres, physiotherapy clinics, disability aids and others (Integrated Programme for Older Persons, 2018). Some of the other schemes under 12th five year Plan were also merged in IPOP. These were Awareness Generation for Maintenance and Welfare of Parents and Senior Citizens Act, Setting up of Helplines for senior citizens at national and district levels and Scheme for implementation of new National Policy on Senior Citizens. In 2018 revision, schemes like day care centres (DCC), Helplines, Multi-service centres, Awareness of MWPSC Act were dropped, renamed or merged with other projects or to be implemented through National Institute of Social Defence. Although IPOP scheme suffers from its low awareness and involves a comprehensive process of selection of projects submitted for grant-in-aid together with their monitoring and auditing, the scheme has many merits (Table 18.3).

(iv) **Maintenance and Welfare of Parents and Senior Citizens (MWPSC) Act 2007**

It was sponsored by Ministry of Social Justice and Empowerment and was enacted in 2007. It is a step towards welfare and dignity of the aged persons and also makes children accountable for care of their aged. Majority of Indian States and Union Territories (UTs) have notified the act and appointed the required Maintenance Tribunals (Implementation of Maintenance & Welfare of Parents & Senior Citizens Act, 2007). The Act provides for limited monetary maintenance support from children for their elderly parents. The Act also provides for States to develop adequate medical facilities (wards and separate queues for senior citizens), expansion of facilities for treatment of chronic, terminal and degenerative diseases for senior citizens and research activities for chronic geriatric diseases and ageing and care by geriatric medical officers. In addition, state governments are required to establish old age homes in each district under this Act. The Act also has a Chapter on Protection of life and property of senior citizens. Limitations of this Act include its low awareness and hesitation by parents to act against their own children. Longitudinal Ageing Studies in India (LASI) in their recent survey found that only 12% of elderly were aware of this Act. Prescribed maximum monetary limit for maintenance support is rather low and moreover, no consolidated information exists on the actual utilization of this act by Senior Citizens. Some amendments to this Act have been suggested for consideration.

(v) **Pradhan Mantri Jan Arogya Yojna (PMJAY) A Health Insurance Scheme**

It was announced in 2018 and was first named the National Health Protection Scheme (NHPS). PMJAY is one of the two components of Ayushman Bharat, a flagship Scheme of the Government of India, to achieve the vision of Universal Health Coverage (UHC) and holistically address the health care system at the primary, secondary and tertiary levels. While PMJAY launched on 23rd September 2018 provides for secondary and tertiary care hospitalization at both public and private hospitals, the other component of Ayushman Bharat Scheme is Health and Wellness Centres (HWCs) which are created by transforming the existing Sub Centres and Primary Health Centres to deliver Comprehensive Primary Health Care (Pradhan Mantri Jan Arogya Yojna (PMJAY), 2018).

PMJAY is the largest health assurance scheme in the world which aims at providing a health cover of Rs. 5 lakhs per family per year to over 10 crores (100 million) of poor and vulnerable families (about 500 million beneficiaries). It is fully funded by the Government. Unlike the earlier health insurance scheme, the Rashtriya Swasthya Bima Yojna (RSBY) launched in 2008 which gave a lower annual cover (Rs.30000/–) and a maximum limit of 5 members per family, PMJAY gives a higher cover and has no cap on family size. PMJAY also covers pre-existing diseases, is cashless scheme and envisions to help mitigate catastrophic expenditure on medical treatment. It also covers up to 3 days of pre-hospitalization and 15 days post-hospitalization expenses such as diagnostics and medicines. PMJAY has subsumed the earlier RSBY insurance scheme.

(vi) National Initiative on Care of Elderly (NICE)

National Institute of Social Defence (NISD) was founded in 1961 and is a nodal training institute in the field of Social Defence, under the Ministry of Social Justice and Empowerment. NISD develops a dedicated cadre of Geriatric Care Givers and generates skilled manpower. A project called NICE (National Initiative on Care for Elderly) from of the Ministry of Social Justice and Empowerment provides geriatric care training in different Indian cities to develop a cadre of skilled caregivers and supervisory level personnel to meet the demand for providing trained personnel in Age Care in NGO sector, Government/Corporate sectors, Academic institutions, etc. This course covers basic and applied geriatrics, social gerontology and geriatric nursing. The institute conducts training courses on Old Age Care by itself and in collaboration with its Regional Resource Training Centres (RRTCs) and others (Table 18.4).

(vii) Miscellaneous Schemes

A Senior Citizens Welfare Fund was created in 2016 to be utilized for some schemes like for promoting financial security of senior citizens, health care and nutrition of senior citizens, welfare of elderly widows, schemes relating to old age homes and day care of senior citizens, etc. and for the promotion of the welfare of senior citizens (Senior Citizens' Welfare Fund, 2019). Recent schemes (2021) for funding

Table 18.4 NISD training programs

1 Year PG diploma in integrated geriatric care
6 Months certificate course of geriatric care
3 Months certificate course on bedside assistance/caregivers
5 Days training on geriatric care for the staff of old age homes
3 Days training on dementia care for old age homes staff
1 Day sensitization programme on intergenerational bonding in schools

include Rashtriya Vayoshri Yojna (RVY-see below), Livelihood and skilling initiatives, Poshan Abhiyan (nutrition support to the indigent elders), promotion of Silver economy, Helplines, Media, Advocacy/Capacity building/research, etc. This Fund comprises the unclaimed amounts from the Central Government Savings Schemes.

Another Central Sector Scheme, Rashtriya Vayoshri Yojna (RVY) was launched by the Ministry of Social Justice and Empowerment on 01.04.2017 for providing physical aids and assisted living devices for age related disabilities among senior citizens in the BPL category. An amount of Rs.16 crore had been released under this scheme during 2016–2017. Another funding of Rs.77 crores from Senior Citizens' Welfare Fund for RVY is under consideration in 2021.

Many other national programs also exist for Indians in general but they are not exclusive for aged persons and will not be discussed here. These are for cancer, diabetes, cardiovascular diseases, stroke, blindness, deafness, mental health, oral health, etc. (National Programme for Prevention and Control of Cancer, Diabetes, Cardiovascular Diseases and Stroke-NPCDCS, National Programme for Control of Blindness-NPCB, National Programme for Prevention and Control of Deafness-NPPCD, National Mental Health Programme-NMHP, National Oral Health Programme-NOHP, etc.).

Different Government Departments also extend income tax exemptions, special interest rates for bank deposits and loans and travel concessions on trains, buses, air travel, etc. to senior citizens.

Several NGOs in the country also provide services to aged persons at their doorsteps and try to link them with institution based public services. They run programs for elderly persons' empowerment, shelter, rehabilitation, income generation, social engagement, respite and palliative care and provide health care to those afflicted with cataracts, dementia, cancer and other ailments. A brief summary of these activities by NGOs and Community-Based Organizations is given below.

- Medical care at home (MMU, camps), linking it with institution based public health services.
- Training of staff & families in home based services (physiotherapy, respite care).
- Special services (cataract, dementia, cancer, palliative care, rescuing, disaster response, partnership with CBOs like Senior Citizens Associations).

- Greater integration of Older Persons into society by fighting ageism and enjoyment of home life (ESHGs, helplines, day care centres, income generation, pilgrimages).
- Scattered services are also rendered by CBOs like charitable hospitals, nursing homes, ESHGs, Senior Citizens Associations, Volunteer bureaus, etc.

Regional Scenario in Indian States and Union Territories

India has significant interregional and interstate demographic diversity based on the state of demographic transition and variations in the onset and pace of fertility transition. Almost every Indian State has been surveyed for socio-economic and health indices for its aged population. These States also participate in national programs and many have their own services for the aged persons as well. All these details can be found in various documents and are outside the scope of this paper. However, following description is provided for India's capital, Delhi in reference to a national perspective. Delhi is unique in as much as it happens to be the smallest state in the country. It has an area of 1484 km^2 and a population of about 20 million people (Fig. 18.3).

Population density of Delhi is almost 11,300 per square kilometre as compared to all India population density of 340 only and is the highest in the country (Government of NCT Delhi, 2021). Overcrowding with huge proportion of dynamic and migrant population due to people coming from other states in search of livelihood is likely to render the aged persons vulnerable in Delhi.

Delhi with its approximately 12 lakh population of aged persons has the second lowest percentage of aged persons among all the Indian states. Delhi also has the second highest percentage of urban aged (97.4%) compared to national average of 29.4% (Census of India, 2011). Recorded crime rate against the aged persons happens to be highest in Delhi compared to national average.

Situation of Aged Persons in Delhi in Reference to National Perspective

(i) Social and health parameters

Comparative analysis reveals that aged persons in Delhi fair better than their average all India counterparts in many social and health parameters. Table 18.5 shows such comparison with respect to literacy rate, old age dependency ratio and percentage of aged persons living alone (Elderly in India, 2016).

Work participation rate among the aged is 24.1% for Delhi and 34.4% for all India average (Key indicators of employment and unemployment in India, 2006)

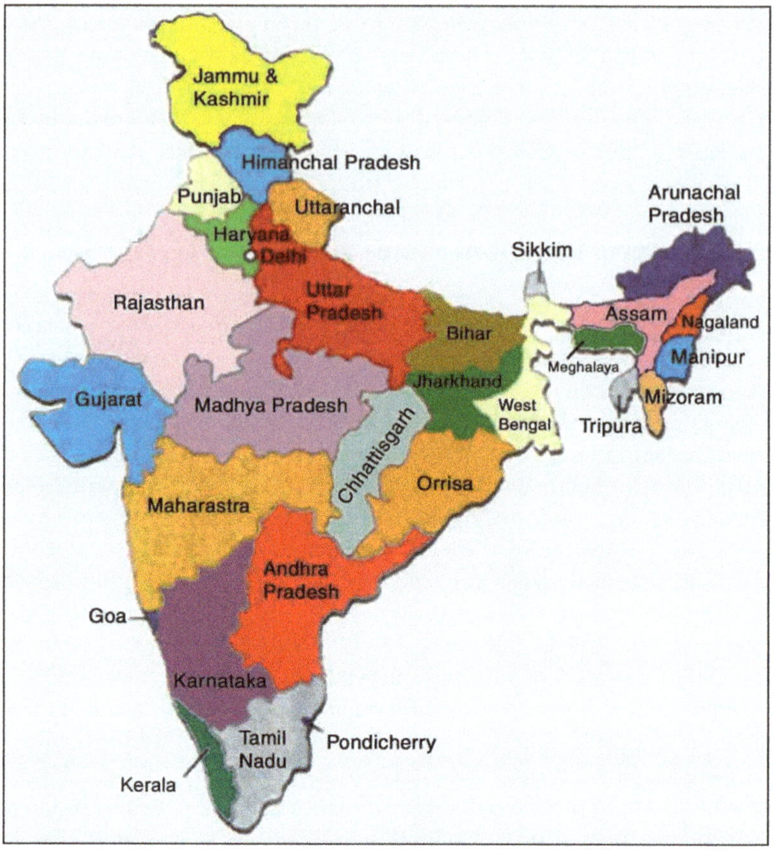

Fig. 18.3 MAP of India depicting Delhi as the smallest state

Table 18.5 Comparative literacy rate, old age dependency those living alone

Place	Literacy rate (%)	Old age dependency	[a]Percent living alone(%)
Delhi	69	10.4	3.6
All India	43.5	14.2	5.2

[a]These figures are higher than 2005–2006 figures of 2.9% for Delhi and 5.0% for all India (National Family Health Survey, 2005)

while their experience of abuse of some kind was 22 and 50% for Delhi and all India respectively (Elder abuse in India, 2014).

Health parameters show similar trends in favour of aged persons of Delhi. Thus all India prevalence of chronic diseases was reported as 45% for rural and 44.8% for urban elderly persons but it was only 38.9% and 35.8% for Delhi's aged (Socio-economic profile of the aged persons, 1987). Life expectancy was also better for Delhi than all India figures (SRS Based Life Table, 2016). Similarly, prevalence of physical immobility in 1986–1987 was 5.4% and 5.5% for all India's rural and urban aged but it was 2.8% for Delhi's urban aged (Socio-economic profile of the aged persons, 1987). Overtime, physical immobility prevalence rose further, overall being 7.8% in 2014 for all India (Key indicators of social consumption in India-Health, 2014), but only 5.25% for Delhi's aged in 2004 (Morbidity, health care and the condition of the aged, 2004b). Pattern regarding life expectancy at age 60, number of ailments experienced during last 15 days and percentage of aged persons having poor perception about current state of their health shows similar trends in favour of Delhi's aged (Table 18.6 and Fig. 18.4).

Table 18.6 Comparative life expectancy, ailments and poor health perception

Place	[a]Life expectancy in years at age 60 (SRS Based Life Table, 2016)		No. of ailments in last 15 days (Key indicators of social consumption in India-Health, 2014)		[b]% of aged persons with poor health perception (Morbidity, health care and the condition of the aged, 2004a)	
	Male	Female	Rural	Urban	Without illness	With illness
Delhi	19.6	20.8	2.6	9.9	10.8	32.9
All India	17.0	19.0	27.0	36.2	15.1	39.7

Note: Shown in brackets are the references listed under the References
[a]Life expectancy for Delhi's aged is second highest among all the states and union territories.
[b]A report of 2016 also observed figures for Delhi as 11% and 34% for those without and with illness and for all India as 13% and 37% for those without and with illness (Elderly in India, 2016)

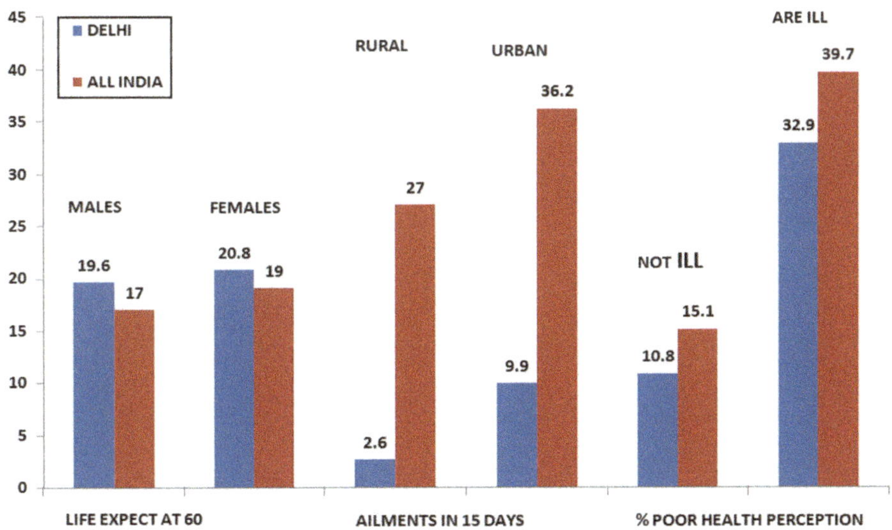

Fig. 18.4 Delhi's aged versus all India-health parameters

(ii) Disease burden

One of the largest studies in India on individual medical problems among elderly was conducted with the support of the Government of India W.H.O. Collaborative Programme in 2007 by trained medical and paramedical personnel who had also undertaken clinical examination and few laboratory tests. The study was done in 10 cities namely, Chennai, Chandigarh, Delhi, Guwahati, Jodhpur, Pune, Raipur, Shimla, Thiruvananthapuram and Vellore (Srivastava Multicentric study to establish epidemiological data on health problems in elderly, 2007).

The study revealed that out of 11 common medical problems, 5 disorders namely ischemic heart disease, chronic obstructive pulmonary disease, falls, arthritis and hearing impairment was most commonly prevalent among Delhi's aged compared to aged persons in any of the other nine Indian cities (Table 18.7). Type of population (rural and urban) and type of gender (males and females) in whom the highest prevalence of these 5 disorders was observed have also been depicted in this Table 18.7.

It was also observed in this study that two out of 11 disorders namely bowel complaints and poor vision had the lowest prevalence among Delhi's aged when compared to any of the other nine cities (Table 18.8). Remaining 4 out of 11 disorders, i.e. diabetes, hypertension, paralysis and urinary complaints had however an intermediate prevalence in Delhi related to other cities (Srivastava Multicentric study to establish epidemiological data on health problems in elderly, 2007).

Table 18.7 Diseases with highest prevalence in Delhi relative to other 9 Indian cities

No	Diseases	Settings where the prevalence is highest	
		Population	Gender
1	Ischemic heart disease	Rural + urban	Males + Females
2	Chronic obstructive pulmonary disease	Rural + urban	Males + Females
3	Falls	Rural + urban	Males
4	Arthritis	Rural	Males + females
5	Hearing impairment	Urban	Males + females

Table 18.8 Diseases with lowest prevalence in Delhi relative to other 9 Indian cities

No	Diseases	Settings where the prevalence is lowest	
		Population	Gender
1	Bowel complaints	Rural + urban	Males
2	Poor vision	Rural	Males + Females

Health Services for Aged Persons in Delhi

Delhi has set up various services for its aged population and also participates in the delivery of services through central government programs. In general, Delhi provides three tier medical services for public at large that include primary care through its Mohalla Clinics (Neighbourhood Clinics), secondary care through Multi-speciality Polyclinics and tertiary care through its Multi-speciality and super-speciality hospitals. For its aged persons Delhi has (i) clinics from 9 AM to 1 PM on Sundays at about 10 major government hospitals to provide services under Medicine, Surgery, Orthopedics, ENT, Eye, etc. supported with pathological tests and radiological diagnostic tests, (ii) all the major hospitals under Delhi government have separate counters for registration and separate OPD rooms for aged persons. Test is done on out of turn basis and (iii) separate queues are there for them in all hospitals and dispensaries (Government of NCT Delhi, 2021).

Other Health Related Services for Aged Persons in Delhi

These include recreation centres, old age homes, services for safety and security for the aged persons, services under MWPSC Act and old age pensions.

(i) Recreation centres: A large number of such centres are run by the Delhi government to provide facilities for relaxation and avenues for social and cultural activities. Geriatric activities include health and yoga camps, entertainment, nutritional seminars and workshops, tours and pilgrimages, walks, lectures by experts, etc. for the aged. Government gives onetime grant of Rs. 75,000/ to senior citizens' or resident welfare organizations and other NGOs having space with a recurring grant of Rs. 20,000/ (Rs. 10,000/ to NGOs having no space) (Government of NCT Delhi, 2021).

(ii) Old age homes: Currently Government runs two old age homes, one at Bindapur in Dwarka which has a capacity of 50 aged persons and is free and the other at Lampur near Narela which is for 100 persons. Half of the seats in this Home are for government nominees, the other half are paid seats (Government of NCT Delhi, 2021). As per provisions under MWPSC Act, 10 more old age homes are in the pipeline (National Human Rights Commission, 2017). As far as old age homes run independently by various non-government agencies is concerned, their growth has been phenomenal. There were only 12 such old age homes reported in 1998 Help Age (India & Directory of Old Age Homes In India, New Delhi, 1988) but in 2016 as many as 73 had come up in and around Delhi (Help Age India, 2018).

(iii) Security and helpline services: are provided by police and sometimes by NGOs. Aged persons who live alone or with their spouses only are surveyed, registered and periodically visited by police staff. Steps for home and neighbourhood security are advised and explained to senior citizens to prevent any untoward injuries and accidents.

(iv) Services under MWPSC Act: Although Delhi has completed all the steps for implementation of this act like setting up of Maintenance Tribunals and Appellate Tribunals in all its eleven districts and has provided for medical care of senior citizens and their protection as prescribed under its Chaps. 4 And 5 but provision for more old age homes (Chap. 3 of the Act) is still in the pipeline. Information on the number of claims settled under this act is not precisely available.

(v) Old age pension: Pension for senior citizens aged 60–70 years has been raised to Rs. 2000/– and for 70 + to Rs. 2500/– compared to Rs. 1500/– earlier (National Human Rights Commission, 2017). An amount of Rs. 500/- as additional amount is for Schedule Casts/Schedule Tribes/Minorities.

Future Directions: Proposals for Innovation for Care of the Aged

It is time to consider establishing national and state level commissions for senior citizens both for their empowerment and for accountability of service providers. There is already one such commission in the Indian State of Madhya Pradesh and one was under consideration for Delhi state. It is also time to consider establishing separate departments at central and state levels dealing exclusively with senior citizens affairs for a better focus on their problems and programs. Following five proposals specifically advocate for a stronger role of government in the delivery of elder health care services not only by its own agencies but also by non-state actors such as not for profit NGOs, for profit private organizations, civil society and senior citizens themselves (Fig. 18.5). These proposals include (i) innovating for better convergence and decentralized delivery of multiple services for the end user, (ii) creating strong public private partnerships (PPPs) as substitute for public services which are not doing so well, (iii) harnessing the benefits of statuary provisions from the corporate world for elderly services under corporate social responsibility (CSR), (iv) capitalizing on the useful services provided by NGOs and (v) tapping the potentials of the aged persons themselves.

These five proposals are now briefly discussed below.

(i) **Innovating for better convergence and decentralized delivery of multiple services**

Although support from Panchayat Raj Institutions (PRIs) to PHCs has resulted in some achievements (Kumar and Jayanta Mishra 2016; Varatharajan et al., 2004), several challenges in public health functioning under the present decentralized system need to be addressed (Fig. 18.6). Panchayats which are required to manage and

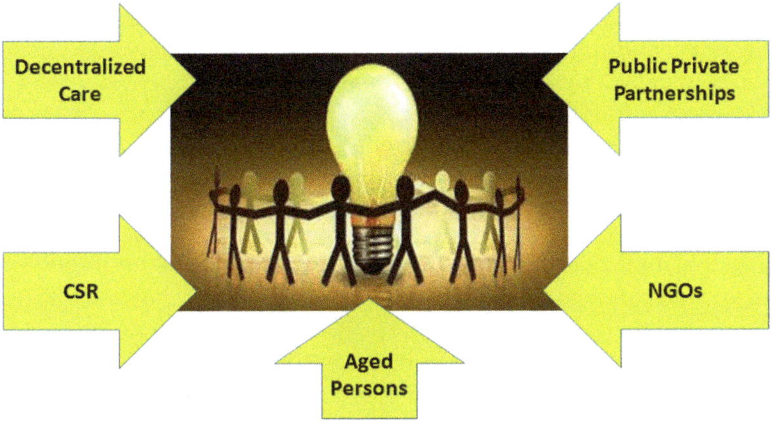

Fig. 18.5 Future directions: proposals for innovations

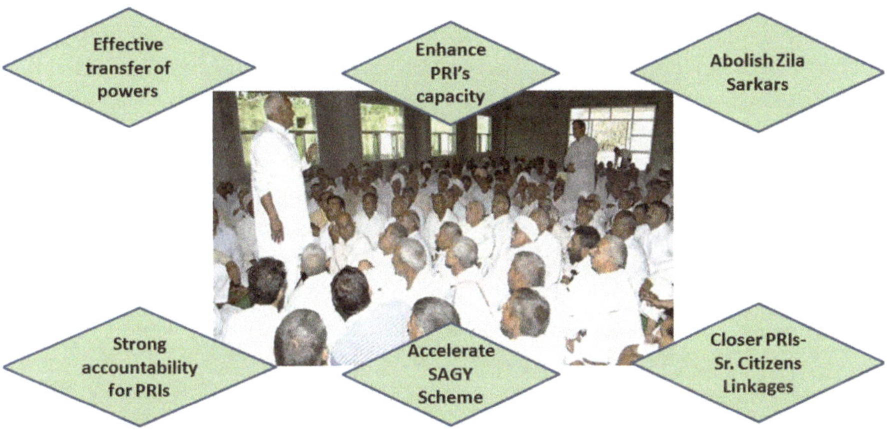

Fig. 18.6 Decentralized care

finance PHCs and coordinate health, social welfare and education activities at village and block levels are not adequately empowered by states through progressive transfer of funds, functions and functionaries or through proper training and equipment. Establishment of Zila Sarkar headed by a Minister and Zila Panchayat President only as its Member at some places probably reflects a lack of will to transfer desired autonomy to PRIs (A study on effectiveness of Panchayat Raj Institutions (PRIs), 2016). Although some of these issues are being addressed, It is suggested that capacity of PRIs may be further increased to achieve convergence of development activities in villages. Sansad Adarsh Gram Yojna (SAGY) is a welcome step that operates through adopting a specified geographic rural area by an elected representative under whose supervision, development work is undertaken for an effective reach to end users.

Kumar and Jayanta Mishra raised the issue about prioritization of service providers and users, coercive unethical work and lack of communication, all of which contribute to non-accountability, non-conducive environment and ineffectiveness of PRIs and hence a negative impact on PHCs' working (Kumar & Jayanta, 2016). It is suggested to address these issues and that PRIs should develop closer linkages with senior citizens and assess their health needs which can be used as feedback for higher authorities in order to forge effective demand driven programs.

(ii) **Creating public private partnerships as substitute for some public services**

Notwithstanding the fact that PPPs involving profit making hospitals and other service providers have at times not succeeded, PPPs offer incentives to commercial agencies including private hospitals and at the same time work under a regulatory legal agreement. Well thought of PPPs should therefore be able to control unbridled and unregulated growth of highly expensive private health sector. Since more hospitals will still be needed in small towns and rural areas due to massive population and also in the light of recently introduced mega PMJAY insurance scheme, PPPs should be encouraged. There are also many non-hospital private agencies like Corporates, NGOs, Foundations, Academic institutions, Associations, or even individual citizens like community leaders and school teachers who can enter into business relationships with government organizations to attain their own objectives and common goals (Fig. 18.7). Health awareness campaigns, training, preventive geriatrics, or even follow-up of the implementation of government health programs at grass root level are good primary care projects for PPPs. Few of the regional examples of PPPs in health care are noteworthy such as located in Tamil Nadu (Emergency ambulance services

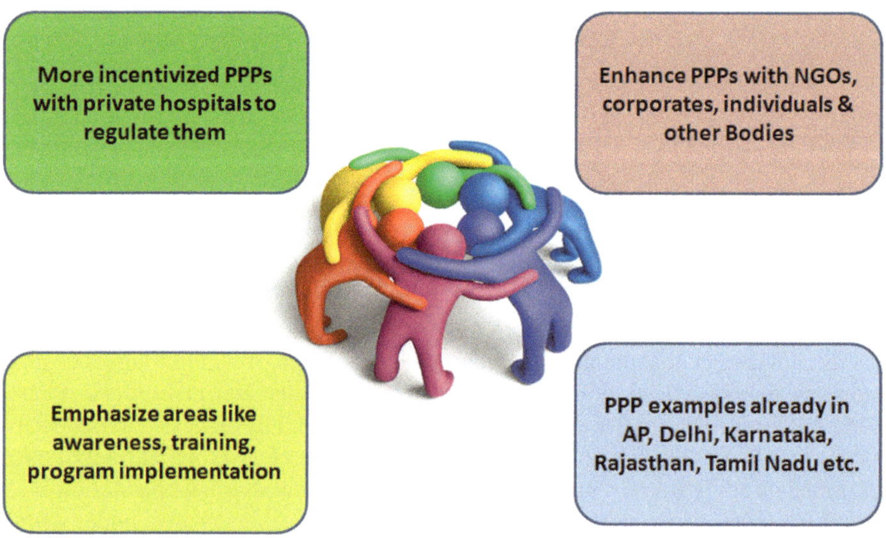

Fig. 18.7 Elderly services through PPPS

partnering with Seva Nilayam Society in association with Ryder-Cheshire Foundation) a Andhra Pradesh (Urban slum health care project partnering with Social Action for Integrated Development Services), Karnataka (Free services to BPL patients at Rajiv Gandhi Super Speciality Hospital, Raichur, partnering with Apollo Hospitals Enterprises Ltd.), Rajasthan (Contracting in Radiological diagnostic services in the public hospitals, provision of quality drugs and supplies cheaper than market rate and all this free for BPL patients, above 70 years of age and freedom fighters, partnering with Medicare Relief Society), Uttarakhand (Mobile health services partnering with Uttarañchal Institute of Scientific Research, Bhimtal (NGO) and Gujarat (Chiranjeevi Yojana partnering with private doctors for deliveries for BPL women) (Sahni, 2007). A detailed document on development of dialysis centres in Delhi hospitals on PPP basis has also been in public domain (Development of dialysis centres in GNCTD hospitals in Delhi on PPP basis, 2013).

(iii) **Harnessing benefits of statuary provisions from the corporate world for elderly services**

Act regarding Corporate Social Responsibility (CSR) is in force since April 1, 2014 (India: Corporate Social Responsibility-Indian Companies Act 2013 and Companies (CSR Policies) 2014). Although old age homes, day care centres and employment enhancing skills for the elderly along with preventive health care is part of the defined schedules of activities that can be supported with CSR, elderly care appears to stand on a low pedestal in the overall ambit of CSR and not much is known how much the corporates have done in this field. It is suggested that Government facilitates in clarifying legal definitions and prioritization of existing schedules of CSR and in providing clear definition of CSR for the purposes of expenditures also. It is suggested that all round awareness about CSR should be created. All India Senior Citizens Confederation (AISCCON) have taken up the issue to sensitize the corporates, senior citizens organizations and others in this regard. What is also needed for the government is to provide better CSR priorities which should change in keeping with changing socio-demographic scenario of the country and determine adequate proportion of different types of activities required in different geographic areas of the country (Fig. 18.8).

(iv) **Capitalizing on the useful services provided by NGOs**

NGOs are the first ones to bring out the problems of elderly in India and often provide health care for the aged in rural and remote areas. Their elder care activities are diverse and include medical and psychiatric care both with modern and alternative forms of medicine. NGOs also run old age homes, day care centres and mobile medical units and arrange provision of food. Awareness generation, health education, counseling and financial assistance through income generation and micro projects are other areas of their work.

Suggestions to enhance the utility of NGOs include their active involvement in (a) empowering the individuals and communities to become responsible for their

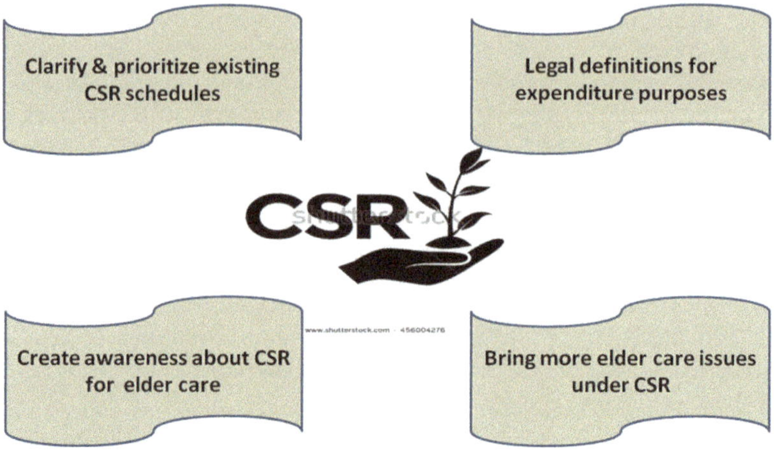
Clarify & prioritize existing CSR schedules
Legal definitions for expenditure purposes
CSR
Create awareness about CSR for elder care
Bring more elder care issues under CSR

Fig. 18.8 Corporate social responsibility

own health, (b) supporting and monitoring national geriatric health programs and (c) collecting feedback from aged persons about their health needs for mid-course correction and incorporation in future health services. Further, in order to avoid duplication of work by different NGOs and consequent wastage of resources, it is important to bring these NGOs into partnerships with each other and with public agencies to disseminate information about their good practice models. A National Policy and a national cell for mainstreaming various NGOs on geriatric care are needed which would also encourage inter NGO communication (Fig. 18.9).

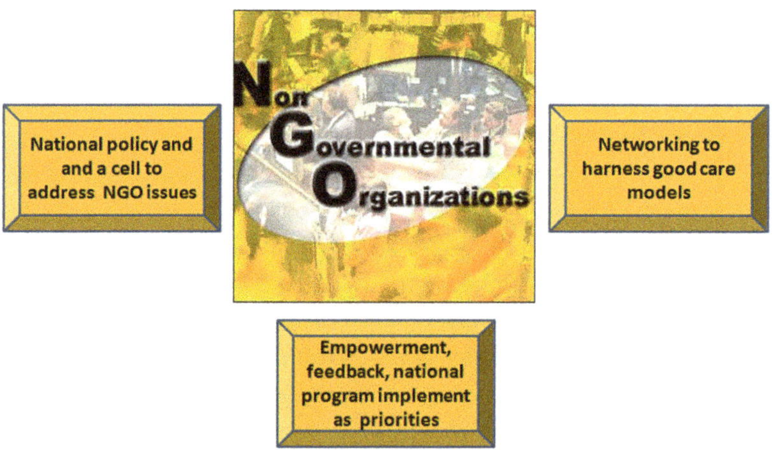
National policy and and a cell to address NGO issues
Non Governmental Organizations
Networking to harness good care models
Empowerment, feedback, national program implement as priorities

Fig. 18.9 Grass root utility of NGOS

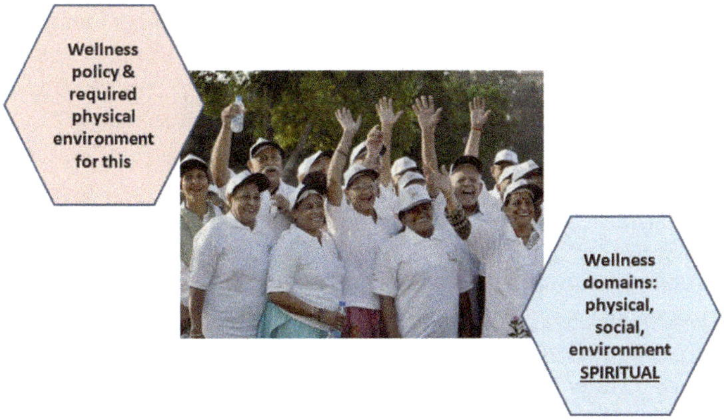

Fig. 18.10 Tapping the potentials of aged

(v) Tapping the potentials of aged persons themselves

Self-caring for one's own health is a time tested affordable way of preventing and controlling diseases. It is also an effective way to preserve one's own health related human rights (Kumar, 2014). Personal hygiene, diet, exercise, tobacco avoidance and mental relaxation are often prescribed and practiced in the physical domain. Determinants of health also encompass social domains like networking and availability of support, environmental domains like housing and climate and spiritual domains like coping ability, resilience, introspection and attitudes of forgiveness, optimism, gratitude and empathy. Spiritual attitudes are scientifically proven to be beneficial for physical and mental health and can be inculcated and strengthened by well-known methods. A separate wellness policy is required for aged persons for overall promotion of health and well-being based on multiple domains mentioned above. Wellness centres, recreation centres, or other types of physical environments should therefore be increasingly created to practice these domains and to especially enhance emotional and spiritual intelligence of aged persons (Fig. 18.10).

Conclusions

This article on policies and programs begins with the note that in addition to pathological morbidity in the ageing population, there should also be an emphasis on the importance of morbidity which occurs due to changes that occur with normal ageing. Burgeoning population of aged persons with rapid rise in the enormous magnitude of multidisciplinary problems among them has been termed as a cascading effect.

Demographic, health and social context of India's ageing population has been expressed with specific situations prevailing in the country's capital city of Delhi. After a brief description of National Policy for Older Persons, various national programs and services for the aged have been discussed under National Social Assistance Programme, National Programme for the Health Care for the Elderly, Integrated Programme for Older persons, Maintenance and Welfare of Parents and Senior Citizens Act, PMJAY (a health insurance scheme), National Initiative on Care of Elderly and several other miscellaneous programs. A description of services available for Delhi's aged persons has been included.

Finally, the article dwells on five proposals for innovations for care of the aged namely Innovating for better convergence and decentralized delivery of multiple services, Creating public private partnerships as substitute for some of the public services, Harnessing benefits of statuary provisions from the corporate world for elderly services, Capitalizing on the useful services provided by NGOs and Tapping the potentials of aged persons themselves.

References

A study on effectiveness of Panchayat Raj Institutions (PRIs) in health care system in the state of Madhya Pradesh. Shri Ram Center, Delhi, May 2016. www.srcirhr.com.

Bhatt TN, James KS, Giridhar G. An appraisal of the functioning of NPHCE in Karnataka and Odisha. Building a Knowledge Base on Population Ageing in India (BKPAI), UNFPA Series II, Working Paper 7, 2016.

Census of India, 2011. Office of the Registrar General and the Census Commissioner of India. Ministry of Home Affairs, Government of India, New Delhi, 2011. www.censusindia.gov.in.

Development of dialysis centers in GNCTD hospitals in Delhi on PPP basis. Request for qualification (24/12/2013), www.delhi.gov.in.

Draft National Policy on Senior Citizens 2011. www.socialjustice.nic.in.

Elder abuse in India. Chapter 4. Personal experience of abuse. In: A Help Age India Report, New Delhi, 2014; 25–47.

Elderly in India, 2016. Ministry of Statistics and Program Implementation, Government of India, New Delhi. www.mospi.gov.in.

Government of NCT Delhi (2021). www.delhi.gov.in.

Help Age India, Personal Communication from CEO, Mr. Matthew Cherian, 2018.

Help Age India, Directory of Old Age Homes In India, New Delhi, 1998.

Implementation of Maintenance and Welfare of Parents and Senior Citizens Act, 2007. Helpage India Report, New Delhi, December, 2017.

India: Corporate Social Responsibility-Indian Companies Act 2013 and Companies (CSR Policies) Rules, 2014.

Integrated Program for Older Persons. Revised as on 01.04.2018. Ministry of Social Justice and Empowerment, Government of India, New Delhi, www.socialjustice.nic.in.

Key indicators of employment and unemployment in India. NSSO 68th Round (July 2011–June 2012). Ministry of Statistics and Program Implementation, Government of India, New Delhi, March, 2006. www.mospi.gov.in.

Key indicators of social consumption in India-Health. NSSO 71st Round (2014, January to June). Ministry of Statistics and Program Implementation, Government of India, New Delhi, June, 2015. www.mospi.gov.in.

Kumar, V. (2015). Geriatric medicine: An overview. In Y. P. Munjal (Ed.), *API textbook of medicine* (vol. 2, pp. 2766–2770, 10th ed.). The Association of Physicians of India. Jaypee Brothers Medical Publishers (P) Ltd., New Delhi.

Kumar, V. (2014). Health and human rights of older persons in India. In: P. K. B. Nayar (Ed.) *Human rights of older persons in Asia Pacific Region* (pp. 255–274). B R Publishing Corporation.

Kumar, V., Jayanta Mishra, A. (2016, May 3). Health care under the Panchayat Raj Institutions (PRIs) in a decentralized health system. Leadership in Health Services, *29*(2), 151–167. https://doi.org/10.1108/lhs-08-2015-0022.

Morbidity, health care and the condition of the aged. NSSO 60th Round (January to June, 2004). Ministry of Statistics and Program Implementation, Government of India, New Delhi, March, 2006. www.mospi.gov.in.

Morbidity, health care and the condition of the aged. NSSO 60th Round (2004, January–June). State Sample. Government of Delhi, November, 2006.

National Family Health Survey, Round 3, 2005/06, Ministry of Health and Family Welfare, Government of India. http://nchiips.org/nfhs/nfhs3.shtml.

National Human Rights Commission. Action taken report of Meeting of Core Group on Protection and Welfare of Elderly Persons held on 13th January 2017. Submitted at the Group's Meeting on 7th February 2018.

National Program for Health Care of the Elderly (NPHCE). (2010). Operational guidelines, Ministry of Health and Family Welfare, Government of India, New Delhi, 2010 www.mohfw.nic.in.

National Social Assistance Program. (2021). Program Guidelines. Ministry of Rural Development, Government of India. www.nsap.nic.in.

Pradhan Mantri Jan Arogya Yojna (PMJAY) (2018). www.pmjay.gov.in.

Pattern of acute and chronic morbidities, care seeking behavior and financing. In: United Nations Population Fund. Report on the status of elderly in selected States of India, New Delhi, 2011 (pp. 124–148).

Prakash I. Directorate General of Health Services. Personal communication through lecture, New Delhi, 2017.

Sahni, A. (2007). Public private partnership in health care: Critical areas and opportunities. medind.nic.in/haa/108/i1/haat08i1p32pdf.

Senior Citizens' Welfare Fund. Journalsofindia.com December 31, 2019.

Srivastava, R. K. (Ed.). (2007). *Multicentric study to establish epidemiological data on health problems in elderly*. Supported by Ministry of Health, Government of India WHO Collaborative Program, 2007.

SRS Based Life Table 2010–2014. Office of the Registrar General and the Census Commissioner of India. Ministry of Home Affairs, Government of India, New Delhi, 2016. www.censusindia.gov.in.

Socioeconomic profile of the aged persons. NSSO 42nd Round (July, 1986–June 1987). Ministry of Statistics, Government of India, New Delhi, September, 1989. www.mospi.gov.in.

Status of NPHCE services 2020. Personal communication from Dr. Gowri N. Sengupta, Asstt Director General, Directorate General Health Services, Ministry of Health and Welfare, Delhi.

The Aged in India. A socioeconomic profile. NSS 52nd Round (July 1995–June 1996). Ministry of Statistics and Program Implementation, Government of India, New Delhi, November, 1998. www.mospi.gov.in.

Varatharajan, D., Thankappan, R., & Jayapalan, S. (2004). Assessing the performance of primary health centers under decentralized government in Kerala, India. *Health Policy and Planning, 19*(1), 41–51.